# Nanotechnology *and* Human Health

# Nanotechnology
## *and* Human
## Health

*Edited by*

Ineke Malsch
Claude Emond

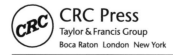

CRC Press
Taylor & Francis Group
Boca Raton  London  New York

CRC Press is an imprint of the
Taylor & Francis Group, an **informa** business

CRC Press
Taylor & Francis Group
6000 Broken Sound Parkway NW, Suite 300
Boca Raton, FL 33487-2742

First issued in paperback 2017

© 2014 by Taylor & Francis Group, LLC
CRC Press is an imprint of Taylor & Francis Group, an Informa business

No claim to original U.S. Government works

Version Date: 20130709

ISBN 13: 978-1-138-07269-5 (pbk)
ISBN 13: 978-0-8493-8144-7 (hbk)

---

**Library of Congress Cataloging-in-Publication Data**

---

Nanotechnology and human health / editors, Ineke Malsch, Claude Emond.
    p. ; cm.
    Includes bibliographical references and index.
    ISBN 978-0-8493-8144-7 (hardcover : alk. paper)
    I. Malsch, Ineke, editor of compilation. II. Emond, Claude, editor of compilation.
    [DNLM: 1. Nanotechnology. 2. Biomedical Technology. 3. Environment. 4. Nanostructures. QT 36.5]

    R856
    610.28--dc23                                                          2013026047

---

**Visit the Taylor & Francis Web site at**
**http://www.taylorandfrancis.com**

**and the CRC Press Web site at**
**http://www.crcpress.com**

# Contents

# Section V  Nanotoxicology Overview and Problems

# Section VI  Life Cycle

# Section VII  Ethical, Legal, and Social Implications of Bionanotechnology

# *Preface*

*Nanotechnology and Human Health* presents scientific and technical developments in nanotechnology for applications in three areas that are expected to lead to impacts on human health: biomedical (pharmaceuticals and medical devices), agrifood and water, and the environment. This technical core is preceded by an introduction including information on current nanotechnology research programs in industrialized countries and emerging economies. Apart from opportunities of nanotechnology for human health, toxicological aspects and life cycle risks and impacts are reviewed. The volume is completed with an analysis of ethical, legal, and social implications of bionanotechnology, and a concluding analysis.

The collection of discussions of current nanotechnology for the above-mentioned three areas together with the environment, health, safety aspects, and ethical and societal implications provides the reader a unique insight into contemporary technological developments and what they may mean for human health. The work has a sound scientific basis, thereby avoiding unrealistic predictions. At the same time, analysis of societal implications is not usually included in most technical books about trends in nanotechnology. By including these aspects, the reader with a technical or natural science background is encouraged to be more responsible in R&D on nanotechnology that will have an impact on human health. The reader with a social science background can benefit because the technical reviews are written for a nonspecialist audience, taking care to explain terminology. The societal aspect chapters are intended to contribute to contemporary debates in social studies of science and at the same time be accessible to nonspecialists.

# Editors

**Ineke Malsch, PhD,** graduated with a degree in physics (Utrecht University, Netherlands, 1991) and holds a PhD in philosophy (thesis: *Ethics and Nanotechnology*, Radboud University, Nijmegen, Netherlands, 2011). She is an expert in ethical and societal aspects of nano- and emerging technologies. She has been the director of her own consultancy—Malsch TechnoValuation (www.malsch.demon.nl) since 1999, including 10 years participating in international and multidisciplinary projects about nanotechnology in its societal context with public and private partners. She is currently involved in the NanoEIS project on Nanotechnology Education for Industry and Society (www.nanoeis.eu) and is coordinating with EthicSchool for workshops and training in Responsible Innovation (www.ethicschool.nl/english). She is the editor of *Biomedical Nanotechnology* (CRC Press, 2005) and has authored extensive publications for academic, professional, and general public audiences. These include peer-reviewed articles such as "Governing Nanotechnology in a Multistakeholder World," (in Nanoethics online first, December 2012, http://link.springer.com/article/10.1007%2Fs11569-012-0163-1) and "The Just War Theory and The Ethical Governance of Research" (in *Journal of Science and Engineering Ethics*, February 2012 http://www.springerlink.com/content/d85w001pj6727512/).

**Claude Emond, PhD,** is a clinical assistant professor in the Department of Environmental and Occupational Health at the University of Montreal, Canada, and an associate professor at the Institute of Environmental Sciences (ISE) at the University of Quebec in Montreal (UQAM). In this capacity, Dr. Emond delivers lectures in toxicology at the university and supervises graduate students. He earned a bachelor's degree in biochemistry in 1987, a master's degree in environmental health in 1997, and a PhD degree in public health (toxicology and human risk assessment option) in 2001 from the University of Montreal in Quebec.

From 2001 to 2004, Dr. Emond received grants from the National Research Council, a branch of the National Academy of Sciences (NAS), to perform postdoctoral studies for two and a half years at the US Environmental Protection Agency (EPA) in North Carolina. At the EPA, Dr. Emond's work focused on describing a developmental physiologically based pharmacokinetic (PBPK) model on dioxins. The research conducted by his team led to recognition from the EPA administration and a presentation of the EPA's Scientific and Technological Achievement Award to the team. The team's research is cited by NAS. His research and consulting interests address problems in toxicology and focus on different chemicals, including polychlorinated biphenyls (PCBs), dioxins, flame retardants (polybrominated diphenyl ether [PBDE] and hexabromocyclododecane [HBCD]), bisphenol A, pyrethroid, and xenoestrogens. Dr. Emond's research interests also focus on the development and improvement of mathematical PBPK models to address and reduce uncertainty for toxicology risk assessment in human health. Much of his research activities focus on toxicokinetic and dynamic effects to further characterize the mode of action between chemicals and biological matrices for individuals or populations. He is also interested in occupational toxicology, mainly on the effects of organic solvents, modeling physiological changes in aging compared to younger workers, and nanotoxicology.

Dr. Emond has also offered his expertise and extensive knowledge on various topics by participating as a peer reviewer for *Health Canada*, as a reviewer of toxicological risk assessments associated with herbicide-spraying operations, and as a consultant on several projects for US universities and for private research institutes. Dr. Emond recently served on EPA's Science Advisory Board Reviewing Committee for Trichloroethylene (TCE). His expertise was recognized and used in the dioxin reassessment by the EPA's National Center for Environmental Assessment. In 2008, Dr. Emond and colleagues founded an international nanotoxicology group called The International Team in Nanotoxicology (www.TITNT.com), which includes collaborators from five different countries. He also recently founded a Delaware-based consulting company called BioSimulation Consulting Inc., which provides services in pharmacokinetics for government by offering analytical data-mining support. He is the president of an Endocrine Disruptor Review Work Group for the French Agency for Food, Environmental, and Occupational Health and Safety (ANSES). He is also a member of a steering committee for a Michigan State University PhD student who is studying the health effects of nanoparticles and PBPK modeling, and he serves as a co-director of a UQAM PhD student who is studying nanoparticles in relation to food. Dr. Emond has published many papers and is often invited to present his research at international meetings on persistent organic chemicals and nanotechnology because his work contributes to the improvement of health, safety, and environmental assessment and regulations.

# Contributors

**Simon Beaudoin**
Institute of Environmental Sciences
University of Quebec
Montreal, Canada

**Tamar Chachibaia**
Responsible Nanotechnology Center
Tbilisi, Georgia

**B. C. Chesnutt**
Department of Biomaterials
College of Dental Science
UMCN St. Radboud
Nijmegen, the Netherlands

**Claude Emond**
BioSimulation Consulting Inc,
Newark, Delaware

**Mahsa Hamzeh**
National Research Council Canada
Montreal, Canada

**Seishiro Hirano**
National Institute for
    Environmental Studies
Ibaraki, Japan

**Danail Hristozov**
Department of Environmental
    Sciences, Informatics and Statistics
University Ca' Foscari Venice
Venezia, Italy

**J. A. Jansen**
Department of Biomaterials
College of Dental Science
UMCN St. Radboud
Nijmegen, the Netherlands

**Olivier Jolliet**
Department of Environmental
    Health Sciences
School of Public Health
University of Michigan
Ann Arbor, Michigan

**Frans W. H. Kampers**
Wageningen University
Wageningen, the Netherlands

**Bernard Lachance**
National Research Council Canada
Montreal, Canada

**Alexis Laurent**
Division for Quantitative
    Sustainability Assessment
Department of Management
    Engineering
Technical University of Denmark
Lyngby, Denmark

**Karim Maghni**
Department of Medicine
University of Montreal
and
Research Centre
Sacred Heart Hospital of Montreal
Montreal, Canada

**Ineke Malsch**
Malsch TechnoValuation
Utrecht, the Netherlands

**Asmus Meyer-Plath**
BAM, Federal Institute for Material
    Research and Testing
Berlin, Germany

**Christian Papilloud**
Department of Sociology
Martin Luther University
Halle-Wittenberg, Germany

**Alireza Parandian**
Delft University of Technology
Delft, the Netherlands

**Ralph K. Rosenbaum**
Division for Quantitative
    Sustainability Assessment
Department of Management
    Engineering
Technical University of Denmark
Lyngby, Denmark

**Florian F. Schweinberger**
Catalysis Research Center
Technische Universität München
Garching, Germany

**Geoffrey I. Sunahara**
National Research Council Canada
Montreal, Canada

**Louise Vandelac**
Department of Sociology
and
Institute of Environmental Sciences
University of Quebec
Montreal, Canada

**X. F. Walboomers**
Department of Biomaterials
College of Dental Science
UMCN St. Radboud
Nijmegen, the Netherlands

**M. van der Zande**
RIKILT Wageningen University
BU Toxicology and Bioassays
Wageningen, the Netherlands

# 1

## Introduction

**Ineke Malsch and Claude Emond**

### CONTENTS

Nanotechnology is expected to bring benefits as well as risks for human health. Most of the discussions on the potential and risks of nanotechnology for health are limited to medical applications, including pharmaceuticals and medical devices, or to toxicology of and exposure to nanomaterials. However, in accordance to the World Health Organization's definition of health as "a state of full physical, mental, and social wellbeing," there are more factors than just modern health care that influence human health: the quality of the environment, agriculture, food, and water. In many of these other factors, nanotechnology may be used to make the living conditions for people more healthy. On the other hand, nanotechnology may also play a role in deteriorating living conditions for humans, through exposure to hazardous nanomaterials or in the form of new or strengthened ethical or societal impacts. The scope of this book is to review and assess recent scientific progress in applications of nanotechnology for medical, environmental, agrifood, and water applications—as well as insight in potential hazards of and exposure to engineered nanostructured materials and in nanobioethical and societal issues. The aim is to enable better insight into the potential benefits and risks nanotechnology may offer for human health.

## 1.1  What Is Nanotechnology?

Definitions of nanotechnology depend on the disciplinary background and professional working environment of the person using the term. The most common and broadest definition is, "Materials and devices having functional features with a length scale between one-tenth and several hundreds of nanometers, in one, two, or three dimensions." One-tenth of a nanometer, or 1 Å, is the diameter of a hydrogen atom, the smallest type of atom ($10^{-10}$ m). Nanotechnology therefore does not deal with subatomic particles. In the 1990s, when nanotechnology emerged as a separate area of research, a hundred nanometers was considered the smallest size of functional features on a microchip. Nanotechnology was seen as a possible way to shrink those features beyond the limits of conventional lithography. Nanotechnology may be rooted in physics and mechanical (or precision) engineering but the research done in nanoscience and technology is inherently interdisciplinary in character, and includes at least parts of chemistry, biology, and materials science, if not more disciplines. Most real applications including nanomaterials and technologies can only be developed by interdisciplinary collaborations involving, for example, chemists and physicists.

Given this variety of subdomains in nanotechnology, one may wonder if nanotechnology exists at all. This vagueness of the term is currently problematic; however, when it was introduced in the 1990s, the same fuzziness of the boundaries of nanotechnology was deemed desirable by the policymakers who invented it. They wanted to stimulate interdisciplinary cooperation between scientists from different disciplines working at the nanometer scale because it was generally believed that innovation takes place at the boundaries between disciplines. The policy makers offered funding for scientists willing to cooperate with colleagues from other disciplines. Since the beginning of the twenty-first century, more and more countries have been active in nanoscience and nanotechnology. Several governments are investing considerable amounts in nanotechnology research, an investment that has gradually been overtaken by private investments according to several business consultants whose methods of data collection are not transparent. According to a survey by the Organization for Economic Cooperation and Development

(OECD) Working Party on Nanotechnology (Palmberg 2009), the United States has invested by far the most in nanotechnology in the period between 2005 and 2010 (~US$1400 million/yr between 2005 and 2009), followed by Japan (~US$730 million/yr between 2005 and 2008), Germany (~US$500 million/yr between 2005 and 2010), France (~US$370 million/yr between 2005 and 2007), and Korea (~US$280 million/yr between 2005 and 2010).

---

## 1.2 Government Funding Programs Worldwide and Main Priorities in Research

### 1.2.1 North America

In the United States, the National Nanotechnology Initiative (NNI) coordinates funding for nanotechnology at the federal level. The budget has steadily increased from US$464 million in fiscal year 2001 to US$2.1 billion in 2012. The cumulative total investment in the NNI was US$16.5 billion in this period. It is complemented by state programs and private funding.*

In Canada, at least until 2008, there was no national nanotechnology strategy; however, there are several provincial nanotechnology initiatives or institutes in Quebec, Alberta, Ontario, British Columbia, and New Brunswick. Since the establishment of NINT (National Institute for Nanotechnology) in 1999, Canada has targeted investment to nanotechnology (OECD 2009).

In Mexico, a national plan for nanotechnology research (2008–2012) is still under construction. Since 2009, the nanoscientific research community in Mexico has joined forces in the national nanoscience and nanotechnology network RedNyN. By 2011, this network had around 280 members, 35% to 45% of nanoscientists in the country. There is a lot of research activity in many universities and research centers in the north and center of the country and in Mexico City, including high-quality research in well-equipped laboratories. The focus of most research is mainly fundamental science. Networking between scientists in different parts of the country or with industry is underdeveloped.† Nanotechnology has been recognized as a strategic research area since 2002, without a dedicated national plan for nanotechnology. CONACYT has invested US$14.4 million in 152 nanotechnology projects between 1998 and 2004, involving 58 research institutes. Since 2007, two national laboratories for nanotechnology have been installed by CONACYT, with an investment of US$20 million each.‡ Recently, new groups of young

---

* *Source*: NNI: http://www.nano.gov/about-nni/what/funding.
† See reports on "Nanotechnology in Mexico" at www.nanoforumeula.eu.
‡ See http://www.economia.gob.mx/?P=944.

researchers have started in remote cities. RedNyN stimulates cooperation between them and more experienced groups.*

### 1.2.2 Europe

The European Commission has been playing a leading and coordinating role in nanoscience and nanotechnology development in Europe, at least from the beginning of this century. The EU policy for nanoscience and technology has been laid down in consecutive documents. Since 2002, nanotechnology is explicitly included as a priority in the thematic programs on Nanotechnology, Materials and Production Process (NMP) in the sixth and seventh Framework Programs for research and technological development (RTD) (FP6, 2002–2006 and FP7, 2007–2013). Before, during the Fifth Framework Program (1998–2002), the corresponding priority was called GROWTH (Competitive and Sustainable Growth). Apart from including nanotechnology as an explicit funding priority, the European Commission has also developed a policy for nanotechnology.

On the European level, funding for nanotechnology RTD is available from several sources, including

- European Union FP7 (NMP program and other thematic priorities).
- Coordination of national funding for RTD of member and associated states through ERANET (FP6 and FP7; e.g., NanoSci-ERA, MNT-ERANET, EuroNanoMed).
- In FP7 ERANET+ schemes, national funding can be topped up by EC funding.

Apart from the European Commission, several EU member states also invest in nanotechnology, including Germany, France, the United Kingdom, Italy, Spain, the Netherlands, Switzerland, Poland, Belgium, Austria, Denmark, Finland, the Czech Republic, and Portugal.

### 1.2.3 Japan

In Japan, nanoresearch was one of four priority areas funded under the third Basic S&T Plan 2006–2010. The budget for nanoresearch was 76.2 billion yen (~€494 million) in fiscal year 2006, 78.6 billion yen (~€510 million) in 2007, and 86.5 billion yen (~€562 million) in 2008.[†]

---

* Interviews with Prof. Dr. Sergio Fuentes and Cecilia Noguez, RedNyN board, Mexico, 2011; see Ineke Malsch, ICPC-NanoNet report Nano in Latin America 2011, www.icpc-nanonet.org.
† *Source:* ObservatoryNANO public funding analysis report 2009, http://www.observatorynano. eu/project/filesystem/files/Economics_PublicFundingAnalysis_final.pdf.

## 1.2.4 BRICS

Several emerging economies are also targeting nanotechnology in their national science, technology, and innovation strategy. The BRICS* countries are often depicted as an upcoming new economic block. In Brazil, the first national nanotechnology networks have been funded since 2001 in the form of four millennium institutes cofunded by the World Bank. Since 2005, the federal government has coordinated investment in nanotechnology in national plans. Currently, the focus is on nano-innovation.

Furthermore, Brazil and Argentina have been collaborating in the Binational Argentinean–Brazilian Nanotechnology Center (CABNN) since 2005.

The Russian government established RUSNANO in 2007, focusing on the commercialization of nanotechnology. The total budget until 2012 is 130 billion roubles (US$4.64 billion). The funding is dedicated to three priorities, including

- Nanoproduct fabrication
- Scientific forecasting and roadmaps, standardization, certification, and safety
- Education and popularization

Most of the funding is reserved for the first priority.[†]

The Indian government's Department of Science and Technology installed the Nanoscience and Technology Mission in 2001. In the period between 2006 and 2011, Rs1000 crore (€177 million) has been allocated to nanoresearch. Funding is available for basic research promotion, infrastructure development for nanoscience and technology research, nano applications and technology development program, human resources development, and international cooperation.[‡] Nanotechnology has been part of the tenth (2001–2005) and eleventh (2006–2010) 5-year plans for science and technology. Funding for nanotechnology was RMB 840 million between 2001 and 2005 (US$100 million) and was expected to be double that amount between 2006 and 2010.[§]

The South African government launched their nanoscience and nanotechnology strategy in 2005 and decided to invest US$74 million. In 2007, they allocated additional investment of €34.8 million for the following 3 years.[¶]

In recent years, nanoscientists in increasing numbers of developing countries have initiated networks, research projects, or education programs in

---

* Brazil, Russia, India, China, and South Africa.

† *Source:* ObservatoryNANO public funding analysis report 2009, http://www.observatorynano. eu/project/filesystem/files/Economics_PublicFundingAnalysis_final.pdf.

‡ http://nanomission.gov.in cited in ICPC-NanoNet Report 2009 on Nanotechnology in Asia (West), http://www.icpc-nanonet.org/content/view/93/46/.

§ http://www.sciencemag.org/cgi/content/full/309/5731/61 cited in ICPC-NanoNet Report 2009 on Nanotechnology in Asia (East), http://www.icpc-nanonet.org/content/view/93/46/.

¶ Cited in ICPC-NanoNet Report 2009 on Nanotechnology in Africa, http://www.icpc-nanonet. org/content/view/93/46/.

nanotechnology. Often, these initiatives are taken in international cooperation, to be able to achieve a critical mass of researchers and share equipment
and infrastructure. Overviews of these initiatives can be found in the annual
reports of the ICPC-NanoNet project, www.icpc-nanonet.org. Table 1.1 gives
an indication of nanotechnology activity by numbers of publications in BRICS
and other emerging economies and developing countries.

## 1.3 State of the Art of Nanoscience and Nanotechnology for Human Health

The diverse chapters in this book contribute to an overview of the emergence
of an ebullient research field offering a variety of benefits as well as risks to
human health in the broad sense. What can we learn from these chapters
about the current state of the art of nanotechnology for human health?

### 1.3.1 Section I: Nanoengineering Overview

In Chapter 2, Asmus Meyer-Plath and Florian Schweinberger discuss the
state of the art in nanomaterials characterization and metrology. They cover
properties of different types of nanoparticles and agglomerates, relations
between nanoparticle characteristics and toxicity, strategies for nanoparticle
characterization, and techniques for nanomaterial characterization. They
make some proposals for further studies.

**TABLE 1.1**

Nanotechnology Publications Published in 2009 in Emerging Economies
and Developing Countries by World Region

| World Region | Nanotechnology Publications in 2009 |
|---|---|
| East Asia | 22,437 |
| West Asia | 6810 |
| EECA | 4089 |
| Latin America | 3528 |
| Mediterranean Partner Countries to the EU | 2046 |
| Africa | 497 |
| Former West Balkan countries | 454 |
| Caribbean | 67 |
| Pacific | 2 |

*Source:* Tobin, Lesley; Dingwal, Keith. *Third Annual Report on Nanoscience and
Nanotechnology in Africa.* ICPC NanoNet 2011, Glasgow, www.icpc-nanonet.org.

### 1.3.2 Section II: Biomedical Nanotechnology Overview

Biomedical nanotechnology is a broad area of research. This volume includes two contributions highlighting interesting developments of medical gold nanoparticles and tissue engineering. Throughout the ages, gold has gained a reputation for its therapeutic properties. In Chapter 3, Tamar Chachibaia explores potential applications of gold nanoparticles in medical and cosmetic products. However, more work needs to be done before nanogold can be considered safe for these applications. In Chapter 4, M. van der Zande, B.C. Chesnutt, X. F. Walboomers, and J.A. Jansen argue that nanomaterials can play an important role in future (bone) tissue engineering applications. They have reviewed literature on nanoceramics, nanofibers, and carbon nanotubes.

### 1.3.3 Section III: Nanotechnology and Agrofood and Water

Pharmaceuticals and medical devices are not the only factors contributing to the health of people. A strong determining factor for human health is the quality of the food and water that is consumed. Nanotechnology may contribute to better quality of food. On the other hand, introducing nanoingredients into food may also bring new unforeseen health risks. Two contributions in this volume explore the potential benefits as well as risks of nanotechnology in agrifood and water. In Chapter 5, Frans Kampers explores opportunities of nanotechnology in all aspects of the value chain "from farm to fork." This includes agriculture, food processing, and food packaging. Progress may be hampered by polarized public debate and a lack of openness in the food industry.

In Chapter 6, Simon Beaudoin, Louise Vandelac, and Christian Papilloud focus on the environmental, health, and socioeconomic risks of nanofoods, taking a critical stance.

### 1.3.4 Section IV: Bionanotechnology and the Environment

In Chapter 7 on benefits of nanotechnology for the environment, Danail Hristozov reviews potential applications of nanotechnology to environmental monitoring, remediation, and treatment, which may contribute to a healthier environment for humans to live in. Even though many of the discussed materials and devices are still in the laboratory phase, their potential for contributing to human health is promising.

### 1.3.5 Section V: Nanotoxicology Overview and Problems

Nanotechnology may improve product safety and offer opportunities for a cleaner environment. However, nanomaterials may also introduce new risks for human health and the environment.

Seishiro Hirano and Karim Maghni review the state of the art of *in vitro* study for nanomaterials in Chapter 8. They explain the role of dose metrics in *in vitro* studies and how nanoparticle suspensions are prepared. They then discuss different cell type-based approaches and compare these with a nanomaterial-based approach, giving implications and recommendations for an *in vitro* study.

In Chapter 9, Claude Emond analyzes toxicokinetics and the interaction of nanoparticles with biological matrices. This subsection of toxicology studies kinetic displacement of nanoparticles in an organism in four steps: absorption, distribution, metabolism, and elimination (ADME). Nanoparticles behave differently in an organism than larger particles and it is important to study their kinetic behavior for understanding their effects on the health of the organism.

In Chapter 10, Bernard Lachance, M. Hamzeh, and Geoffrey Sunahara review studies on environmental fate and ecotoxicological effects of nanomaterials. Whereas some nanomaterials may adversely affect different environmental receptors, it is not clear how this toxic potential can be influenced by environmental factors. They pinpoint a number of knowledge gaps that should be addressed.

### 1.3.6 Section VI: Life Cycle

In Chapter 11, Olivier Jolliet, Ralph K. Rosenbaum, and Alexis Laurent present a framework for analyzing the trade-offs between risks and benefits of nanotechnology-enabled alternatives to conventional technologies. This framework takes a life cycle perspective and focuses on impacts on human health.

### 1.3.7 Section VII: Ethical, Legal, and Social Implications of Bionanotechnology

In this part of the volume, the technical trends in nanotechnology for medical, agrifood, and environmental applications and the state-of-the-art in risk assessment of engineered nanomaterials discussed in earlier chapters are placed in a broader societal picture, including socioeconomic dynamics in the innovation chain, ethical aspects of risk assessment such as different interpretations of the precautionary principle, and a general governance framework for nanotechnology in the context of international development cooperation.

As shown in earlier chapters in this volume, nanotechnology promises many benefits for human health, not least by applications of nanotechnology in pharmaceuticals and medical devices, and in monitoring the health status of patients. However, these benefits do not come about all by themselves but must be taken up by a network including research organizations, companies, hospitals, health insurance companies, government bodies, patients and health-care professionals, etc. In Chapter 12, Alireza Parandian examines current gaps in the innovation chain for the case of Body Area Networks for health monitoring.

In Chapter 13, Ineke Malsch applies the capability approach proposed by philosopher Martha Nussbaum to case studies of nanotechnology policies in three middle-income countries in Latin America. This approach offers potential for a new, more integrated governance of nanotechnology in the interest of global human health, by taking into account interests of people in developing countries, and potential risks as well as benefits to human health.

### 1.3.8 Conclusions

Claude Emond summarizes the main findings of the different chapters in the volume.

## References

OECD, *Inventory of National Science, Technology and Innovation Policies for Nanotechnology 2008*. OECD Working Party Nanotechnology, Paris, July 17, 2009, http://www.oecd.org/dataoecd/38/32/43348394.pdf.

Palmberg, Christopher; Dernis, Hélène; Miguet, Claire. *Nanotechnology: An Overview Based on Indicators and Statistics*. STI Working Paper 2009/7. Statistical Analysis of Science, Technology and Industry. OECD, Paris, June 25, 2009, www.oecd.org/sti/nano.

Tobin, Lesley; Dingwal, Keith. *Third Annual Report on Nanoscience and Nanotechnology in Africa*. ICPC-NanoNet 2011, Glasgow, www.icpc-nanonet.org.

# Section I

# Nanoengineering Overview

# 2

## Nanomaterial Characterization and Metrology

**Asmus Meyer-Plath and Florian F. Schweinberger**

## CONTENTS

## 2.1 Introduction

The nanoscale world with structures smaller than 250 nm remained unob-
served for a long time owing to limitations in the resolution of classic optical
microscopy as described by Abbe in 1873* [1]. However, already at that time,
synthetic nanomaterials and nanoparticles were manufactured. An example
is colloidal gold nanoparticles. If synthesized in dispersion, they form a ruby
fluid, which was studied by Faraday in the 1850s. He concluded that it was
composed of gold in very fine metallic form not visible under any microscope
available [2–3]. With the use of electrons as probe particles and the invention
of transmission electron microscopy (TEM) by Knoll and Ruska in 1932, it
became possible to overcome optical resolution limits and to observe and
study nanoscaled structures [4]; early samples were of natural origin: viruses
[5], the endoplasmic reticulum [6], and exfoliated graphites [7]. Soon, a new
quality of material research became possible by the control and manipulation
of structures at the nanometric level. This new quality of control is the central idea behind what is called "nanotechnology" today. Its prospects were
outlined in 1959 in Feynman's famous lecture, "There's plenty of room at the
bottom."† Structure optimization at the nanometer scale turned out to be an
astonishingly successful strategy. Nowadays, new nanoscaled materials are
being designed at a steadily increasing rate. The speed of nanotechnological innovation can safely be predicted to increase even further. It is stimulated by nanostructured materials showing a broad range of surprising or
even revolutionary new properties. Prominent examples in this context are
carbon nanotubes. Their extreme material properties stem from a number
of size- and structure-related phenomena emerging solely at the nanoscale.
Already simple geometrical considerations predict an increase in surface-
to-volume ratio with decreasing particle size. This is linked to an increasing
fraction of surface or grain-boundary atoms of the nanoparticle that exhibit
modified and generally enhanced reactivity. Other astonishing material
properties can be predicted from more complicated arguments of quantum
theory, which are commonly applied to small atom clusters or atom lattices:
size-constrained effects allow for tuning absorption and emission properties
of nanoscaled pigments and semiconducting quantum dot dyes. Band-gap
tailored nanoscaled solid-state structures revolutionize microelectronics and
optics. In composites, nanoparticle additives can dramatically enhance surface hardness of paints by modifications of the particle–matrix interphase.

During the last decades, a close relation between nanotechnological innovation speed and analytical capabilities became apparent. However, the

---

* For visible light, this law limits the resolution to $d = \lambda/(n \sin \alpha)$, where $\alpha$ is the half opening angle of the microscope objective, $n$ is the diffraction index of medium, and $\lambda$ is the
wavelength.
† http://calteches.library.caltech.edu/47/2/1960Bottom.pdf.

development and proper application of new nanomaterial characterization techniques is an urgent issue also for another reason: the successes and prospects of nanostructured material developments create new potential sources of emission of nanoparticles during synthesis, processing, and use. The widely unknown hazards and generally unquantified emission probabilities of most of the new nanomaterials must be of great concern to nanotoxicology. This underlines the importance of reliable nanoparticle characterization techniques and motivates to review its state in the present chapter.

The spectrum of nanomaterials under contemporary research is very broad and incoherent. Consequently, the International Organization for Standardization (ISO) is developing a systematic and hierarchic set of definitions for nanomaterials.* Other sets of nanomaterial definitions have been or are being developed for various regulatory contexts. As a widely accepted feature, nanomaterials are composed of or contain discrete structural parts below 100 nm in one or more spatial dimension: a thin film (nanoplate), a nanorod or nanotube, or a nanoparticle. Furthermore, with a spatial extension in-between molecules and extended bulk materials, nanoparticles[†] are already too complex to be simple objects. Being confronted with a large but heterogeneous ensemble of single, distinguishable complex objects, the characterization of nanomaterials is a challenge. In contrast to simple molecules, nanomaterials already possess a multitude of material characteristics. For instance, even well-synthesized carbon nanotubes, known for their extended cage structure of–theoretically–high symmetrical perfection, exhibit in real-life a large number of individual characteristics such as length, diameter, wall number, chirality, defect density, etc., as depicted in Figure 2.1. Carbon nanotubes will serve as a representative example of nanoparticles also in the following sections.

Even determinate closed-cage molecular structures, such as that of $C_{60}$ fullerenes or silsesquioxanes, obtain a high degree of complexity if chemical side-group functionalization is present. Nanostructured bulk materials, such as nanocomposites containing nanoparticles or nanostructured domains, exhibit an even higher degree of material complexity. This complexity leads to an extremely high variability of nanostructured materials, which allows for synthesis of new, optimized materials. On the other hand, due to the multitude of material characteristics, comprehensive characterization is a demanding and painstaking task. It requires involving different advanced analysis techniques and will be unaffordable in most cases. Therefore, minimum sets of characterization techniques have to be identified that are capable of providing the information relevant for material development and nanotoxicological testing.

---

* ISO/TS 27687.
† Instead of the core term "nano-object" introduced by ISO/TC 229, the term "nanoparticle" will be used throughout this chapter for nanoplate (2D), nanorod (1D), or nanoparticle (0D) nano-objects.

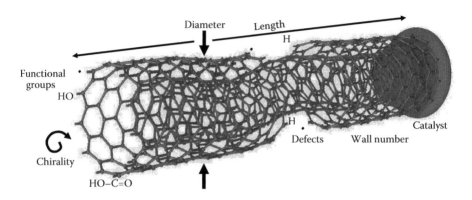

**FIGURE 2.1**
Schematic of double-walled carbon nanotube (DWCNT) with individual characteristics, such as defects, functional groups, and impurities.

The present chapter therefore introduces analytical concepts and techniques for nanomaterials and derives recommendations for a qualified selection of characterization techniques for specific types of samples.

Future nanomaterial research should aim at the synthesis of carefully selected and narrowly distributed material properties. This will remain a demanding task for many years to come and will require closed feedback loops between nanomaterial synthesis and characterization. However, only such well-synthesized nanomaterials with narrow property distributions will allow studying comprehensively characterized nanomaterials. Such well-defined materials are of fundamental importance to achieve an efficient nanotoxicological research on structure–response relations. Also possible toxicity of nanocomposites, that is, nanomaterials containing nanoparticles, will predominantly be related to the action or release of nanoparticles in or from the material's bulk or surface. This chapter therefore focuses on the characterization of nanoparticles and their agglomerates or aggregates.

## 2.2 Properties of Nanoparticles

Nanoparticles range from indistinguishable molecules with a well-defined structure, such as fullerenes, to in principle distinguishable macromolecules and atom clusters with a large number of individual material properties. For such complex particles, their atomic arrangement can no longer be described by conventional chemical notations. Instead, for a complete description, a complex set of atom coordinates with atom type and bond state would be necessary. It could allow numerical computing-derived particle properties such as chemical composition, impurities, structure, structure defects, crystallinity, size, shape, diameter, length, layer number, chirality, surface chemistry, specific surface area, to mention only a few. However, to compile such a complete atomic particle data set for a disperse many-particle ensemble is practically impossible for most materials and contemporary analytical techniques.

Analytical techniques for nanoparticles can be classified into individual (single) particle analysis (IPA) and ensemble-averaging (integral) analysis (EAA) techniques. They derive material information of nanoparticle ensembles in two principally different ways.

Individual particle analysis techniques rely on small random subsamples of an ensemble, consisting of a few particles only. These are prepared and analyzed in detail on a particle-by-particle basis. Individual properties of the observed particles are then compiled into distributions. However, this approach may produce unreliable property distributions if laborious analysis impedes characterization of a sufficiently large number of particles; that is, lacks an adequate amount of statistical significance. In addition, subsample preparation artifacts may affect the resulting property distributions; for instance, if large particle agglomerates are filtered off the ensemble or are omitted during microscopic analysis.

Ensemble-averaging techniques, on the other hand, allow determination of material property distributions of large ensembles. This may help improve statistical significance of ensemble averages. Because of their integral, non-microscopic character, however, they may fail to detect unexpected morphological features of individual particles or particle subsets of the ensemble. For instance, they may fail to unambiguously distinguish porous large particles from similar-sized small particle aggregates. For a complete and meaningful analysis, which should be the basis of any nanotoxicological study aiming at reliable and traceable results, a combination of both approaches is recommended here, in order to avoid systematic misinterpretation of ensemble-averaging results owing to unexpected individual particle features or shapes.

## 2.2.1 Primary Nanoparticles

The characterization of nanoparticulate matter requires answering basic questions on its nature. First, whether it is composed of primary particles or of so-called secondary particles, which are themselves composed of several primary particles, called agglomerates or aggregates, as it will be discussed in Section 2.2.2. The second important question is that of primary particle size, which is closely related to particle shape and is subject of the following subsections.

### 2.2.1.1 Particle Structure, Shape, and Size

Only ensembles of nonagglomerated compact spherical particles allow a *complete* morphological description solely on the basis of a particle diameter distribution. For ensembles containing nonspherical, polydispersed, or partially agglomerated particles, more descriptive parameters and their according distributions have to be determined for a comprehensive morphological characterization. For example, for nonspherical particles such as nanorods and nanoplates, more than one distribution is required for a complete ensemble description, for example, distributions for diameter and length, or thickness and two lateral extensions. Sometimes particle symmetries allow for a simplified description. For hierarchically constructed objects such as multiwalled nanotubes, for instance, data on the number of walls and their according chirality provides complex structure information in a compact, numeric form.

Achieving a complete description of a nanoparticle ensemble is only possible with data from further parameter distributions, including porosity, pore size, defect density, chirality, crystallinity, and surface-crystallographic orientations. However, the dominance of surface atoms of unknown binding state may prohibit efficient information reduction, for instance by crystallographic classification of nanoscale crystallites. Already the structure description of a nanoparticle ensemble requires a large number of parameter distributions and thus significantly complicates the nanotoxicological identification of structure–effect relations. Further, the characterization of the chemical composition, as described below, will add additional material descriptors.

To reduce the necessary information for structure description, and since many nonmicroscopic characterization techniques are unable to measure shape parameters, nanoparticles are frequently *assumed* to be spherical and then described by *equivalent* diameters. Such equivalent diameters correspond to spherical particles showing the same behavior as the (possibly) nonspherical particles under investigation. For instance, gas mobility analysis determines aerodynamic diameters, centrifugation determines sedimentation diameters, dynamic light scattering (DLS), and nanoparticle tracking analysis (NTA) determines hydrodynamic diameters, whereas BET (Brunauer-Emmett-Teller) analysis allows for the analysis of porosity and specific surface area that can be used to derive an averaged diameter (per weight) for nonporous spherical model particles. However, even for truly spherical particles, these *apparent* diameters do not necessarily correspond to the geometric particle diameter and must be treated with care. The aerodynamic diameter, for instance, depends on the orientation of the particles during flight, whereas the hydrodynamic diameter is affected by a pH-dependent ion sheath, which may surround surface-charged particles. The reduced information content provided by equivalent particle diameters must be kept in mind if particle size data are used for particle ensemble characterization. Any research on structure–toxicity relations must therefore comprise particle size assessment and particle shape analysis.* Small-angle

---

* For elongated particles, for example, the extension of the particle in one dimension may exceed a critical threshold and could render it into a toxic fiber-like particle that may cause frustrated phagocytosis [8].

x-ray scattering (SAXS) can provide first ensemble-averaged indications of deviations from spherical shape and initiate subsequent shape inspection by microscopic techniques. Other methods for particle size or mass determination include static light scattering, differential mobility analysis, and mass spectrometric techniques such as time-of-flight mass spectrometry (ToF-MS, MALDI-ToF-MS, ESI-ToF-MS) and asymmetric flow-field flow fractionation (AF4). The shape and size of individual nanoparticles can be analyzed by scanning probe microscopic techniques (SPM) such as scanning tunneling microscopy (STM) and atomic force microscopy (AFM), as well as electron beam-based microscopic techniques such as scanning electron microscopy (SEM) or TEM. The latter also allows investigation of individual crystallite structures, whereas x-ray diffraction (XRD) can determine crystallographic data of particle ensembles.

### 2.2.1.2 Particle Composition and Impurities

The chemical composition of a nanomaterial is of utmost importance, in particular for any toxicological assessment. Individual nanoparticles may be chemically analyzed by SEM or scanning transmission electron microscopy (STEM) paired with energy dispersive x-ray analysis (SEM/EDX, STEM/EDX). Common and important methods for the characterization of the elementary composition of nanoparticle ensembles are inductively coupled plasma mass spectrometry (ICP-MS) and ICP optical emission spectrometry (ICP-OES), atomic absorption spectrometry (AAS),* x-ray fluorescence analysis (XFA), x-ray photoelectron spectroscopy (XPS), and other less frequently used elemental analysis techniques.

For nanoparticles, the release rate of soluble material not only depends on the type, composition, and pH value of the immersing medium, but will also show significant particle size dependence. In addition, particle solubility is strongly related to its surface chemistry, as discussed below. For a proper toxicity assessment, the surface properties of persistent nanoparticles and the release rate of soluble toxic nanoparticles need to be studied in detail. Special care is further required for the characterization of soluble impurities, which may have toxic effects that must not be falsely attributed to the parent nanoparticle. An example is the observed toxicity of catalyst metals in chemically inert carbonaceous materials [9].

### 2.2.1.3 Surface Composition and Chemistry

The surface of a nanoparticle governs all particle–medium interactions. Considering their high specific surface area, nanoparticles require devoting

---

* Using methods such as ICP-MS, ICP-OES and AAS, the samples with the analyte will be atomized before measurement, limiting the obtained data exclusively to the elementary composition of the sample.

special attention to the surface composition and chemistry. The stoichiometry and structure of a nanoparticle's surface may significantly differ from its bulk material. Most importantly, missing binding partners of surface atoms may cause enlarged crystal lattice spacings, affect crystal plane orientations, and induce secondary surface reactions such as oxidation or the formation of radical surface states. This generally leads to the formation of enhanced surface polarity and/or reactivity, which tend to affect dissolution processes acting on the particle.

The chemical nature of surface groups also determines pH-dependent formation of surface charges and governs particle agglomeration propensities and surface adsorption phenomena. Surface chemistry therefore plays an important role in biological systems, in particular with respect to particle transport and biological interactions. Especially the presence of radical surface sites on nanoparticles may induce reactive oxygen species and lead to biological stress [10]. Polar or chemically reactive surface groups may interfere with biological systems in many ways, for instance, by immobilizing toxic chemicals, nutrients, or biomolecules such as proteins and enzymes on their surface.

The importance of a comprehensive characterization of the particle surface chemistry must therefore not be underestimated. However, the reliability of state-of-the-art techniques for the identification and quantification of functional groups on nanoparticle surfaces requires further improvement. Determination of the chemical composition of nanoparticle surfaces relies on traditional analytical tools, originating from surface science. These techniques generally require compact, laterally extended surfaces of known orientation, conditions that are not necessarily satisfied by nanoparticles. Furthermore, the information depth of those analysis methods may lie in the order of the particle size.

For example, XPS probes core electrons of atoms and collects information from a depth of a few nanometers below the surface. This may render XPS a volume-sensitive technique if applied to nanoparticles. The same holds for SEM/EDX, confocal microscopy, and Fourier-transform infrared (FTIR) spectroscopy, which exhibit an analysis depth of several micrometers. For TEM/EDX, the information depth equals the sample thickness. Therefore, cross-sectional views of surface layers are required for EDX analyses. Laterally and vertically resolved surface chemical analysis is achievable by complex and time-consuming high-resolution (HR) scanning TEM (HR-STEM) in combination with electron energy loss spectroscopy (EELS). Also, advanced AFM techniques that explore nanoparticle surfaces with functionalized tips by force–distance curve measurement allow surface chemical analysis. Titration measurements and functional group labeling by chemical derivatization techniques, including fluorescence staining and calorimetry, exhibit analysis depth profiles that critically depend on, for instance, particle solubility, porosity, as well as reagent size and permeability. Surface chemical analysis therefore requires expertise for proper sample preparation and precise interpretation of results.

## 2.2.2 Nanoparticle Agglomerates and Aggregates

Assemblages of nanoparticles are firmly attached at their faces by fusion, sintering, or growth. They form so-called aggregates that are not readily dispersed. The specific surface area of an aggregate is smaller than that of the primary particles.

Agglomerates, on the other hand, are formed by particles that are loosely attached by contact at their corners and edges and exhibit a surface area comparable to that of the particles. However, due to the large specific surface of nanoparticles, even small electrostatic or van der Waals dispersion forces can result in considerable agglomeration strength. Therefore, also agglomerates and little interacting but geometrically entangled nanofibers can, in many cases, not readily be dispersed. As described above, the two terms agglomerates and aggregates are not synonymous; unfortunately they are not used consistently in the literature [11].

In many cases, it is necessary to know not only the size of a particle but also whether a nanoparticle is a primary particle or an agglomerate composed of several primary ones. Agglomerates may, for example, show significantly different biological effects because of reduced mobility, delayed dissolution, and reduced clearance, etc. Since agglomeration generally is a dynamic phenomenon, the question of nanoparticle agglomeration in biological media may be a surprisingly complicated one. Agglomeration forces strongly depend on the composition and properties of the immersing medium. Whether agglomerates are detected in a nanoparticle ensemble also critically depends on the sample preparation and measuring technique.

Electron microscopic techniques that allow reliable agglomeration analysis typically require a drying preparation step that may cause agglomeration by capillary forces during solvent evaporation. Cryogenic preparation for TEM (Cryo-TEM) analysis, on the other hand, using shock-frozen samples, can give valuable insights into the dispersion state of nanoparticles [12]. X-ray or light scattering techniques are important for biological samples since they can be directly applied to cell culture or biological liquids. In such media, numerous agents affect the agglomeration or deagglomeration propensity of nanoparticles. Surface-attaching biomolecules, such as proteins and glycoproteins, can show surfactant effects that may, dependent on the system, both stabilize dispersions or induce agglomeration. In any case, biomolecule coating of nanoparticles or agglomerates can affect cell–membrane interactions. A deagglomeration of nanoparticle assemblages in biological liquids may also be triggered by pH change or enzymes. The agglomerate size of the test sample therefore has to be determined under suspension conditions as similar as possible to the toxicity testing conditions.

## 2.2.3 Nanoparticle Suspensions

As introduced, the problem of agglomeration is a fundamental one with respect to the question of nanoparticle toxicity, as it is directly related to the stability of nanoparticle suspensions used for toxicological studies and material characterization. Since agglomeration shifts particle size distributions to higher medians and may result in microparticle formation, it affects the stability of suspensions and may lead to sedimentation. Larger particles may show less nano-size-specific toxicity and sedimentation may become a clearance effect that changes the effective dose. This underlines the importance of a comprehensive characterization of nanoparticle suspensions.

Further, it has to be considered that nanotoxicological studies working with the most dispersed nanomaterials may represent worst-case scenarios that may not be representative for nanoparticles in their usual agglomeration state. The preparation step for the separation of agglomerates or aggregates into primary nanoparticles may require very high energies or shear forces and may be able to affect the nanoparticle's properties.* Especially, breaking of aggregates by sonication may generate surface radicals that would not have been created under milder dispersion conditions. Such radicals may be quantified by means of electron paramagnetic resonance (EPR) spectroscopy.

Many researchers add surfactants to facilitate dispersion and stabilization. Such additives coat nanoparticles with a film of nanometric thickness that generally change the character of the nanoparticles by suppressing surface-chemical features. Their application therefore requires elaborate control experiments to understand their effects and verify the nontoxicity of the additives themselves.

### 2.2.4 Morphology and Porosity

Experimental techniques for the determination of the structure, shape, and size of primary particles, agglomerates, and aggregates have been discussed in Section 2.2.1.1. Here, methods to determine their porosity will be briefly presented.

The porosity of a nanomaterial can either be an intrinsic particle property or a collective property of particle aggregates. High porosity reduces the apparent density of the nanomaterial and enhances its surface area. Nanoscale and mesoscale pores may induce trapping of molecules, as known from molecular sieves. Surface-functionalized porous materials were successfully used for selective sorption of contaminants from waste streams. The toxic effects of molecule trapping in biological environments are to be studied.

---

* Grinding or ultrasonic treatment may create radicals on particles and fiber fragments [13].

The size distribution of macropores and mesopores can be investigated by mercury porosimetry and from gas adsorption isotherms by the BJH (Barrett-Joyner-Halenda) method. Nanoscale poresize distributions are accessible by SAXS or small angle neutron scattering. TEM or SEM studies should be used additionally to investigate the appearance of the pores.

## 2.2.5 Substance Properties

The chemical composition and crystallinity of the bulk of a nanomaterial determines toxicologically critical properties such as radical formation propensity and release of toxic substances. Crystalline materials may exhibit higher surface radical activity but reduced solubility. The weakly bound surface states exhibit enhanced solubility and reactivity. Therefore, particle size and surface area play a central role for interactions and substance release or dissolution rates of nanoparticles. Solubility increases with decreasing particle size but is also strongly dependent on the surrounding medium and its pH value. Even macroscopically insoluble materials may evolve significant dissolution rates in nanoscale form. Dissolution may also lead to deagglomeration of nanoparticle clusters and thus induce accelerated dissolution rates or release of smaller fragments.

The dissolution rate can, analogue to the chemical composition of nanomaterials, be determined by means of standard chemical analysis techniques such as elemental analysis, ICP-MS, AAS, x-ray fluorescence, and nuclear magnetic resonance (NMR). An alternative approach to dissolution rate determination is particle size monitoring in light or x-ray scattering experiments in solution.

If the structure of a nanomaterial exhibits regularities, such as crystallites, this can be analyzed by XRD or Raman spectroscopy. More important from the toxicological point of view are structure irregularities and defective sites in nanomaterials that may drastically enhance their reactivity.

Reactive radicals, for instance, formed during nanomaterial synthesis or processing, generally lead to functional group formation by oxidation. They disturb the chemical homogeneity of the material and can strongly affect its surface chemistry. Defective radical surface sites can be quantified by colorimetric measurement of the deactivation of free stable radicals such as diphenyl picrylhydrazyl. Surface radicals are known to be a possible source of reactive oxygen species. They cause stress to cells in biological environments. Radical defects are quantifiable by EPR. which does, however, not allow distinguishing surface from volume radicals. The latter may be released upon dissolution of the particle.

## 2.2.6 Surface Properties

The interaction probability of nanosized materials scales with their surface area and reactivity. Determination of the surface area therefore plays a central role for nanomaterials. BET measurement is a well-established standard technique. However, geometrical calculations of the surface area as a substitute for BET may be valid only for regularly shaped, similar-sized, nonporous particles such as spheres.

The tendency of adsorption and agglomeration of nanoparticles is governed by the surface free energy and the polarity of the particles. As the reactivity of the surface, they all depend on the surface chemistry. However, investigation of the surface chemistry of nanoparticles is the most challenging task in nanomaterial sciences. For comprehensive analysis, a number of different techniques have to be combined. Practical characterization is therefore often limited to surface charge estimations by particle charge sizers (PCS) and zeta potential measurement, surface polarity assessment by dynamic vapor sorption or inverse chromatography, and surface free energy determination by tensiometry. For the identification and quantification of surface functional groups, a number of surface analytical techniques have to be combined. XPS is a valuable tool for chemical composition and oxidation state determination. It can be combined with surface group labeling by derivatization reactions. Also, fluorescent staining, coupling of isotope-enriched reagents for NMR spectroscopic quantification, or radioactive markers can be employed to label reactive surface groups. Potentiometric titration has been employed successfully for acid-base quantification. Temperature-induced cleavage of surface functionalities coupled to a balance and to infrared absorption spectroscopy or mass spectrometric detectors (TGA/FTIR, TGA/MS) is used frequently for qualitative group analysis by thermogravimetry. Ion-beam induced surface fragmentation patterns are subject of time-of-flight scanning ion-beam mass spectroscopy (ToF-SIMS) and may allow to derive surface-chemical information. Individual particle surface-chemical investigations have been performed by scanning probe microscopy with functionalized tips or electrochemical measurements by a SPM tips.

## 2.2.7 Aging of Nanoparticles

The characterization of nanoparticles is further complicated by aging phenomena. For the example of carbon nanotubes (CNTs), it has been reported in the literature that similar aging-related decreases in three unrelated properties (surface area and pore volume, surface oxygen, and structural defects) in multiple CNT samples were observed [14]. It is therefore suggested that (certain) physicochemical properties for this particular class of nanoparticles can be characterized with reliability only after the samples have sufficiently aged (9–15 months).

Knowing about the possibility that certain nanoparticles alter in various properties with time, makes the postsynthesis stability, storage (humidity, temperature, exposure to light and atmosphere conditions) and aging of materials under nonequilibrium and under ambient conditions an important issue [15], which has to be tested and investigated before applying the samples in further studies, in order to exclude effects from aging of samples [16].

---

## 2.3 Relations between Nanoparticle Characteristics and Toxicity

For a given amount of granular matter, the number of particles increases with decreasing particle size; additionally, finer granularity changes the material properties. Smaller particles tend to show enhanced diffusivity, permeation propensity, reactivity, and solubility. These observations raise concerns that nanoscaled material may show unanticipated *specific* toxicity (i.e., toxicity per mass), in comparison to microscaled particles.

### 2.3.1 Possible Origins of Nanoparticle-Specific Toxicity

There are various possible origins of enhanced nanoparticle toxicity, which will be discussed in the following. Nanoparticles show higher motility and higher-frequency Brownian motion, which lead to enhanced diffusivity and reduced sedimentation. Their nanometric size can increase permeation and lead to effective dissemination and thus enable nanoparticles to reach new sites of action. For example, in contrast to larger objects, airborne nanoparticles may reach alveolar cavities of the lung, may show enhanced vascular permeability via cell junction passage, and may cross cell membranes via endocytosis.

Also, the reactivity and solubility of nanoscaled matter may be significantly enhanced. Accumulation and clearance processes from cells, organs, or the body will generally be affected by particle size. It is a general geometric feature that with decreasing particle size, the specific surface area (i.e., surface per mass) becomes larger. This increases the specific number of incomplete or less-tightly bound surface atoms or molecules, and gives rise to enhanced surface reactivity. Reactions at the nanoparticle surface can lead to the formation of functional surface groups with enhanced reactivity or polar character, and affect immobilization and transport properties. Both are closely related to clearance, accumulation, and toxic properties. In addition, increased reactivity may accelerate the dissolution rate of surface constituents, and enhance the bioavailability of a substance in nanoscale form. Persistent insoluble nanoparticles, on the other hand, are potentially toxic if they either exhibit or generate radical surface sites that induce oxidative stress to cells, or they initiate frustrated phagocytosis [8]. Unprecedented toxic effects may therefore arise if their surface functionality enables toxic nanoparticles to reach new sites of action, for example, the cytoplasm or the cell nucleus. In this respect, receptor-mediated phagocytosis of functionalized nanoparticles emerge as a critical scenario.

## 2.3.2 Characterization-Related Problems of Toxicological Assessment

As was pointed out before, the size and agglomeration state of an ensemble of anoparticles is a dynamic property and sensitively depends on the characterization medium. In liquid phase, soluble particles may dissolve and insoluble particles may dynamically agglomerate or deagglomerate in accordance to the medium composition and pH value. For most classes of nanoparticles, there is still insufficient understanding of dissolution and agglomeration dynamics in biological environments. These complex dynamics are governed by particle composition and, especially, its surface chemistry. Surface-chemical groups can form pH-dependent surface charges and control immobilization of molecules as well as of proteins present in the biological testing environment.

The characterization of nanoparticles for nanotoxicology, due to the described observations, requires careful adaptation of measurement conditions. The physicochemical characterization of particle size and surface charge should be preferably performed *in situ*; that is, directly inside the biological testing environment. If this is not possible, both setups should resemble as much as possible in order to be sensitive for the complexity of nanoparticle–medium interaction. These interactions of medium constituents and nanoparticles are also far from being fully understood. They may result in profound new effects that are unknown from testing of chemicals and can hardly be perceived. Nanoparticles may exhibit new transport properties through cell membranes or the blood–brain barrier. It is even possible that the surface of inert particles may act as adsorbent for toxic substances or nutrients. Soluble nanoparticles may release toxic ions, as this has been described for silver nanoparticles [17]. This way, nanoparticles may act as vectors (i.e., transport vehicles), inducing local accumulation or release. With their large surface-to-volume ratio, surface interactions of functional groups on nanoparticles introduce an additional degree of complexity to the interaction of nanoparticles with biological systems. Their understanding, especially in environments of complex composition such as cell culture media and biological systems, will be a scientific challenge for many years to come. Any significant progress in this field will require interdisciplinary cooperation of nanotoxicologists together with material scientists, chemists, biologists, and medicines.

## 2.4 Strategies for Nanoparticle Characterization

Only comprehensive and reproducible nanomaterial characterization can provide the basis for a reliable understanding of relations between material properties and biological effects. However, comprehensive characterization of nanomaterials is time consuming, expensive, and complex. As was pointed out in Section 2.2, there are two different approaches to characterize nanoparticles: individual (IPA) and ensemble-averaging (EAA) characterization. The two approaches differ in accuracy and reliability and therefore need to be discussed in detail in the following. As a general rule, a reliable interpretation of the particle properties will require applying both characterization approaches whenever possible. Table 2.1 provides a list of analytical methods for nanomaterials together with their statistical character and information content.

### 2.4.1 Characterization Techniques for Individual Nanoparticles (IPA)

Individual particle characterization is based on signals acquired from distinct particles. This can be achieved either by nanometrically resolving microscopy or by nonresolving techniques applied to spatially separated particles (SSP). However, individual particle analysis is generally accompanied by low strength of the measurement signals, and thus not all analysis techniques may therefore be sensitive enough for individual particles. Examples of microscopic techniques that are able to resolve features of individual nanosized particles include, for example, STM, AFM, and TEM.

The spatial separation required for nanometrically nonresolving techniques can, for instance, be achieved by dilution of suspensions, mobility-related separation in gases (scanning mobility particle sizer [SMPS]) or liquids (AF4 [18,19]), or low-density seeding of particles on substrates. For nonresolving techniques, a subsample must be microscopically characterized in order to elucidate the nature of the particles and to verify spatial separation. Examples of nonresolving analysis techniques include Raman microscopy of individual carbon nanotubes [20] and NTA, which determines hydrodynamic particle diameters by analyzing the Brownian motion of individual particle tracks [21]. Dispersion of particles by gases into aerosols is a frequently used technique for particle counting or size-related transport properties by SMPS.

Characterization of many individual particles allows compiling of a number of distributions of the respective particle property. This does not only provide more detailed information but, more important, allows discovering unexpected structures that may result from artifacts during particle synthesis or dispersion. In addition, individual particle analysis can be a model-free approach, not based on assumptions on the mechanism of collective signal synthesis, as is the case for ensemble-averaging techniques. However, for state-of-the-art technology, individual characterization is still time consuming. The number of analyzed individual particles will therefore generally be small with regard to the nanoparticle ensemble size. This requires that the representativeness of a subsample must be assessed by statistical methods. The property distributions obtained from individual characterization must therefore be tested for normality and pathologic minorities, which, as a benefit of the approach, are not averaged-out, and can be studied in detail. Future developments will focus on automated data acquisition and evaluation in

**TABLE 2.1**

List of Acronyms for Analytical Methods and Statistical Character of the Method

| Acronym | Method | Type | Information |
|---|---|---|---|
| AAS | Atomic absorption spectroscopy | EAA | Atom concentrations [21] |
| AF4 | Asymmetric flow-field flow fractionation | EAA | Size separation for subsequent size determination [18] |
| AFM | Atomic force microscopy | IPA | Size, morphology, topography, chirality [22,23] |
| AFM/FDC | AFM with force distance curve measurement | IPA | Stiffness; for functionalized AFM tips: surface functionality [24] |
| BET | Brunauer, Emmett, Teller method | EAA | Specific surface area, purity and porosity [25] |
| BJH | Barrett, Joyner, Halenda method | EAA | Pore volume and area [26] |
| CM | Confocal microscopy | IPA | Microscopy with subwavelength resolution |
| CPC | Charged particle counter | IPA | Particle number |
| Cryo-TEM | TEM with cryogenic sample preparation | IPA | Particle morphology and agglomeration in (liquid) matrix |
| DLS | Dynamic light scattering | EAA | Apparent particle size (hydrodynamic radius), agglomeration [27] |
| DSC | Differential scanning calorimetry | EAA | Thermal properties, fundamental thermodynamic values, stability |
| DVS | Dynamic vapor sorption | EAA | Surface adsorption and wetting properties |
| EELS | Electron energy loss spectroscopy | | Atomic composition, chemical bonding |
| ESR | Electron spin resonance spectroscopy | EAA | Radical concentration, temperature dependency [28] |
| Fluorescence | Fluorescence spectroscopy | SSP | Detection of fluorescent structures and immobilized markers |
| FTIR | Fourier-transform infrared absorption spectroscopy | EAA | Chemical structure and functionalities |
| HR-TEM | High-resolution TEM | IPA | Morphology, crystal lattice, and atomic structure |
| ICP-MS/OES | Inductively coupled plasma mass or optical emission spectroscopy | EAA | Atom concentrations |
| NMR | Nuclear magnetic resonance spectroscopy | EAA | Chemical structure, solubility |
| NTA | Nanoparticle tracking analysis | IPA | Particle mobility and hydrodynamic size [22,23] |
| PCS | Photocorrelation spectroscopy, see DLS | EAA | Apparent particle size (hydrodynamic radius) [27] |
| PCS | Particle charge sizer | EAA | Surface charge |

*(continued)*

**TABLE 2.1 (Continued)**

List of Acronyms for Analytical Methods and Statistical Character of the Method

| Acronym | Method | Type | Information |
|---------|--------|------|-------------|
| Raman | Raman spectroscopy | SSP | Chemical bonding, defects, fingerprint spectra |
| SAXS | Small-angle x-ray scattering | EAA | Particle core/shell sizes and form factor [2,18] |
| SEM/EDX | SEM with energy dispersive x-ray spectroscopy | SSP | Chemical composition for heavier elements, not quantitative |
| SIMS | Secondary ion mass spectrometry | EAA | Surface composition profile |
| SLS | Static light scattering | EAA | Apparent particle size [27] |
| SMPS | Scanning mobility particle sizer | IPA | Apparent particle size (aerodynamic radius) [29] |
| Solubility | Solubility testing | EAA | |
| STEM | Scanning TEM | IPA | Chemical material analysis with nanometer resolution |
| STM | Scanning tunneling microscopy | IPA | Size, morphology, topography |
| STS | Scanning tunneling spectroscopy | IPA | Chemical composition and band structure |
| TEM | Transmission electron microscopy | EAA | Size, morphology |
| TEM/ED | Electron diffraction | IPA | Crystal structure, chirality |
| TEM/EDX | STEM with energy dispersive x-ray spectroscopy | IPA | Chemical composition for heavier elements, purity |
| TEM/EELS | STEM with EELS | IPA | Atomic composition, chemical bonding |
| TEM/XRD | STEM with XRD | IPA | Local crystalline structure |
| TGA | Thermogravimetric analysis | EAA | Oxidation stability, ash content, elemental/organic carbon, surface chemistry (MS coupled) |
| Titration | Potentiometric acid–base titration of solid particles (Boehm titration) | EAA | Surface acidity/basicity |
| TPD | Temperature programmed desorption | EAA | Adsorption sites and reactivity fingerprint |
| USS | Ultrasonic spectroscopy | EAA | Concentration in suspension |
| UV/Vis/NIR | Ultraviolet/visible spectroscopy, near-infrared spectroscopy | EAA | |
| XFA | X-ray fluorescence analysis | EAA | Atom concentrations |
| XPS | X-ray photoelectron spectroscopy | EAA | Chemical composition and oxidation state |
| XRD | X-ray diffraction | EAA | Crystallinity, domain sizes, lattice spacing |

*Note:* EAA, ensemble–averaging analysis; IPA, individual particle analysis; SSP, IPA is possible only for spatially separated particles with a mutual distance exceeding the spatial resolution of the analysis technique used, see Section 2.4.1.

order to improve counting statistics and reduce (personnel) costs. However, automated analysis requires high-quality spectra or micrographs that are rich in contrast. The automation algorithms must be carefully tested with appropriate reference samples, including variant particle morphologies. Only both reliable algorithms and larger datasets will help improve the reliability of data obtained from individual analysis.

### 2.4.2 Ensemble-Averaging Characterization Techniques for Nanoparticles (EAA)

Ensemble-averaging techniques determine nanoparticle property distributions by integrating the collective response of a particle ensemble to a stimulus. The main advantage of ensemble-averaging techniques is the size of the ensemble that is analyzed with high acquisition speed owing to collective signal generation. The interpretation of data from ensemble-based analysis generally requires model assumptions for the individual particle response to the stimulus in order to derive particle property distributions. For example, in DLS for stimulus, a laser beam is focused on the sample, scattered by individual particles and results in collective interference that shows fluctuations due to Brownian particle motion. Theoretical models are then used to describe individual light scattering and particle motion. Intensity fluctuation interpretation requires complicated data deconvolution in order to obtain the particle size. The validity of the underlying model assumptions can sometimes not be easily tested by the nonexpert user. The interpretation of measurement data of ensemble-averaging analysis techniques therefore requires awareness for possible experimental error sources. Especially, unexpected particle features such as exotic shape, spontaneous agglomeration, or surface charging effects may result in systematically misinterpreted data. Therefore, the applied model assumptions generally require verification by microscopic analysis of a representative set of individual particles.

### 2.4.3 Sample Preparation Issues

Sample preparation for toxicological studies and material characterization is a very demanding task and a crucial basis for reliable results. Artifacts and severe systematic errors can arise from incorrect sample preparation procedures. Insufficient stability of nanoparticle dispersions and accuracy of material dosing are closely related, omnipresent problems. Aging phenomena of nanoparticles, such as accelerated surface oxidation, imply additional complications for reliable and reproducible studies. Incomplete dispersion and uncontrolled reagglomeration makes primary particle size determination from nonmicroscopic methods invalid. Controlled suspension concentration by means of dilution will not be successful in case of unexpected sedimentation or dish wall adherence. The practical determination of particle concentration in liquid fractions taken from dispersions is not easily achieved with high accuracy at low absolute mass content. As a result, it may be difficult to accurately determine nanoparticle doses. Air-to-liquid interfaces have been developed for controlled transfer of nanoparticle aerosols to *in vitro* assays [33].

Also, a reproducible transfer from suspended particles to dry, substrated particles suffers from incomplete dispersion and uncontrolled suspension concentration. In addition, evaporation-related convection and capillary forces can induce reagglomeration on the substrate. Resulting agglomerated material, such as highly entangled nanotubes or large particle agglomerates, may not be accessible to microscopic or individual analysis and thus deteriorate the representativeness of the analyzed sample fraction by systematic omission. Likewise, sedimenting fractions may escape from ensemble-averaging characterization of suspensions and thus will bias property distributions. Also, orientation effects and incorrect viewing angle may bias particle shape and fiber length determination. Sample preparation for TEM, especially preparation of tissue samples containing nanoparticles, requires profound experience and great care to preserve relevant details.

Owing to these complications, toxicological testing of nanoparticles must be based on very carefully designed tests with respect to particle selection, characterization, preparation, dosing, and tracing. Whenever possible, particle concentrations and property distributions should be determined under conditions as relevant as possible to the specific testing conditions. It has to be considered that dynamic interactions in test media will generally affect the agglomerate size. Double-layer expressing salts, pH-dependent surface charge, and proteins such as albumin can induce agglomeration or dispersed nanoparticles. The dynamics of adsorption and agglomeration can be studied experimentally by light or x-ray scattering (SLS, DLS, SAXS).

The use of dispersants may help study the effect of individualized nanoparticles. However, individualized nanoparticles are a limiting case and perhaps a worst-case scenario that does not necessarily reflect naturally occurring agglomeration. In addition, interference effects of the dispersants with the assay have to be studied carefully.

The particle concentration "as dosed" and "as exposed" may differ significantly. Which dose unit is relevant for toxicity testing is still under controversial discussion. Up to now, the most frequently used unit for concentration is the mass of nanomaterial per testing medium volume. However, also the dosed particle number concentration, surface area of nanoparticles, and even the number of nanoparticles per area of lung tissue or culture dish may be suited to assess the significance of nanoparticle effects. Therefore, both mass concentration and particle size distributions must be determined in order to allow for dose unit conversions and comparability of different studies.

### 2.4.4 Importance of Reference Materials

A reliable nanotoxicological understanding of fundamental structure–response relations can only be obtained from systematic studies under well-defined testing conditions. Most important, this requires most complete characterized nanomaterials with properly chosen sample fractions showing narrowly distributed material properties. The selection of appropriate reference materials plays a crucial role for many aspects of nanomaterial research. Their synthesis will therefore remain a demanding task for the next decade. Establishing nanoscale reference materials goes hand in hand with progress in nanometrology, which requires reference materials suited for method calibration.

In addition, reference materials have not only to be well defined with respect to physical properties, such as primary particle size, surface area, and porosity; for the determination of doses and size distributions applied during nanotoxicological testing, detailed knowledge of agglomeration dynamics in dispersion is needed. This imposes the requirement of well-defined particle surface chemistry and working concepts for dispersion stabilization. Recently, nanoscaled gold became available as the first certified reference material for applications in metrology and preclinical biomedical testing [34].

---

## 2.5 Techniques for Nanomaterial Characterization

This section focuses on analytical methods relevant for determination of the most important material characteristics. It does not provide a complete overview of all available techniques.

### 2.5.1 Minimum Set of Nanomaterial Characteristics

The scientific community aims at identifying correlations between nanomaterial properties and biological or ecological responses. For the identification of the nanomaterial under study and for study comparison purposes, any nanotoxicological testing therefore requires precise determination of relevant material characteristics [35–39]. The characteristics given in Table 2.2 are general recommendations for a minimum set required for nanotoxicological studies. The given suggestions may be modified for a particular nanomaterial sample, if part of the methods are not applicable or do not provide relevant information.

In any case, selecting a set of techniques to characterize a nanomaterial sample needs to respect the requirements of the scientific community that a retrospective interpretation of toxicological data in the light of new findings must be possible [16]. Therefore, all relevant information on all potentially significant material characteristics must be provided.

For comparable toxicological studies, every processing step used for preparation of nanomaterial suspensions has to be reported in detail. This includes additives, dispersion, or sonication setup and applied dispersion

**TABLE 2.2**

Set of Minimum Nanomaterial Information Required for Nanotoxicological Studies with Applicable and Recommended (in bold) Characterization Techniques

| Information | | Information Source |
|---|---|---|
| Nanomaterial identity | Manufacturer name | Supplier |
| | Batch number | Manufacturer |
| | Method of synthesis | Manufacturer |
| | Age and storage conditions | Manufacturer and own handling |
| | Sample preparation | Documentation of guideline or operational procedure for testing |

| Information | | Characterization Technique |
|---|---|---|
| Agglomerate or aggregate properties | Morphology | |
| | Agglomerate shape | SEM, TEM, COM |
| | Size distribution | **DLS**, SEM, **TEM**, NTA |
| | Pore size distribution | **BJH**, SAXS |
| Primary particle properties | Morphology | |
| | Particle shape and aspect ratio | **TEM**, SEM, AFM |
| | Size distribution | **TEM**, **DLS**, SEM, NTA |
| | Presence of surface coating | TEM, SIMS-ToF, SAXS, TGA (for organic coatings) |
| | Porosity | TEM, SEM, SAXS, BJH |
| | Crystalline phase | **XRD**, TEM/XRD, HR-TEM |
| | Chemistry | |
| | Chemical composition and levels of impurities | Elemental analysis (**ICP-MS/OES**, AAS, CHN-analysis), SEM/EDX, TEM/ EDX, XFA, FTIR, UV/Vis, NMR, Raman |
| | Solubility | Solubility testing in different media: water, cell culture medium, serum, etc. |
| Surface properties | Physical properties | |
| | Specific surface area | BET |
| | Surface charge | **Zeta potential**, PCS, tensiometry |
| | Chemistry | |
| | Surface chemical composition | **XPS**, STEM/EDX, SIMS |
| | Surface functionality and basicity/acidity | **Titration**, fluorescence staining, AFM/FDC |
| | Surface reactivity | **Derivatization** reactions with XPS or fluorescence detection |

energies (power, duration). Otherwise, reproducible dosing and testing will be impossible. Nanomaterial suspensions generally exhibit highly dynamic properties that must be studied in detail. It is therefore mandatory to study and report the following properties:

- Particle surface charge under testing conditions
- Agglomeration or deagglomeration propensity under testing conditions
- Stability and sedimentation propensity of suspensions used for dosing
- Applied nanomaterial dose in units of surface area and mass

Any study published without providing such crucial data will be of little value for the scientific community. A number of additional nanomaterial characteristics may be relevant for toxic properties and should be studied whenever possible, including

- Apparent density
- Solubility in cytosol for cell toxicological studies
- Surface wettability and surface free energy
- Molecule adsorption dynamics in test medium
- Radical concentration and photocatalytic properties

### 2.5.2 Example: Characterization of Carbon Nanotubes

Carbon nanotubes exhibit fascinating and exceptional material properties. With various applications under development, they are at the brink of becoming ubiquitous nanomaterials. CNT will therefore serve as an example for the following brief presentation of a possible approach to nanoparticle characterization for a toxicological assessment.

To begin with, a literature study should be performed focusing on characterization methods, synthesis and purification methods, as well as material particularities such as chirality and defects of CNT. With the gained insights, a material choice with respect to the synthesis method has to be made between more facile characterizable samples of high purity, structural regularity and ensemble homogeneity, and "real-world" material samples that are used in applications. All material data should be made available, including material supplier, production process, batch number, storing conditions and sample age (see Section 2.2.7). A fraction of the sample should be stored under dark and inert conditions for possible future studies.

For tests of CNT specific toxicity, additional purification steps might be required and should be adapted to the purity requirements of the sample and the test with respect to remaining metal catalysts, amorphous carbon, chemical functionalization, etc. Generally, a multistep purification protocol might be required using both physical and chemical methods. The most important issue of CNTs is the removal of catalytic metals from the production process. Otherwise, toxicity assessment may reflect toxic effects of by-products or residues of CNT synthesis rather than of the CNT material.* On the other hand, any postsynthesis treatment may alter the material characteristics of a sample, especially the CNT sample's length distribution and surface reactivity. Thus, purification must be balanced against modification.

Another challenge is the dispersion of CNT samples for *in vivo* or *in vitro* toxicological assessment. Research on fundamental interactions of CNTs and cell or organs may require fully dispersed (high purity) CNTs. Overall toxicity assessment may require more realistic exposition scenarios using unpurified, as-produced samples with dispersion degrees adapted to the emission source.

Next, an appropriate choice of characterization methods must be made in order to cover the following metrics necessary to determine relevant physicochemical properties of CNTs: size (aspect ratio, distribution), shape, surface area (area/mass ratio), composition (element analysis), surface chemistry (functionalization), crystallinity, agglomeration (dispersion), porosity, heterogeneity, stability (thermal), impurities, defects, solubility, chirality, and conductivity. The selection of techniques should consider the fact that previously acquired data on CNT material properties must be comparable at least with reference to the chosen technique. Minimal requirements for characterization and the commonly used methods should be extracted from the literature, e.g. [30,31]; however, other classes of nanoparticles may require different sets of techniques. In particular, Raman spectroscopy, SEM, and TEM can be considered as base techniques for CNT characterization. Additionally, TGA, UV-Vis/NIR, and XPS are necessary assets for a complete characterization. Electron diffraction and EDX are usually included in advanced TEM devices and may thus be available for elemental analysis without additional instrumentation. Local probe techniques that characterize CNTs on an individual basis, such as AFM, STM, and STS, appear not suitable for routine characterization of CNTs and thus are not considered in this selection.

Last, not least, comparative assessment of CNT standard materials, whenever available, will set a nanotoxicological study into a broader context, allow comparability of results, and promote the understanding of observed effects [32].

## 2.6 Conclusion and Perspectives

The characterization of nanoparticles for toxicological testing is an essential but complex task. Owing to the manifold characteristics of nanoparticles

---

* Frustrated phagocytosis in macrophages resulting from the physical CNT characteristics [8] must be distinguished from chemical effects [9].

that may be of relevance for possible toxic properties, some of them being still unknown, the characterization of a nanomaterial may require as much effort as its toxicological testing. Progress in the understanding of structure–relation properties of nanoparticles will therefore require close collaboration of material scientists and toxicologists. This requires additional costs; however, if characterization is omitted in order to avoid extra costs, the whole study will be worthless if nonstandardized materials were studied.

The development of standardized characterization procedures will progress with the availability of nanoscaled reference materials, which are an important topic of contemporary material research. For missing nanomaterial characterization standards, multimethod characterization should be applied to the nanomaterials under study whenever possible [22].

The release of manufactured nanoparticles from synthesis, compounding, product handling, or end-of-life processes may have important implications for environmental and human health. Assessment of the related risks requires methods to detect and trace nanoparticles in the environment and organisms [22,40]. Determination of nanoparticle release rates, persistency, concentrations and distribution kinetics requires careful design of laboratory tests or strategies to distinguish nanoparticles of natural sources from that of synthetic origin during field testing. In the latter case, such a distinction may require advanced labeling strategies for nanoparticles, for instance by isotopes or fluorescence markers.

## References

1. E. Abbe, "Beiträge zur Theorie des Mikroskops und der mikroskopischen Wahrnehmung," *Arch. Mikrosk. Anat.*, vol. 9, 1873, pp. 413–418.
2. J. Polte, R. Erler, A.F. Thünemann, S. Sokolov, T.T. Ahner, K. Rademann, F. Emmerling, and R. Kraehnert, "Nucleation and growth of gold nanoparticles studied via in situ small angle X-ray scattering at millisecond time resolution," *ACS Nano*, vol. 4, 2010, pp. 1076–1082.
3. M. Faraday, "The Bakerian lecture: Experimental relations of gold (and other metals) to light," *Philos. Trans. R. Soc. Lond.*, vol. 147, 1857, pp. 145–181.
4. M. Knoll and E. Ruska, "Das elektronenmikroskop," *Z. Physik*, vol. 78, 1932, pp. 318–339.
5. B. von Borries and E. Ruska, "Bakterien und Virus in übermikroskopischer Aufnahme," *Klin. Wochenschr.*, vol. 17, 1938, p. 64.
6. K.R. Porter, A. Claude, and E.F. Fullam, "A study of tissue culture cells by electron microscopy: Methods and preliminary observations," *J. Exp. Med.*, vol. 81, 1945, pp. 233–246.
7. G. Ruess and F. Vogt, "Höchst lamellarer Kohlenstoff aus Graphitoxyhydroxyd," *Monatsh. Chem.*, vol. 78, 1948, pp. 222–242.

8. C.A. Poland, R. Duffin, I. Kinloch, A. Maynard, W.A.H. Wallace, A. Seaton, V. Stone, S. Brown, W. MacNee, and K. Donaldson, "Carbon nanotubes introduced into the abdominal cavity of mice show asbestos-like pathogenicity in a pilot study," *Nat. Nanotechnol.*, vol. 3, 2008, pp. 423–428.

9. L.M. Jakubek, S. Marangoudakis, J. Raingo, X. Liu, D. Lipscombe, and R.H. Hurt, "The inhibition of neuronal calcium ion channels by trace levels of yttrium released from carbon nanotubes," *Biomaterials*, vol. 30, 2009, pp. 6351–6357.

10. E. Park and K. Park, "Oxidative stress and pro-inflammatory responses induced by silica nanoparticles in vivo and in vitro," *Toxicol. Lett.*, vol. 184, 2009, pp. 18–25.

11. G. Nichols, S. Byard, M.J. Bloxham, J. Botterill, N.J. Dawson, A. Dennis, V. Diart, N.C. North, and J.D. Sherwood, "A review of the terms agglomerate and aggregate with a recommendation for nomenclature used in powder and particle characterization," *J. Pharm. Sci.*, vol. 91, 2002, pp. 2103–2109.

12. R. Bandyopadhyaya, E. Nativ-Roth, O. Regev, and R. Yerushalmi-Rozen, "Stabilization of individual carbon nanotubes in aqueous solutions," *Nano Lett.*, vol. 2, 2002, pp. 25–28.

13. C. Damm and W. Peukert, "Kinetics of radical formation during the mechanical activation of quartz," *Langmuir*, vol. 25, 2009, pp. 2264–2270.

14. L. Yang, P. Kim, H.M. Meyer, and S. Agnihotri, "Aging of nanocarbons in ambient conditions: Probable metastability of carbon nanotubes," *J. Colloid Interface Sci.*, vol. 338, 2009, pp. 128–134.

15. R. Hurt, M. Monthioux, and A. Kane, "Toxicology of carbon nanomaterials: Status, trends, and perspectives on the special issue," *Carbon*, vol. 44, 2006, pp. 1028–1033.

16. G. Oberdörster, A. Maynard, K. Donaldson, V. Castranova, J. Fitzpatrick, K. Ausman, J. Carter et al, and A report from the ILSI Research Foundation/Risk Science Institute Nanomaterial Toxicity Screening Working Group, "Principles for characterizing the potential human health effects from exposure to nanomaterials: Elements of a screening strategy," *Part. Fibre Toxicol.*, vol. 2, 2005, p. 8.

17. J. Liu, D.A. Sonshine, S. Shervani, and R.H. Hurt, "Controlled release of biologically active silver from nanosilver surfaces," *ACS Nano*, vol. 4, 2010, pp. 6903–6913.

18. A.F. Thünemann, S. Rolf, P. Knappe, and S. Weidner, "In situ analysis of a bimodal size distribution of superparamagnetic nanoparticles," *Anal. Chem.*, vol. 81, 2009, pp. 296–301.

19. M.H. Moon and J.C. Giddings, "Extension of sedimentation/steric field-flow fractionation into the submicrometer range: Size analysis of 0.2–15 μm metal particles," *Anal. Chem.*, vol. 64, 1992, pp. 3029–3037.

20. G. Duesberg, "Experimental observation of individual single-wall nanotube species by Raman microscopy," *Chem. Phys. Lett.*, vol. 310, 1999, pp. 8–14.

21. L.C.J. Thomassen, A. Aerts, V. Rabolli, D. Lison, L. Gonzalez, M. Kirsch-Volders, D. Napierska, P.H. Hoet, C.E.A. Kirschhock, and J.A. Martens, "Synthesis and characterization of stable monodisperse silica nanoparticle sols for in vitro cytotoxicity testing," *Langmuir*, vol. 26, 2010, pp. 328–335.

22. R.F. Domingos, M.A. Baalousha, Y. Ju-Nam, M.M. Reid, N. Tufenkji, J.R. Lead, G.G. Leppard, and K.J. Wilkinson, "Characterizing manufactured nanoparticles in the environment: Multimethod determination of particle sizes," *Environ. Sci. Technol.*, vol. 43, 2009, pp. 7277–7284.

23. I. Montes-Burgos, D. Walczyk, P. Hole, J. Smith, I. Lynch, and K. Dawson, "Characterisation of nanoparticle size and state prior to nanotoxicological studies," *J. Nanopart. Res.* vol. 10, 2009, pp. 47–53.

24. H. Butt, B. Cappella, and M. Kappl, "Force measurements with the atomic force microscope: Technique, interpretation and applications," *Surf. Sci. Rep.*, vol. 59, 2005, pp. 1–152.

25. S. Brunauer, P.H. Emmett, and E. Teller, "Adsorption of gases in multimolecular layers," *J. Am. Chem. Soc.*, vol. 60, 1938, pp. 309–319.

26. E.P. Barrett, L.G. Joyner, and P.P. Halenda, "The determination of pore volume and area distributions in porous substances. I. Computations from nitrogen isotherms," *J. Am. Chem. Soc.*, vol. 73, 1951, pp. 373–380.

27. J. Holoubek, "Some applications of light scattering in materials science," *J. Quant. Spectr. Rad. Transfer*, vol. 106, 2007, pp. 104–121.

28. J.F. Reeves, S.J. Davies, N.J. Dodd, and A.N. Jha, "Hydroxyl radicals (OH) are associated with titanium dioxide ($TiO_2$) nanoparticle-induced cytotoxicity and oxidative DNA damage in fish cells," *Mutat. Res. Fundam. Mol. Mech. Mutagen.*, vol. 640, 2008, pp. 113–122.

29. V.H. Grassian, P.T. O'Shaughnessy, A. Adamcakova-Dodd, J.M. Pettibone, and P.S. Thorne, "Inhalation exposure study of titanium dioxide nanoparticles with a primary particle size of 2 to 5 nm," *Environ. Health Perspect.*, vol. 115, 2007, pp. 397–402.

30. R.H. Hurt, M. Monthioux, and A. Kane, "Toxicology of carbon nanomaterials: Status, trends, and perspectives on the special issue," *Carbon*, vol. 44, 2006, pp. 1028–1033.

31. G. Oberdörster, A. Maynard, K. Donaldson, V. Castranova, J. Fitzpatrick, K. Ausman, and J. Carter et al. "Principles for characterizing the potential human health effects from exposure to nanomaterials: Elements of a screening strategy," *Part. Fibre Toxicol.*, vol. 2, 2005, pp. 8–42.

32. F.F. Schweinberger and A. Meyer-Plath, "Status of characterization techniques for carbon nanotubes and suggestions towards standards suitable for toxicological assessment," *J. Phys.: Conf, Ser.*, vol. 304, 2011, p. 012087.

33. A. Lenz, E. Karg, B. Lentner, V. Dittrich, C. Brandenberger, B. Rothen-Rutishauser, H. Schulz, G. Ferron, and O. Schmid, "A dose-controlled system for air–liquid interface cell exposure and application to zinc oxide nanoparticles," *Part. Fibre Toxicol.*, vol. 6, 2009, p. 32.

34. D. Kaiser and R. Watters, *Reference Material 8011–8013—10, 30, 60 nm Gold Nanoparticles*, http://www.nist.gov/msel/ceramics/gold-standard.cfm. NIST, 2007.

35. W. Catenhusen and A. Grobe (Eds.), *Responsible Use of Nanotechnologies—Report and recommendations of the German Federal Government's NanoKommission for 2008*, http://www.bmu.de/files/english/pdf/application/pdf/nanokomm_abschlussbericht_2008_en.pdf

36. D.R. Boverhof and R.M. David, "Nanomaterial characterization: Considerations and needs for hazard assessment and safety evaluation," *Anal. Bioanal. Chem.*, vol. 396, 2010, pp. 953–961.

37. D.B. Warheit, "How meaningful are the results of nanotoxicity studies in the absence of adequate material characterization?" *Toxicol. Sci.*, vol. 101, 2008, pp. 183–185.

38. M. Hassellöv, J. Readman, J. Ranville, and K. Tiede, "Nanoparticle analysis and characterization methodologies in environmental risk assessment of engineered nanoparticles," *Ecotoxicology*, vol. 17, 2008, pp. 344–361.
39. C.M. Sayes and D.B. Warheit, "Characterization of nanomaterials for toxicity assessment," *Wiley Interdiscip. Rev. Nanomed. Nanobiotechnol.*, vol. 1, 2009, pp. 660–670.
40. K. Tiede, A.B.A. Boxall, S.P. Tear, J. Lewis, H. David, and M. Hassellöv, "Detection and characterization of engineered nanoparticles in food and the environment," *Food Addit. Contam. Part A Chem. Anal. Control. Expo. Risk Assess.*, vol. 25, 2008, p. 795.

# Section II

# Biomedical Nanotechnology Overview

# 3

# Nanoparticles: New Medical Potential—Today and Tomorrow

**Tamar Chachibaia**

## CONTENTS

## 3.1 Introduction

The history of drug formulations that rely on nanoengineering is quite modern. The launch of products incorporating nanostructure particles is showing clear differentiation across sectors. Materials and products based on nanotechnology are regulated today within the existing network. Nanostructures are evaluated as "chemicals with new uses" or as "new chemicals."

Health-care and life sciences applications, such as nanostructured medical devices and nanotherapeutics, have the longest time to market due to sector-specific regulation. In 2004, the US Food and Drug Administration (FDA) estimated that the proportion of all new drugs entering first-phase trials that ultimately gain approval had fallen to 8% from a historical average of about 14%. The most common factors resulting in project failure are lack of efficacy (25%), clinical safety concerns (12%), and toxicological findings in preclinical evaluation (20%). Proposed Investigational New Drug Application (IND) needs to follow the way to FDA and EC approval, passing through all stages of investigations lasting up to 10 to 15 years, starting *in vitro* and ending with the third phase of clinical trials with subsequent approval of medication and pharmaceutical market entry.

The current applications of nanotechnology span a wide range of sectors. The current niche for such applications is in the areas where there is an overlap between the medicine and cosmetic sectors. Many products are marketed as a means to enhance performance for different lifestyles and age groups, as an aid to health, beauty, and wellbeing. Although such applications are relatively new and emergent, they appear to have started to make a global impact. The number one question is if the quality of life will improve thanks to the synthesis of new materials with new properties. How should people benefit from achievements of nanotechnology and nanoengineering? The answers to these and related questions are controversial, owing to the different approaches of regulation rules before the market entry of new products.

While FDA requirements are strict for novel medications, conversely, regulatory mechanisms for cosmetic products allow earlier market entry. Unlike the medical and health-care sectors, the cosmetic industry outpaces the commercial potential of nanoparticle-containing products. To compare with the rate of released cosmetics, widely distributed worldwide, the situation is quite unequal. Drugs, food packaging, and new chemical compounds require premarket review and approval, whereas in cases related to cosmetics and the majority of consumer products, postmarket surveillance and monitoring are sufficient.[1]

Although the constituent materials used in cosmetic and personal care products should be approved by the FDA, at the same time there is no need for conducting long-running clinical trials, as in the case of pharmaceutical drugs. However, regulatory mechanisms require revision when dealing with ingredients processed to nanoscale dimension, where absolutely diverse chemical and physical properties are revealed. Of particular interest are cosmetics and personal care products. Recently, there is widespread use of nanoparticle gold-containing cosmetics such as skin creams that are used on the whole body surface for the "shining glow" appearance, lipsticks, antiaging face creams, and many other products. Despite the large interest and widespread investigations performed for safety and efficacy studies for nanoparticle gold utilization in medical diagnostics and treatment, it is obvious that few, if any, are approved for these purposes. An overview of the state-of-the-art exploration of nanoparticle gold compounds will provide us with special knowledge about the differences in physical and chemical properties of nanogold, dependent on size, shape, charge, and even the solvent used in processing of this metal.

Gold nanoparticles are widely used in biomedical imaging and diagnostic tests. On the basis of their established use in the laboratory and their chemical stability, gold nanoparticles are expected to be safe. The recent literature, however, contains conflicting data about the cytotoxicity of gold nanoparticles.

## 3.2 Health Monitoring Issues Concerning Nondestructive Use of Nanoparticle Gold Compounds in Medicine and Cosmetology

"All is not gold that glitters"

The postindustrial gold rush reflects the hype of nanotechnologies, already ubiquitous in a wide range of consumer products, as diverse as electronics, medicine, environmental remediation, cosmetics, and solar energy. Discovering distinctive properties that many materials display at the extremely minuscule scale opens new opportunities for their conventional use.[2] Of particular interest to most nanotechnology applications are engineered nanoparticles (ENPs), which have much larger surface-to-mass ratios. Nanosized ENPs have also been claimed to have a greater uptake, absorption, and bioavailability in the body compared with their bulk equivalents. This makes it possible to reduce the use of solvents in certain applications, such as certain cosmetics and personal care products, to allow the dispersion of water-insoluble colors, flavors, and preservatives in low-fat systems. Nanosized water-insoluble substances can enable their uniform dispersion in aqueous formulations. This aspect alone has attracted a lot of commercial interest in the use of nanosized ingredients.[3]

Among other ENPs, interest in gold has not diminished; on the contrary, it has increased enormously in recent years, particularly since the early 1980s, when the mass production of nanoscaled chemical substances started, owing to the invention of the scanning tunneling microscope and the atomic force microscope. IBM scientists have enabled the manipulation of even individual atoms to design and synthesize materials for attaining desired features. Later in the 2000s, IBM scientists, by precisely placing atom-by-atom 20,000 gold particles, each about 60 nm in diameter, reproduced an image of Robert Fludd's seventeenth century drawing of the sun—alchemists' symbol for gold. IBM scientists demonstrated a new nano "printing" bottom-up technique, which will lead to breakthroughs in ultratiny chips, lenses for optics, and biosensors for health care.

As gold is the most studied chemical element, it is characterized as having the most predictable behavior. However, gold nanoparticles may act absolutely diversely. Bulk gold, which is usually characterized by its yellow color, while being processed to a nano-dimensional scale, transforms its color to orange, purple, red, or a greenish tinge owing to different particle sizes. The most well-known cultural artifact in nanotechnology is housed in the British Museum—the Lycurgus Cup (dated fourth century AD), which is a glass cup of ruby red color due to its colloidal gold content and changes to a greenish color upon light exposure. Nanogold was used in medieval times in stained glass materials to attain almost all the colors of the rainbow. Today, nobody will argue that nanosized gold particles do not act like bulk gold.[4]

Traditionally, bulk gold was considered a chemically inert and biocompatible material; owing to these features, it is utilized widely in medical applications, for example, in dental prosthesis and eyelid implants. Throughout history, gold has been used to cure diseases. Finely ground gold particles in the size range of 10–500 nm can be suspended in water. Such suspensions were used for medical purposes in ancient Egypt over 5000 years ago. In Alexandria, Egyptian alchemists used fine gold particles to produce a colloidal elixir known as "liquid gold," which was intended to restore youth.[5] Dating back to the Roman Empire, colloidal gold was thought to have healing properties. A colloid refers to a substance in which many fine particles are suspended in a stable condition with another substance. Gold nanoparticles were traditionally used in the Indian remedy "curcumin."[6] The German bacteriologist Robert Koch showed that gold compounds inhibit the growth of bacteria. He was awarded the Nobel Prize for medicine in 1905.

With the developments in the pharmaceutical industry, first in 1935, gold salt-containing drugs were reported to be effective for the treatment of rheumatoid arthritis. It is thought that gold affects the entire immune response (phagocytes, leukocytes, T cells) and reduces its potency and limits its oxidizing nature on joint inflammation and erosion. This effect is explained by the fact that administered gold compounds accumulate within the body once absorbed into the cells and are linked to antimitochondrial activity, inducing the apoptosis of proinflammatory cells. The World Health Organization classified gold salt-containing compounds as antirheumatic agents and included such compounds in the basic treatment scheme of the disease.

Because of the long history of the use of gold inside the body, the safety issues seem to have been somewhat easier to assume, despite becoming more and more challenging owing to achievements in the synthesis of new materials enabled by nanotechnology.

The properties of gold molecules processed to nanometer dimension are thoroughly studied. Gold attains divergent physical and chemical characteristics while its molecules are being processed to nanoscale dimension. Scientists have revealed the diverse properties of nanoparticle gold, which is dependent on various factors. Particularly, such properties are dependent not only on the size of the gold nanoparticle but also on other characteristics such as particle shape, charge and composition, or surface coating, which are also important. Consequently, the health monitoring aspects are of greater concern than before.

When dealing with constraints of size <100 nm, the laws of quantum physics supersede those of traditional physics, resulting in changes in a substance's properties. Quantum size effects begin to significantly alter material properties, such as transparency, color of fluorescence, electrical conductivity, magnetic permeability, and other characteristics. All these properties are of great interest for the industry and society, as they enable new applications and products. Consequently, more attention is focused on determining the ratio of efficiency versus toxicity, or harm versus benefit. There are some examples of conventional use of nanoscaled gold particles. For instance, the Japanese scientist Dr. Masatake Haruta discovered that while the particle diameter is turned in the size range of 3–5 nm, gold exhibits unique catalytic performance, for example, carbon monoxide ($CO$) oxidation and direct peroxide ($H_2O_2$) production at a temperature as low as $-77°C$.[7] In practice, this invention was tested to prevent bad odor in rest rooms and are already in use in Japan. Thus, gold nanoparticles can eliminate odors produced by bacterial action. This is an unusual feature for bulk gold but characteristic for nanoscaled gold particles. Another application for the catalytic properties of nanosized gold particles is for fuel cells of hydrogen batteries.

One hundred and fifty years after one of the founders of chemistry, Michael Faraday, first created gold nanoparticles in the 1850s and observed that these nanoparticles absorb light, researchers in the twentieth century rediscovered that a mere flash of light can cause gold particles to melt. Absorbed light is efficiently turned into extreme heat, which is capable of killing cancer cells. The externally applied energy may be mechanical, radiofrequency, laser, optical, or near-infrared light, but the resultant therapeutic action is the same. Gold nanoparticles are also recognized by their ability to bind to DNA, which may be exploited for the treatment of diseases, for example, as anticancer agents or gene therapy agents; however, they may also contribute to genotoxicity, or block transcription.[8] Hamad-Schifferli et al.[9] have demonstrated that transmitted radiosignals influence the integrity of the DNA strand while it is bound to nanoparticle gold molecules. This discovery opens up the possibility of controlling more complex biological processes of living cells, such as enzymatic activity, protein folding, and biomolecular assembly. Furthermore, the ability of gold nanoparticles to bind to DNA is of concern, owing to their potential cytotoxic or genotoxic consequences, which may be exploited for anticancer drugs or gene therapy, and warrants further investigation. In addition, the ability of gold nanoparticles to interrupt transcription is of concern.[10]

Naomi Halas of Rice University (Houston, TX) developed gold nanoshells in the 1990s. According to the study's lead authors, Rebekah Drezek and Jennifer West, nanoshells have a core of silica and a metallic outer layer of gold, or may be exchanged by copper or iron. Nanoshells will preferentially concentrate in cancer lesion sites. In her interview with Nova, Naomi Halas describes a nanoshell as "essentially a nanolens" that captures light and then focuses it around itself.[11] A near-infrared laser aimed at the tumor site from outside the body (light can travel through tissue more than 10 cm) induces the nanoshells to absorb the light and focus it on the tumor. The area around the nanoshells heats up and the tumor "cooks" until it is ablated. Halas points out that the nanoshells leave no "toxic trail" in the body the way conventional chemotherapeutic agents do, and stated that "long-term studies have not indicated any toxicity or effect on the immune system."

The structure and properties of gold nanoparticles make them attractive for a wide range of biological applications. Nanoparticle gold is considered a low-toxicity material and is currently widely used in cosmetology.

Actually, nanostructured gold particles possess various properties that are under investigation and need longer time to final approval. Few if any of the fabricated nanoparticle gold-containing medications are yet approved by the FDA. In August 2009, a report of the EU Seventh Framework Program, "Engineered Nanoparticles: Review of Health and Environmental Safety," was released.[12]

Particle size has been demonstrated to influence the dermal penetration of gold nanoparticles.[13] Therefore, in general, greater effects are observed for smaller particles. The size of particles has been proven to have a large influence on their behavior. Accordingly, smaller particles have a wider tissue distribution, penetrate further within the skin and become internalized to a greater extent, and have a larger toxic potency. However, more extensive investigations in the future are required to more fully understand the tissue distribution and fate of metal particles after exposure.

It was estimated that the optimal size of nanoparticles for interaction with the skin would be in the range of 50 nm. Smaller particles tend to penetrate the skin more easily than large particles, sometimes being taken up by the lymphatic system and becoming localized in the lymph nodes.[14] Among other factors that should also be considered are particle concentration and charge state, which are in causal relation with their influence on living cells. Goodman et al.[15] demonstrated gold cationic particles of 2 nm size as moderately toxic, whereas anionic particles were relatively nontoxic; their observation data coincide with those obtained in different studies.[16] Toxicity, however, has been observed at high concentrations of these systems.

In one study, the research group headed by Dr. Shuguang Wang[17] demonstrated a cytotoxic effect on human skin keratinocytes of gold nanomaterials of different sizes and shapes. It was shown that spherical gold nanoparticles of different sizes are not inherently toxic to human skin cells; conversely, gold nanorods are highly toxic due to the presence of the coating material cetyltrimethylammonium bromide (CTAB), which is used in the manufacturing process. This toxicity factor caused a limitation on the commercialization of gold nanorods for *in vivo* and *in vitro* applications. It is unreasonable to make generalizations from just a few studies because in recent years the company Nanopartz has found a new manufacturing method, replacing the undesirable organic molecule CTAB with polyethylene glycol (PEG). PEG has low toxicity and is used in a variety of products. Nanorods from one supplier may not be necessarily representative of the toxicity of the physical characteristics of all manufactured nanorods. Furthermore, other nanocoating molecules, such as liposomes, dendrimers, biodegradable polymers, or albumin, are capable of reducing the toxicity of the incorporated agent.

The major promise lies on the discovery of thiol (a compound with a functional group composed of a sulfur atom and a hydrogen atom—SH), which protects colloidal gold nanoparticles bound to the cytokine tumor necrosis factor (TNF). Diminishing the extreme activity of free TNF, an enhanced antitumor effect is attained by assembling TNF molecules into a complex structure with PEG linked with colloidal gold nanoparticles.[18] This new approach has significant advantages over other alternatives and is under development by the company CytImmune, elaborating the results to achieve final approval.

Gold nanoparticles are also more biocompatible than other types of optically active nanoparticles, such as cadmium-containing quantum dots.

Owing to its toxicity, the use of cadmium is restricted in living cells. This is why the process of nanofabrication, in particular the preparation of gold nanodots or quantum dots, is well known. In 2007, the National Medal of Science, the United States' highest honor in the field, was awarded to the Egyptian-American chemist Professor Mostafa El-Sayed, director of the Laser Dynamics Laboratory of the Georgia Institute of Technology, for his many outstanding contributions, among which using gold nanorods in cancer tumor treatment was the most recent. Gold nanoparticles are very good at scattering and absorbing light. For example, nanoparticles that are 36 nm wide absorb light over 10,000 times better than conventional organic dyes, making them potential candidates for optical imaging applications of small tumors. In the study, researchers found that gold nanoparticles have 600% greater affinity for specific overexpressed surface receptors in cancer cells than in noncancerous cells.

As nanotechnology tended to progress in a most responsible manner from the moment of its foundation, when the US National Nanotechnology Initiative (NNI) was established in 2000, it seems to have the most number of regulatory mechanisms for greener development than any other known technology, and social scientists have been involved from the very beginning.

Green nanotechnology is developed to be environmentally friendly. Dr. Jim Hutchinson's research group at the University of Oregon works at the cleaner and greener production of gold nanoparticles, a process that also reduces the cost of synthesizing these materials from 300,000 to 500 dollars per gram.[19] Actually, cost is one of the determining factors for manufacturing, next to safety and effectiveness.

Recent studies have enabled the synthesis of gold nanoparticles by means of certain bacterial strains; for example, *Stenotrophomonas maltophilia* was incubated for 8 h in a gold salt-containing solution, resulting in the synthesis of gold nanoparticles that were about 40 nm in size.[20] The opportunity of this way of synthesis is that it produces gold nanoparticles that are free of solvent and have hydrophilic properties, and may attain particles of various sizes in industrial quantities. This is a new approach to green technology development.

A recent report by J. Davies, from the Woodrow Wilson International Center of Scholars, strongly criticized the current approach in cosmetics regulation as wholly inadequate in dealing with the risks posed by nanotechnologies: "Although the Food, Drug and Cosmetic Act (FDCA) has a lot of language devoted to cosmetics, it is not too much of an exaggeration to say that cosmetics in the USA are essentially unregulated."[21]

David Rejeski, director of the Project on Emerging Nanotechnologies, Woodrow Wilson International Center of Scholars, gives recommendations: "for building confidence in nanotechnologies it is necessary to achieve greater transparency and disclosure; compulsory requirement is also pre-market testing, as well involvement of third party for additional testing and further research."[22] Although some cosmetic manufacturers may differ with regard to such conclusions, based on unpublished propriety research, due diligence is needed in tracing assertions back to primary sources.[23]

In 2007, the United States listed gold and silver nanoparticles among a number of new chemicals and materials that the FDA had asked the National Toxicology Program (NTP) to study. This will seek to determine whether their use causes specific health problems. The NTP should test gold nanoparticles and determine what types of tests are warranted.

## 3.3 Summary

Although bulk gold is considered to be intact and the most inert material used safely for centuries, in addition to being considered the most nontoxic material by chemists, nanoparticulated gold poses certain risks for human health, mainly due to the many aspects of modifications enabled by nanotechnology. Particle shape and the solvent used to obtain gold nanoparticles present some danger to safety. Experiments have shown that gold nanoparticles can result in uptake via the relevant exposure routes. Their properties and the cell types used for their exposure are likely to influence the uptake, subcellular distribution, and toxicity of gold nanoparticles. That is why scientists work to obtain safe and nontoxic forms of nanoparticle gold—examples include ultrasound exposure for the production of gold nanoparticles and the use of certain bacterial strains capable of producing gold nanoparticles that are free of solvent. However, the charge and particle shape characteristics remain a cause for concern with regard to consumer safety. From a thorough analysis of the scientific literature, investigating the divergent features of gold nanoparticles, the concept that some gold nanoparticles pose human health risks can be obviated, as information about the exact physical and chemical properties of gold nanoparticles used in certain cosmetic or health-care products need to be strictly regulated. Until now, relevant control mechanisms are under development. As cosmetic products achieve market acceptance earlier than drugs, there are currently available personal care items in the market that are positioned as nanoparticle gold containing and safe. Actually, many of them must be safe, as manufacturers sell nanogold-containing fluids, the chemical and physical properties of which are presented in product certificates.

However, investigations on metal particulates are still in their infancy at this time and have concentrated on revealing the toxicity, safety, tissue distribution, antibacterial properties, and cellular uptake of gold nanoparticles. Consequently, more comprehensive studies are required to more fully understand the risks associated with metal particulate exposure.

Inevitably, any emerging technology requires extensive safety assessment before coming to market, including diagnostics, medications, and cosmetics. While comparing and evaluating newly established properties at the nanoscale, consumers may experience confusion concerning safety issues. Mass production and the uncontrolled release of products containing gold nanoparticles may reveal the same consequences as any irresponsible application of a new technology. The twenty-first century "gold rush" may result in worse consequences than any other emerging technology.

Fortunately, in recent years, the control and regulatory mechanisms for the utilization of nanoparticles in cosmetic products have increased. For instance, on March 24, 2009, the European Parliament (EP) approved an update of the EU legislation on cosmetics. As requested by the EP, the new regulation introduces definition, safety assessment procedure, and labeling requirements for all nanomaterials that are used in cosmetics.

## References

1. Roco MC. Nanotechnology: Societal Implications—Maximizing Benefit for Humanity. Report of the National Nanotechnology Initiative Workshop. *Setting New Targets for Responsible Nanotechnology*. Arlington, Virginia, 2003:22–32.
2. Technology review published by MIT of nanotech developments in 2005 (http://www.technologyreview.com/Nanotech-Materials/wtr_16096,318,pl.html).
3. Chaudhry Q, Castle L, and Watkins R. Nanotechnologies in the Food Arena: New Opportunities, New Questions, New Concerns. In Nanotechnologies in food. *RSC Nanosci. Nanotechnol.* 2010, n. 14(1):1–18. (Royal Society of Chemistry: www.rsc.org).
4. Ratner M and Ratner D. *Nanotechnology*. Upper Saddle River, NJ: Prentice Hall, 2003.
5. Amer MS. Nanotechnology, the Technology of Small Thermodynamic Systems. In Raman spectroscopy, fullerenes and nanotechnology. *RSC Nanosci Nanotechnol.* 2010, n. 13(1):1–42. (Royal Society of Chemistry: www.rsc.org).
6. Jagannathan R et al. Functionalizing gold nanoparticles for biomedical applications: From catching crystals at birth to mature activity. In: 5th Int. Conf. Gold Sci., Technol. & Appl., 2009.
7. Haruta M. Catalyst surveys of Japan 1:61 and references therein, 1997; M. Haruta. *Catal. Today* 1997;36:153.
8. Pan Y et al. Size-dependent cytotoxicity of gold nanoparticles. *Small* 2007;3(11):1941–9 (http://www.virlab.virginia.edu).
9. Hamad-Schifferli K, Schwartz JJ, Santos AT, Zhang SG, and Jacobson JM. Remote electronic control of DNA hybridization through inductive heating of an attached metal nanocrystal. *Nature* 2002;415:152–5.
10. Goodman CM et al. DNA-binding by functionalized gold nanoparticles: Mechanism and structural requirements. *Chem. Biol. Drug Design* 2006;67(4):297–304.
11. Halas N. Working with nanoshells: A conversation with Naomi Halas (Nova interview, February 3, 2005: http://www.pbs.org/wgbh/nova/sciencenow/3209/03-nanoshells.html).

12. Engineered Nanoparticles: Review Environmental Safety (International Collaborative Review—Project's co-coordinator Prof. Vicki Stone), 2008–2009 (http://nmi.jrc.ec. europa.eu/project/ENRHES.htm).

13. Savanone G et al. *In vitro* permeation of gold nano particles through rat skin and rat intestine: Effect of particle size. *Colloids Surf. B Biointerfaces* 2008;65(1):1–10.

14. Oberdorster G et al. Nanotoxicology: An emerging discipline evolving from studies of ultrafine particles *Environ. Health. Perspect.* 2005;113:823–39.

15. Goodman CM, McCusker CD, Yilmaz T, and Rotello VM. Toxicity of gold nanoparticles functionalized with cationic and anionic side chains. *Bioconjug. Chem.* 2004;15:897–900.

16. Hainfeld JF, Slatkin DN, and Smilowitz HM. The use of gold nanoparticles to enhance radiotherapy in mice. *Phys. Med. Biol.* 2004;49:309–15.

17. Wang S, Lu W, Tovmachenko O, Rai US, Yu H, and Ray PC. Challenge in understanding size and shape dependent toxicity of gold nanomaterials in human skin keratinocytes. *Chem. Phys. Lett.* 2008;463:145–9.

18. Paciotti GF, Meyer L, Weinreich D, Goia D, Pavel N, McLaughlin RE, and Tamarkin L. Colloidal gold: A novel nanoparticle vector for tumor directed drug delivery. *Drug Deliv.* 2004;11:169–83.

19. Ritter SK. Planning nanotech from the ground up. *Chem. Eng. News* 2006;84(16):37–8.

20. Nangia Y, Wangoo N, Goyal N, Shekhawat G, and Suri CR. Bacterial strain used to synthesize gold nanoparticles. *Microbial Cell Factories* 2009;8:39.

21. Davies J. *Managing the Effects of Nanotechnology*. Washington, DC: Woodrow Wilson International Center for Scholars: Project on Emerging Nanotechnologies, 2006.

22. Rejeski D. *Nanotechnology: How Much EH&S Research Is Enough?* Washington, DC: Woodrow Wilson Center for Scholars: Project on Emerging Nanotechnologies, 2005.

23. Bell TE. *Understanding Risk Assessment of Nanotechnology*, 2006. (www.nano.gov/Understanding_Risk_Assessment.pdf).

# 4

## Nanomaterials for Bone Reconstructive Composites

M. van der Zande, B. C. Chesnutt, X. F. Walboomers, and J. A. Jansen

### CONTENTS

In a natural environment, the cells of our body interact with the extracellular matrix (ECM) that is surrounding them. When examined from a topographical point of view, it becomes apparent that the ECM is structured as a mixture of pores, ridges, and fibers, which all are sized in the nanoscale range.[1–3] From this perspective, it has been suggested that it could be worthwhile to develop man-made materials of similar dimensions. Such biomimetic nanomaterials could harbor great promise in advanced medical applications, and in this chapter we will focus on the relation between such nanomaterials and the tissue engineering procedures for bone reconstructive purposes. The placement and subsequent tissue integration of a bone implant or tissue-engineered construct requires symbiosis between a biological and a nonbiological system. Nanotechnology that is applied to create biomimetic features can serve as a "lubricant" to enhance the reactions between both systems. In this, it is vital to understand that nanomaterials have physicochemical and biological properties that can be totally different from their "macroscopic" counterparts. Various nanomaterials are currently described in the literature; however, not all materials possess the appropriate criteria to be incorporated into, or placed onto, a bone implant or tissue-engineered construct. Ongoing research on nanomaterials for bone implants is mainly focused on three materials: nanohydroxyapatite (nHA), nanofibers, and carbon nanotubes (CNTs). Some of these materials are already proven materials on a microscale level, while others are fairly new in the bone tissue engineering field.

## 4.1 Nanohydroxyapatite

Natural bone tissue consists of a high percentage of nanosized needle-like calcium phosphate crystals of approximately 5–20 nm in width and 60 nm in length, combined with a poorly crystallized nonstoichiometric apatite phase, containing $CO_3^{2-}$, $Na^+$, $F^-$, and other ions, embedded in a collagen matrix.[4] Resembling the naturally occurring calcium phosphate crystals, nHA might be a perfect material to use in bone implant materials (Figure 4.1). Microscale HA, previously used for this purpose, has already shown to be osteoconductive.[5,6] However, the use of nHA has several advantages over the conventional ceramic microsized HA formulations; it enhances proliferation and differentiation of bone-forming cells, as well as the synthesis of the mineralized matrix. These beneficial features of nHA are a direct effect of

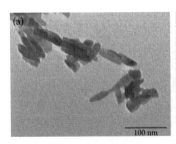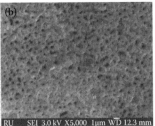

**FIGURE 4.1**
(a) Transmission electron micrograph of nHA. (b) Scanning electron micrograph of an nHA coating.

the nanometer grain size and surface wettability. On top of this considerable impact on osteoblast function, the nanometric dispersion has also been shown to induce absorption of specific proteins important for osteoblast adhesion.[7–10]

nHA can be used in two configurations, as a coating material or mixed in a composite material, and both approaches improve the osteoconductivity of implant materials. When used as a coating material, nHA can be applied onto implant materials by electrostatic spray deposition (ESD) of a nHA precursor solution, direct precipitation using a biomimetic depositing technique, or an electrocrystallization technique from dilute electrolytes.[6,11–14]

### 4.1.1 Preparation of Nanohydroxyapatite

Several techniques for preparing HA nanocrystals are known, all based on precipitation reactions. In the following sections, all techniques for the production of nHA powders as well as nHA coatings are described.

One of the methods to create nHA powders is wet chemical deposition. For this method, the characteristics of the nHA created depend on the reaction formula, temperature, time, and addition rate of the reactant. The most commonly used reaction formula is the one defined by Bouyer et al.[15]

$$10Ca(OH)_2 + 6H_3PO_4 \rightarrow Ca_{10}(PO_4)_6(OH)_2 + 18H_2O$$

The purity can be controlled by the reactant addition rate, while the crystallinity is determined by the reaction temperature, where low temperatures ($T \leq 60°C$) result in monocrystallinity and high temperatures ($T > 60°C$) result in polycrystallinity. The $Ca^{2+}$ ion concentration was found to play a dominant role on the final morphology of the synthesized nHA, as described by Kumar et al.[16] Another wet chemical deposition formula is based on the reaction between calcium nitrate ($Ca(NO_3)_2 \times 4H_2O$) and ammonium hydroxide ($NH_4HPO_4$).[5] Here, the nHA grain size can be controlled by changing the reaction time and temperature.[8,9] Further, Janackovic et al.[17] reported on a wet chemical precipitation reaction according to the following formula:

$$Ca(EDTA)^{2-} + 3/5HPO_4^{2-} + 2/5H_2O \rightarrow 1/10Ca_{10}(PO_4)_6(OH)_2$$
$$+ HEDTA^{3-} + 1/5OH^-$$

Urea is added instead of NaOH, which leads to a more homogeneous monetite precipitation, followed by transformation to HA due to pH changes. Crystal growth can be modified by changing the reaction temperature between 125°C and 160°C, changing the reaction time, or changing the precursor concentration. A final method to produce nHA by wet chemical deposition is by mixing $H_3PO_4$ with $Ca(OH)_2$ and $C_3H_6O_3$ at pH 10 under continuous stirring at room temperature until a Ca/P ratio of 1.67 is reached.

This is followed by the addition of $NH_4OH$ to start the crystallization reaction. After 24 h, the final product is sintered at 1100°C for 1 h to obtain nHA.[18]

Besides wet chemical precipitation, a second method to create nHA is by the sol–gel process. This technique is also based on a precipitation reaction, but the densification of the HA is achieved at lower temperatures. These temperatures are dependent on the calcium and phosphorus precursor solutions that are used. Pure HA phases can be formed by mixing calcium diethoxide $(Ca(OEt)_2)$ and triethyl phosphate $(PO(OEt)_3)$ solutions at temperatures above 600°C, with aging times longer than 24 h.[19,20] Also, solutions of calcium acetate and triethyl phosphate can be blended at 775°C, creating a mixture of HA and CaO. Subsequent purification of the HA is performed by leaching the mixture with hydrochloric acid.[21] A final and more recent sol–gel technique to produce HA is a two-step procedure. In this procedure, triethyl phosphate is hydrolyzed with water for 24 h, followed by the addition of an aqueous nitrate solution. The resulting gel is transformed into a low-crystallized nanoscale apatitic structure at temperatures between 300°C and 400°C.[22]

### 4.1.2 Nanohydroxyapatite Composite Materials

To obtain optimal composite materials for bone tissue engineering purposes, several natural and synthetic-derived materials have been mixed with nHA. For instance, a porous scaffold of gelatin–starch enriched with nHA was fabricated through a microwave vacuum-drying process, followed by cross-linking with trisodium citrate. Addition of nHA increased the biocompatibility and mechanical properties of the material.[23] Another composite material of chitosan mixed with nHA was prepared by a chemical method in which nHA formed *in situ*. This preparation method ensured the nHA to be tightly bound to the scaffold, and the scaffold was shown to be biocompatible.[24] Also, collagen matrices with embedded nHA were fabricated and proved to be biocompatible and osteoconductive; however, the weakness of these scaffolds was the mechanical strength.[25] Furthermore, silk fibroins were mixed with nHA into a composite material by a coprecipitation and freeze-drying method. The nHA provided the material an excellent compressive modulus and strength, especially after adding high amounts of nHA (up to 70% w/w).[26]

Besides natural materials, nHA has also been combined with synthetic materials. Porous composite materials of the synthetic polymers poly(lactic-acid) (PLLA) and poly(glycolic-acid) (PLGA) were mixed with nHA by *in situ* polymerization and thermally induced phase separation methods. Both scaffolds had a high ability to absorb water and excellent mechanical properties.[27,28] Another composite material, fabricated of polyamide (PA) and nHA, resulted in a porous scaffold material with good biocompatibility and a compressive strength equal to the upper limit of cancellous bone.[29] Finally, mixing poly(caprolactone) (PCL) with nHA by a layer manufacturing process also produced biocompatible scaffolds, with a high porosity and well-interconnected microsized pores.[30]

In addition to these solid preshaped materials, a bone filler based on nHA has also been developed, that is, Ostim® (aap Biomaterials GmbH & Co, Dieburg, Germany). This synthetic paste consists of nHA and 40% water and is biocompatible and fully degradable after hardening. The possibility to inject and shape the paste inside bony defects and to mix it with other materials such as morselized bone grafts and tricalcium phosphate-HA to provide better handling of the granules are the major advantages of this material.[31]

### 4.1.3 Nanohydroxyapatite Coatings

A common method to prepare nHA coatings on biomaterials is by spontaneous nucleation and growth of nanosized "bone-like" HA in metastable synthetic body fluid (SBF). SBF contains an inorganic salt composition similar to that of human blood plasma, which facilitates the growth of nHA at physiological pH and temperature over time.[32–35] This biomimetic coating technique can be used to evenly coat porous or smooth implants or scaffolds, and the major advantages of this technique are the possibility to incorporate biologically active agents in the coating by coprecipitation and to control the release of the factors. Potential incorporated biological agents are antibiotics to prevent local infections after surgical procedures or osteoinductive (growth) factors.[36–38] SBF with a modified composition containing calcium nitrate tetrahydrate and diammonium hydrogen phosphate salts can also be used in a chemical precipitation technique to produce nHA powders. Precipitation takes place at 37°C and pH 7.4, and the precipitate is transformed into HA with submicron sizes after sintering at 1200°C for 6 h.[35]

Electrocrystallization from dilute electrolytes ($Ca^+$ and $PO_4^{3-}$) is another method to create ultrafine-grained nHA coatings. The electrolytes are prepared by dissolving $Ca(NO_3)_2$ and $NH_4H_2PO_4$ in deionized water, and the deposition takes 2 h at a physiological pH and at a temperature of 85°C. With this technique, the nHA is deposited directly onto the cathode when using very low calcium and phosphate concentrations.[39]

As a final example, the ESD technique can be used to create nHA coatings. This technique requires a precursor solution containing nHA that is pumped through a metal nozzle. Under the influence of a high voltage between the nozzle and the substrate, a spray of highly charged droplets is formed, which is attracted to the grounded substrate (Figure 4.2).[40–45] By this technique, monodisperse and even porous coatings can be created. As an example, Huang et al.[46] described the electrospraying of a nHA precursor solution that resulted in a biocompatible coating composed of nHA particles with a hexagonal shape and a particle size below 80 nm. The compositional and morphological properties of the coating can be tailored by choosing the appropriate deposition parameters. For instance, the flow rate and voltage

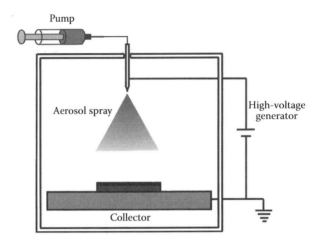

**FIGURE 4.2**
Experimental set-up of the ESD technique.

applied over the nozzle, control the droplet size, which can vary between hundreds of micrometers and several tens of nanometers, and the applied voltage also controls the motion of the droplets.[40,41,46] Next to the ability to control the properties of the coating, this technique also allows the incorporation of biological agents.

## 4.2 Nanofibers

A second category of nanomaterials, extensively studied by bone tissue engineers, comprises nanometric fibers of natural and synthetic polymers. Synthetic polymers can be divided into two groups, that is, degradable and nondegradable polymers. For tissue engineering purposes, degradable polymers are favored as they can be resorbed over a period of time, thereby avoiding the long-term complications of a foreign substrate in the body.[47] Both natural and degradable synthetic polymers have already found applications in the field of tissue engineering, and the choice of polymer type depends on the characteristics the construct should possess. Natural polymers mostly resemble the ECM compounds; however, occasionally, they are immunogenic or exhibit unsuitable mechanical properties.[48] Synthetic degradable polymers, on the other hand, possess higher mechanical strength and are mostly nonimmunogenic. Polymers can easily be shaped into porous scaffolds by several techniques such as self-assembly, phase separation, solvent casting and particulate leaching, freeze drying, melt molding, template synthesis, gas foaming, and solid free forming. Most of these techniques, however, are incapable of synthesizing scaffolds with nanosized features. Therefore, researchers are recently focusing on fabrication of such materials into nanosized fibrous scaffolds. These nanofibrous constructs provide, besides their morphological similarity to natural matrices, a high porosity with controlled pore size and pore geometry, and a controlled fiber dimension and spatial orientation. The high surface-to-volume ratio offers a good environment for cell contact.[3,48]

The conventional technique to produce fibers is by mechanical spinning. However, this technique produces fibers with a low specific surface area and relatively large diameters (above 2 microns in diameter), which are much larger than the diameters of ECM components encountered in nature. Also, melt-blowing techniques can be used to produce fibers, but they too have large diameters (slightly below 1 μm) that are, aside from their large diameter, also discontinuous or highly nonuniform. Actual nanofibers can be produced by electrospinning, self-assembly, or phase separation techniques, with the electrospinning technique being favored, for it is the only technique that consistently produces continuous polymeric nanofibers.[3,49]

### 4.2.1 Fabrication of Nanofibrous Scaffolds by Electrospinning

Composite, hollow, and liquid-containing nanofibers, electrospun from natural or synthetic polymers with diameters ranging from a few microns to tens of nanometers, can be tailor-designed to create a tissue-matching mechanical compliance.[50–52] By collecting fibers after continuous spinning, layers with a porosity of >90% and a pore diameter up to 110 μm can be created. The disadvantages of this technique are that it is time consuming and that it is still not possible to create very thick three-dimensional scaffolds.[53]

Electrospinning is based on the ejection of a fine charged jet of polymer solution by gravity or mechanical pumping from a nozzle of a capillary tube. The jet moves subsequently into an external electric field and elongates according to the applied forces. Finally, the jet segments are deposited onto a collector in the form of random or (partially) aligned nanofibers, depending on the collector type.[54] Three types of collectors are known: the plate type, on which fibers are deposited randomly; the cylinder type, on which fibers are deposited partially aligned; and the disc type, on which fibers are deposited in a highly aligned manner (Figures 4.3 and 4.4). This last collector type, however, still poses problems for trying to produce high-quality nanofibrous constructs.[53]

To date, >200 synthetic or natural polymers have been successfully electrospun into nanofibers, and >30 have been used for a variety of tissue-engineered applications (Figure 4.5).[54,55] Some of the frequently used synthetic polymers are listed in Table 4.1.

The diameter and morphology of electrospun polymers can be accurately controlled by varying the concentration and the molecular weight of the polymer. Other properties influencing the jet flow, and thereby the

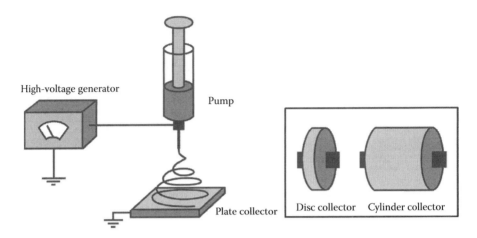

**FIGURE 4.3**
Experimental set-up of the electrospinning technique, with three different types of collectors (plate, disc, and cylinder collector).

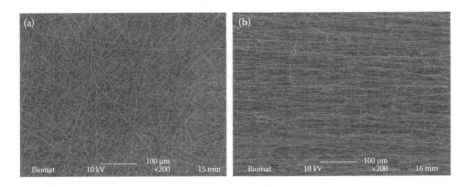

**FIGURE 4.4**
Scanning electron micrographs of (a) random and (b) aligned deposited PLLA electrospun nanofibers.

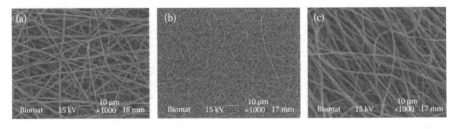

**FIGURE 4.5**
Scanning electron micrographs of randomly aligned electrospun (a) PLGA, (b) PCL blended with gelatin, and (c) PCL.

**TABLE 4.1**

Natural and Synthetic Biodegradable Polymers Used in Electrospinning Scaffold Tissue Engineering

| Naturally Derived | Synthetic |
|---|---|
| Collagen | Poly(lactic acid) |
| Gelatin | Poly(glycolic acid) |
| Chitosan | Poly(lactic-co-glycolic acid) |
| Chitin | Poly(ε-caprolactone) |
| Cellulose | Poly(lactide-co-caprolactone) |
| Elastin | Poly(vinyl alcohol) |
| Starch | |
| Silk fibroin | |
| Fibrinogen | |
| Hyaluronan | |

**TABLE 4.2**

Physical Properties of Some Polymers Used for Electrospinning of Tissue Engineering Constructs

| Material | Fiber Diameter (nm) | Stress (MPa) | Tensile Modulus (MPa) |
|---|---|---|---|
| Collagen type I[56] | 250 | – | – |
| Collagen type I 1:50 polyethyleneoxide[57] | 100–150 | 037 | 12 |
| Gelatin[58] | 200 | 5.77 | 499 |
| Poly(lactide-co-glycolic acid) (85:15)[59] | 500–800 | 22.67 | 323.15 |
| Poly(lactide-co-glycolic acid) (75:25)[60] | 550 | 4.67 | 110.78 |
| Poly(ε-caprolactone)[61] | 200–600 | – | – |
| Poly(lactide-co-ε-caprolactone)[62] | 470 | 6.3 | 44 |

morphology, of the fibers are the nozzle size, surface tension, quality of the solvent, diffusion coefficient, flow rate, and temperature. Some of these properties may be altered by the addition of salt or surfactant.[48] In Table 4.2, an overview is given of the physical properties of some frequently used polymers for electrospinning.

## 4.2.2 Modification of Nanofibrous Scaffolds

Considering the everlasting demand for further innovation of scaffold materials, there is a possibility to improve nanofibrous scaffolds to a greater extent by several modifications. For instance, mechanical strength and stability of the scaffolds can be improved by cross-linking the polymers, and biocompatibility of the construct might be improved by introducing proteins and ligands into the scaffold. As an example, addition of poly(ε-CBZ-L-lysine) to PLLA scaffolds resulted in increased binding of collagen type II, which is a component of the ECM, by exposure of free $NH_2$ adherence groups.[63] Incorporation of collagen itself and glycosaminoglycans (GAGs) has been shown to improve cell growth on the scaffold.[64] GAGs are, like collagen, ubiquitous components of the ECM that exert various biological effects. Besides collagen, there is little focus in the literature on incorporation of other proteins since denaturation of macromolecules occurs rapidly. Nevertheless, two other proteins, bovine serum albumin and human β-nerve growth factor, have been successfully blended into poly(vinyl-alcohol) (PVA) and PCL scaffolds, respectively.[65,66] Another possibility to modify the fibrous matrices is by the incorporation of bioactive agents, such as drugs and plasmid DNA. Successful incorporation of the low molecular weight drugs ibuprofen, cefazolin, rifampin, paclitaxel, itraconazole, mefoxin, and tetracycline hydrochloride has already been reported. Usually, these drugs are released in a "burst release mode," meaning an instant release of the total amount of incorporated drugs. Therefore, current research is focusing on controlling this release.[67–73]

Finally, blending different types of polymers or blending polymers with substances such as nHA amorphous tricalcium phosphate (ATCP), bioactive glass, calcium carbonate ($CaCO_3$), or polysaccharides might be useful in producing scaffolds with superior properties compared with the pure materials, that is, by increased mechanical properties or biocompatibility.[47,74–77]

## 4.3 Carbon Nanotubes

With regard to nanomaterials in (bone) tissue engineering, a third material that is attracting a lot of attention are CNTs. The unique physical–chemical properties of CNTs might enhance the mechanical, electrical, and thermal characteristics of tissue engineering constructs extremely.[78,79] Subsequently, CNTs might also be used as a carrier system for drug delivery, or as a cell tracking system to expand our knowledge on cell behavior.[80–82] Already, many reports on the effects of CNT incorporation into composite materials, regarding the mechanical properties and biological behavior, can be found in the literature.[83,84]

There are two groups of CNTs: single-walled CNTs (SWNTs) and multi-walled CNTs (MWNTs) (Figures 4.6 and 4.7).[85] Sometimes, fullerenes are also listed among the CNTs; however, their closed ball-shaped structure excludes them from further discussion in this chapter. SWNTs are composed of only one sheet of graphene, while MWNTs contain a multiple coaxial structure. Different existing chiralities, that is, the armchair, the zigzag, and the chiral chirality (Figure 4.8), of the graphene sheet in SWNTs determine the electrical properties as a function of helicity and tube diameter.[86] Aside from these basic structural features, defects present in the tube walls were found to determine the Young's modulus of the CNTs, and they also provide the possibility for covalent or noncovalent functionalization of the tubes.[87]

(a)  (b)

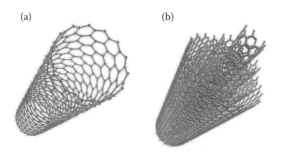

**FIGURE 4.6**
(a) Single-walled and (b) multiwalled CNTs.

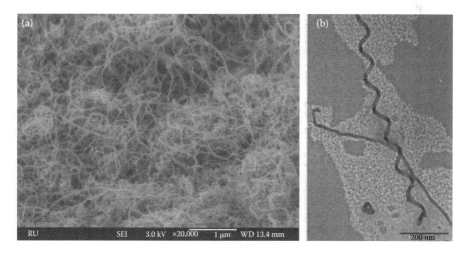

**FIGURE 4.7**
(a) Scanning electron micrograph and (b) transmission electron micrograph of CNTs.

Until now, the most common functionalization for CNTs is to decrease their hydrophobicity otherwise they tend to aggregate into bundles. Aggregated CNTs are difficult to handle and also result in loss of function.[88] A study by Shi et al.[82] demonstrated this by reporting on much better dispersion of fluoride functionalized SWNTs throughout poly(propylene fumarate) (PPF) scaffold materials resulting in increased reinforcement of the materials. However, there are also other reasons for functionalizing CNTs. For instance, functionalization with gadolinium has been shown to result in an excellent contrast agent for magnetic resonance imaging (MRI).[89–91] In the near future, it may also be interesting to functionalize the CNTs with biological agents, in order to gain biocompatibility or osteoconductivity of scaffold materials to prevent immune responses at the site of implantation, or to use the nanotubes as drug delivery systems.

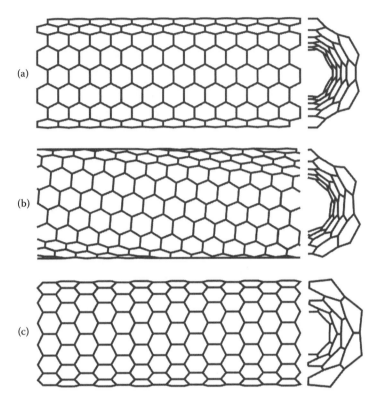

**FIGURE 4.8**
Models of SWNTs at molecular level with different chiralities. (a) Armchair chirality; (b) chiral conformation; and (c) zigzag arrangement.

## 4.3.1 Preparation of Carbon Nanotubes

Fullerenes were discovered in 1970 by Richard E. Smalley at Rice University in Houston, Texas. With this discovery, he was granted the 1996 Nobel prize in chemistry. After fullerenes, nanocages (also termed graphitic onions) were presented in 1980, followed by MWNTs in 1991, and lastly, SWNTs were discovered.[86,92]

At present, there are several methods to produce MWNTs and SWNTs. The first described was the arc–discharge method. This method is based on the self-assembly (growing) of CNTs in an inert gas atmosphere between carbon, or catalyst-containing carbon, electrodes.[93–95] Highly crystalline MWNTs with diameters ranging from 2 to 30 nm, and a length up to 30 μm can be grown on the cathode, at a pressure of 500 torr.[86] SWNTs can be synthesized by arcing graphite electrodes containing a metal catalyst in a methane–argon or helium atmosphere.[96] As metal catalysts, Fe, Co–Ni, Gd, Co–Ru, Co, Ni–Y, Rh–Pt, and Co–Ni–Fe–Ce are optional choices.[86]

Later, other CNT manufacturing procedures were discovered, such as laser vaporization, chemical vapor deposition (CVD), and pyrolytic methods.

Production of MWNTs by the laser vaporization method is achieved by firing a high-power laser toward a graphite target inside a furnace at 1200°C.[97,98] Addition of Ni or Co to the graphite target, or using a $CO_2$ laser focused on a graphite-metal target, results in the production of SWNTs.[86,99] Ultrafast laser pulses were found to be most effective in increasing the produced quantities of SWNTs.[100]

The CVD method is used to produce well-aligned MWNTs and SWNTs with good uniformity in size. Besides these advantages over the arc–discharge and laser vaporization methods, this production process can also be scaled up.[101] CVD is based on exposure of metal particles to a medium containing hydrocarbon gases, in which the formation of CNTs is catalyzed. In the near future, there will hopefully be precise control over the nanotube orientation, position, density, and joining.[102]

Finally, the pyrolytic method is based on heating hydrocarbons, or any organic precursor containing carbon, in the presence of a transition metal catalyst such as nickel, cobalt, or iron. This method is used to produce MWNTs, as well as SWNTs, and the production process depends strongly on the type and dimension of the metal particles, the temperature, the amount of hydrocarbons, and the type of gases involved in the process.[86] A well-characterized pyrolytic production process is the HiPco process. Here, SWNTs are produced by thermolysis of $Fe(CO)_5$ in the presence of CO at elevated pressures (<10 atm) and temperatures (800°C–1200°C). This extremely efficient method is very applicable for producing bulk amounts.[103]

## 4.4 Nanomaterial–Cell Interaction: Health Issues

To conceive a better understanding of the interactions between cells and nanomaterials created for bone tissue engineering, it is important to know that there are three levels of structures in bone: the first is the nanostructure, which consists of noncollagenous organic proteins, fibrillar collagen, and embedded minerals with an average grain size of 20–50 nm in length and 2–5 nm in diameter; this is followed by the microstructure, consisting of lamellae, osteons, and the Haversian systems; and finally the macrostructure, which consists of the cortical and cancellous bone.[104]

After contact of a tissue-engineered construct with body fluids, proteins are immediately adsorbed onto the surface. These proteins determine the cell type that interacts with the construct since the proteins interact with specific cell membrane receptors. This interaction is dependent on the type, concentration, and conformation of the proteins. The surface chemistry, hydrophilicity, hydrophobicity, charge, topography, roughness, and energy determine the type of protein that absorbs to the implant. Smooth surfaces have been shown to favor fibrous tissue integration, which ultimately encapsulates implants. Therefore, a bone-like surface topography is often regarded as being of great importance when designing implant materials.[7,105–109]

### 4.4.1 Nanohydroxyapatite–Cell Interaction

Considering the nanostructured bone surface, it is best to mimic this situation, thereby invoking the correct proteins to adsorb and avoiding fibrous tissue encapsulation. Cellular responses to HA particles have been demonstrated to depend on physical and chemical properties such as particle size, morphology, crystallinity, and chemical composition. A nanostructured topography increases the surface space enormously, thereby increasing protein and cell attachment. Better adherence of osteoblasts was reported with the use of several types of nanomaterials (i.e., nHA and CNTs) either deposited onto the surface or mixed into composite materials.[53] Regarding particle size, the ability of nanophase ceramics to promote bone cell function was found to be limited below 100 nm.[8] The nanometer HA grain size topography, in combination with the high surface wettability, promotes increased selective vitronectin adsorption, and also affects the protein conformation, thereby enhancing osteoblast functions.[4,8] This conformational change implies unfolding of the proteins to a greater extent, presenting more epitopes for osteoblasts to adhere to. Other proteins that are known to particularly increase osteoblast functions are fibronectin, laminin, and collagen.[7,8,104]

#### 4.4.1.1 In Vitro *Studies on Nanohydroxyapatite*

Many coated and composite bone tissue engineering materials have been investigated with regard to their *in vitro* and *in vivo* biocompatibility. Here, some *in vitro* study results of different nHA composite or coated materials are summarized, starting with a porous chitosan/nHA composite scaffold, seeded with MC 3T3-E1 cells. Compared with a porous chitosan scaffold, the composite scaffold showed a better cytocompatibility, in terms of cellular proliferation and morphology.[24] Addition of nHA to porous silk fibroin scaffolds seeded with MG63 cells resulted in an elevated cytocompatibility as well, as determined by an MTT assay.[26] The addition of nHA to collagen scaffolds increased proliferation and redifferentiation of cells, originating from rat bone fragments, toward osteogenic lineages. Migration of the cells throughout the network of the porous scaffold was also increased.[110]

Synthetic materials can also be improved by the incorporation of nHA, as demonstrated by PLGA/nHA and PCL/nHA scaffolds seeded with mesenchymal stem cells (MSCs), which obtained better cytocompatibility compared with their counterparts without nHA. They showed a higher alkaline phosphatase (ALP) activity and an increased rate of matrix mineralization.[27,30] Seeding polyamide/nHA (PA/nHA) scaffolds with MSCs did not result in an increase, nor a decrease, in cell proliferation and differentiation.[29]

Besides nHA composite materials, nHA-coated scaffolds have also been studied. nHA coated onto collagen beads did not alter the proliferation of MG63 cells but increased ALP activity and expression of osteocalcin (a component of the ECM) compared with noncoated collagen beads. Thus, nHA seemed to switch the MG63 cells from the proliferation stage to the differentiation stage.[6] Other studies, comparing nHA coatings with conventional microsized HA coatings, showed an increased osteoblast adhesion. The underlying mechanism was supposed to be an increase in specific protein absorption, thus increasing osteoblast adhesion.[8,9] However, a study contradicting these positive findings on nHA was reported by Zhu et al.[111] who observed that cell attachment and spreading was decreased when smooth titanium implants were coated with nHA compared with noncoated implants. In addition to the Zhu study, Ostim was also shown to have a negative effect on cells *in vitro*, as primary osteoblasts were not able to grow on the material. This, however, was hypothesized to be primarily due to the high amount of free water in the product and not to the presence of nHA.[112]

Although there is no complete uniformity between all studies, the data show that in an *in vitro* situation, the addition of nHA into, or onto, bone tissue engineering constructs, mostly provides the construct with an increased cytocompatibility, as confirmed by increased adhesion and differentiation of the cells.

### 4.4.1.2 In Vivo *Studies on Nanohydroxyapatite*

In an *in vivo* situation, nHA was reported to improve the performance of bone tissue engineering constructs as well. PA/nHA constructs, produced by Wang et al.[29] showed adequate bone ingrowth in rabbit mandibles, with a bone density almost equal to the host bone. Enriching the construct with rabbit mesenchymal cells before implantation resulted in even more and earlier bone formation. The commercial product Ostim also proved to be biocompatible in most *in vivo* studies, in contrast to disappointing results from *in vitro* studies. After injecting Ostim in the dorsal skin chambers of hamsters, biocompatibility was shown by the absence of leukocyte activation, a more pronounced angiogenic response and an increased microvessel density, when compared with a synthetic hydroxyapatite bone substitute.[113] Injecting Ostim in a critical-sized defect in the calvaria of minipigs resulted in bone formation in the defects, which also indicates the biocompatibility of the material.[114] On the other hand, a study with Ostim injected in fresh extraction sockets in dogs revealed a remaining gap up to 0.2 mm in the graft surrounding tissue, which indicated that the use of this material does not always lead to positive results.[112,115] Also, in a study of Meirelles et al.[116] in which titanium nHA-coated implants were compared with noncoated implants, no obvious positive effect of nHA was observed. The implants were implanted in a gap healing model in rabbit tibia, and for both implants there was no difference in gap closure. This proves that not all results from *in vitro* studies can be extrapolated to an *in vivo* situation.

## 4.4.2 Nanofiber–Cell Interaction

Electrospun materials facilitate, or even enhance, cell growth and differentiation, thereby qualifying these fibers as an excellent material for tissue engineering purposes. The interaction between cells and scaffold material is dependent on material properties such as the degradation rate and the flexibility. Slow-degrading polymers provide scaffolds with a longer-lasting stability. Flexibility of the materials allows cells to migrate through the matrix by pushing the fibers aside, which is important since the pores created in nanofibrous materials are often smaller than the size of a single cell.[13,47,77]

### 4.4.2.1 In Vitro *Studies on Nanofibrous Constructs*

Many nanofibrous materials from nature-derived, as well as synthetic, polymers have been elaborately tested for their suitability as tissue engineering scaffolds. For example, collagen type I, electrospun into a fibrous scaffold, showed excellent proliferation and infiltration of smooth muscle cells in several studies, even though the pore diameter was smaller than the cell diameter.[53,56] These studies were followed by seeding chondrocytes onto a collagen type II scaffold, on which the cells proliferated and were evenly distributed, after 1 week.[47,117] The disadvantage of using collagen, however, is the possibility of immunogenic reactions.[48]

A second material of choice is chitosan because of its known biocompatibility, degradability, and even an antimicrobial and antifungal activity. The physical characteristics provide this material with favorable plasticity and adhesiveness for many applications.[48] When blended with nHA and seeded with human fetal osteoblasts, this scaffold significantly stimulated proliferation and mineral deposition after 15 days.[118]

In addition, fibrous gelatin scaffolds are biocompatible and bioresorbable, and when blended with nHA and PCL, good attachment and proliferation of bone marrow stromal cells was shown.[47,48,119]

Finally, the natural material silk has also been shown to be cytocompatible. Seeding electrospun silk/polyethyleneoxide scaffolds with human MSCs resulted in proliferation of the cells, and addition of nHA and bone morphogenetic protein 2 (BMP-2) to the scaffold resulted in high calcification values. It was therefore concluded that the addition of nHA and BMP-2 significantly improves the osteoconductivity/inductivity of this specific type of scaffold.[47,77]

PLLA is one of the synthetic polymers often used for bone tissue engineering purposes because it is biocompatible, biodegradable, and has a high tensile strength. When seeded with 3T3-E1 osteoblastic cells, nanofibrous PLLA films showed an increase in differentiation of the cells, as evidenced by higher ALP activity, an increase in bone sialoprotein (BSP) gene expression, and a decrease in proliferation of the cells, compared with flat PLLA films.[120] To overcome the low pore size and lack of interconnectivity that is present in conventional electrospun PLLA scaffolds, Leong et al.[121] created

PLLA nanofibrous scaffolds with large interconnected pores by using a low-temperature electrospinning technique first described by Simonet et al.[122] with ice crystals serving as removable templates. Subsequently, the scaffolds were seeded with 3T3/NIH fibroblasts, and as a result good infiltration of the cells up to 50 μm thickness was observed.[121] PLLA fibers can also be blended with other substances. For instance, in a study by Kim et al.[123] PLLA fibers were mixed with fibers spun from bioactive glass. The scaffold created exhibited an even distribution of both fibers. When seeded with 3T3-E1 osteoblasts, the cells showed favorable attachment and proliferation, as well as an improved differentiation and mineralization behavior, as compared with cells seeded onto pure PLLA scaffolds.

Also, PLGA is a biocompatible material and has a tunable biodegradability, depending on the ratio of lactic to glycolic acid.[53,59] Seeding fibrous PLGA scaffolds with MSCs was found to result in good proliferation in the first week of culturing. However, after this week, no further effect of the scaffolds on the cells was noted.[48,53] Like PLLA, PLGA can also be blended with other substances, for instance with αTCP nanoparticles as described by Schneider et al.[124] After immersing the scaffolds in SBF and subsequent seeding of the scaffolds with human MSCs, an increase in proliferation and differentiation of the cells was seen, as compared with pure PLGA electrospun scaffolds.

Another frequently used synthetic polymer for electrospinning is PCL. MSCs seeded onto electrospun PCL microporous scaffolds were reported to migrate through the entire scaffold, to differentiate into osteoblastic cells, and to form a calcified matrix.[53,61] Blending PCL with a high $CaCO_3$ content during the electrospinning procedure and subsequent seeding of the material with osteoblasts resulted in low proliferation of the cells and high mineralized matrix formation.[125] Another material blended into PCL nanofibrous constructs was nHA. Seeding of these scaffolds with human osteoblasts, however, was not successful and resulted in comparable proliferation to plain PCL scaffolds.[126]

### 4.4.2.2 In Vivo *Studies on Nanofibrous Constructs*

In addition to *in vitro* studies, several *in vivo* experiments with nanofibrous constructs have been performed. Implanting electrospun scaffolds of silk fibroin material in critical-sized calvarial defects in New Zealand white rabbits showed complete healing of the defects without observing any inflammatory reaction, thereby proving the material to be osteoconductive as well as biocompatible.[127]

Synthetic electrospun PLLA scaffolds with large interconnected pores were produced by low-temperature spinning with ice crystals serving as removable templates and were also tested *in vivo*. As a control, conventional spun PLLA scaffolds with small nonconnected pores were used. After 14, 28, and 56 days of subcutaneous implantation in rats, the scaffolds were histologically examined. Both materials showed good biocompatibility but the scaffold with large interconnected pores showed higher cell infiltration and proliferation.[77]

Another synthetic scaffold, produced from PLGA, with or without incorporation of nHA and BMP-2, was implanted in the long tibia bone of nude mice. Both scaffolds were biocompatible, and the best bone healing was observed for the scaffolds with added nHA and BMP-2.[128]

PCL fibrous scaffolds were also tested *in vivo*. Before implantation into the omenta of rats, the scaffolds were seeded with MSCs. Histological examination after 4 weeks showed collagen type I formation throughout the scaffold and mineralization of the scaffold. This indicated that the scaffold was biocompatible, and that the preseeded cells provided the scaffold osteoinductivity, since ectopic mineralization of the scaffold was observed.[129] Finally, electrospun scaffolds of PCL, with or without the incorporation of the bone formation–stimulating drug simvastatin, were implanted in 8 mm critical-sized cranial defects in rats. Histological examination after 1, 3, or 6 months showed biocompatibility and osteoconductivity of all scaffolds, with a significant increase in bone formation for the drug-containing scaffold.[130]

The *in vitro* as well as the *in vivo* studies often show increased cytocompatibility or biocompatibility of electrospun nanofibrous scaffolds in comparison with the bulk polymer. Therefore, these nanomaterials are considered very promising in future bone tissue engineering applications.

### 4.4.3 Carbon Nanotubes–Cell Interaction

Nanomaterials produced from natural or synthetic polymers are often degradable materials that are broken down and systemically removed from the body.[131,132] Nanoceramic materials are remodeled and also generally regarded as nonhazardous since they are naturally occurring materials in the body. CNTs, however, might pose a problem for future applications. Therefore, many recent research studies focus on the interaction between cells and CNTs in *in vitro* and *in vivo* situations. In light of this emphasis in the literature, the current review will mainly describe CNTs with regard to risks involved (not necessarily only on bone cells or tissue since incorporation of CNTs into bone implants and tissue-engineered constructs may also introduce the possibility of exposure to other tissues).

CNTs are nondegradable and foreign to the body; however, the vast applications of this material make it still very popular. Various toxicity issues proved to be related to the properties of this material, such as structure, length, surface area, degree of aggregation, extent of oxidation, surface topology, and bound functional groups. It can be argued that these are the same physical and chemical properties that make the use of CNTs so interesting. Besides the physico–chemical properties, also the concentration or dose to which cells and tissues are exposed to this material were found to be of great importance concerning safety risks.[78,83]

Safety aspects start with the production process of the material, which may already be hazardous, since CNT containing aggregates might become airborne during production and remain airborne for long periods, causing health risks to the lungs and dermis. The HiPco process, for instance, forms aerosols that easily break down into smaller particles, leading to higher airborne concentrations. In contrast, laser vaporization forms compact aerosols that are more difficult to break down into smaller particles.[85,133] Another hazard of CNTs is the accumulation along the food chain. Oberdorster et al. studied the possible accumulation of SWNTs ingested by round worms (*Caenorhabditis elegans*). In this model, SWNTs were shown to move through the digestive tract and were not absorbed by the animals.[134] Another study, in compliance with these results, reported detection of unsolubilized SWNTs, ingested by fish, in fecal material.[135] However, even though these studies indicate that SWNTs are not absorbed by these animals, there is still a possibility of CNTs moving up the food chain.

### 4.4.3.1 In Vitro *Studies on Carbon Nanotubes*

Initial studies examining the toxicity of CNTs involved mainly unpurified and nonfunctionalized CNTs. One of the first studies reported exposure of human epidermal keratinocytes to pristine SWNTs to result in accelerated oxidative stress, as indicated by the formation of free radicals and accumulation of peroxidative products, depletion of total antioxidant reserves, an increase of lipid peroxidation products, and loss of cell viability.[136] In another study, addition of unpurified MWNTs to dermal keratinocytes resulted in reduced cell viability and an undesirable increase in interleukin-8 (IL-8) up to six times.[137] When added to skin fibroblasts, cell cycle arrest was induced, and apoptosis and necrosis were increased.[138] Also, nonfunctionalized aggregated SWNTs and (raw) aggregated MWNTs incubated with murine lung alveolar macrophages resulted in severe toxic effects, even comparable with those of asbestos, within a short term of 48 h.[139] According to studies by other research groups, this toxicity, however, was indicated to be mainly resulting from the metal catalysts present in the used unpurified CNTs. Metal catalysts are known to lead to the formation of hazardous reactive oxygen species.[137,138,140–142]

In time, knowledge of not only purification but also of functionalization of CNTs increased. Owing to their extreme hydrophobic nature, CNTs aggregate almost immediately, which makes them difficult to handle and increases their toxicity on cells.[143,144] Therefore, CNT functionalization, by surface treatments and coatings, is being investigated with great interest. In a biological model system, it was shown that well-dispersed SWNTs were less cytotoxic than micrometer-sized aggregates.[144] However, the effect of functionalization on cell behavior is difficult to predict, since these treatments do not only alter their solubility, but also their cell interaction. In most cases, as reported in several studies, functionalization increases the solubility of CNTs, and therefore decreases their toxicity, as mainly the hydrophobic character is associated with their toxicity.[145] For instance, addition to neurons of functionalized MWNTs with an increased hydrophilic character increased the number of branches grown per neuron, compared with pristine MWNTs.[146] A study by Nimmagadda et al.[147] hypothesized that the toxicity of nonfunctionalized, hydrophobic CNTs is linked to their high potential to penetrate and aggregate within the hydrophobic cell membrane, leading to rupture and cell death. Zanello et al.[148] stated that neutrally charged CNTs resulted in optimal osteoblast proliferation and bone matrix-forming functions, compared with sidewall functionalization that introduced a positive or negative net charge. Besides the type of sidewall groups, the amount of sidewall groups also influences the cytotoxicity, for there is an inverse relation between the toxic potential and the degree of sidewall functionalization.[78,85,149] Another important parameter related to toxicity appeared to be the mass of the CNTs. Short MWNTs showed higher cytototoxicity than long ones. Also, short SWNTs displayed a higher toxic behavior than short MWNTs.[150,151] Finally, even though toxicity decreases with an increase in purification and sidewall functionalization, the toxic behavior of CNTs is still concentration, dose, and time dependent, as shown in a study by Cui et al. Here, cell proliferation of human embryo kidney cells was inhibited, and cell adhesive ability decreased, in a dose- and time-dependent manner after addition of suspended SWNTs.[85,137,140]

However, we should stress that the literature is not consistent, and frequently contradictory results are described. Ingestion of MWNTs and SWNTs by macrophages, for instance, leads to necrosis and degeneration, as described in a study by the group of Jia et al.[150] while it does not lead to any signs of toxicity in a study by the group of Cherukuri et al.[152] Also, the addition of three types of SWNTs, namely purified SWNTs, SWNTs functionalized with 4-*tert*-butylphenylene, and ultrashort SWNTs, to a fibroblast culture did not result in any cytotoxicity in a study by Shi et al.[153] Another noticeable report is the favorable positive cellular interaction, as well as the sustained cell viability, of macrophages and leukemia cells, after the addition of functionalized SWNTs in suspension.[152,154] Finally, Bottini et al.[155] found an increase in toxicity to be correlated to a decrease in hydrohobicity of CNTs, thus contradicting the earlier reported opposite correlation.

### 4.4.3.2 In Vivo *Studies on Carbon Nanotubes*

The large surface area of nanoparticles allows easy entrance to the body, and makes them more biologically active than their larger counterparts.[135] Potential routes for CNTs to enter the body are by inhalation, through the skin, by ingestion, or by injection/infusion. Although we mainly focused on nanomaterials incorporated into bone constructs in our *in vivo* experiment sections, for a full overview of the pathological effects of CNTs, it is necessary to mention data on inhalation toxicity, which is the most studied administration route.

*In vivo* studies with MWNTs, as well as with SWNTs, show pulmonary responses after inhalation to be of immediate concern. Intratracheal instillation of MWNTs and SWNTs in mice, guinea pigs, and rats lead to a dose-dependent formation of granulomas, fibrosis or necrosis, inflammation, and lethality. Additionally, instillation of MWNTs also lead to a nonspecific interstitial pneumonia-like reaction, and instillation of SWNTs lead to a decreased bacterial clearance and a loss of pulmonary function.[83,85,156–159] A study by Lam et al.[160] proved these pathologic reactions to be independent of metal impurities. In contrast, an earlier study by Huczko et al.[157] reported no evidence of inflammatory reactions, or perturbation of lung function, after instillation of MWNTs in guinea pigs. However, this study is also disputed due to the absence of lung pathology examination.

Since intratracheal instillation is not a correct representation of the natural entrance of materials into the lungs, Li et al.[161] compared instillation of SWNTs in the lungs with systemic inhalation, and showed less severe effects from inhalation of the material. This is probably due to an altered aggregation size and distribution in the lungs. This theory is further supported by other studies, in which administration of agglomerated nanotubes led to the mechanical blockage of airways.[156,159] On the other hand, pharyngeal aspirated SWNTs caused severe granulomatous inflammations and accumulation of oxidative stress markers.[162] In addition to the administration route of CNTs, physico–chemical and environmental factors, such as the particle size, the free particle life, and the residence time in the lungs, were also found to determine toxicity to a great extent.[13,135,163] One of the studies investigating the effects of the particle size on toxicity was performed by Muller et al.[151] who instilled grinded and nongrinded MWNTs intratracheally in rats. The nongrinded MWNTs remained longest in the airways and resulted in granulomas in the bronchi, while the grinded MWNTs were better dispersed in the lung tissue and showed a higher degree of pulmonary inflammation with fibrotic granulomas in the alveolar space. Since there are many other administration routes besides instillation and inhalation, toxicity studies were performed for these routes as well. It is very likely that CNTs will be in contact with the bloodstream, after degradation or remodeling of a bone tissue–engineered construct. When entered into the bloodstream, CNTs were found to induce thrombosis by platelet aggregation and to provoke vascular effects related to mitochondrial oxidative modification and accelerated artheroma formation.[164] However, implantation of degradable PPF scaffolds with incorporated ultrashort SWNTs in a rabbit model showed no toxic effects of the released ultrashort SWNTs, as compared with animals that received pure PPF scaffolds. In contrast, a drastic favorable increase in bone ingrowth was reported.[165]

While toxicity is being investigated elaborately, there is almost no knowledge on the distribution of CNTs in the body after release from scaffold materials. Part of the problem is that the small size of the particles makes it impossible to visualize them microscopically unless they are agglomerated. Oberdorster et al.[135] reported that nanoparticles located in the lung translocate into the pulmonary interstitium, which indicates that the particles might also damage other tissues in the body. Also, translocation of nanosized $TiO_2$ and iridium-192-labeled particles from the lung into the bloodstream and to secondary organs was reported.[166,167] To gain insight into the CNT distribution, iodine-125-labeled SWNTs were injected into mice. They were shown to be distributed throughout the whole body, except the brain, and accumulated in bone.[158] However, a contradictory result was reported by Singh et al. who administered diethylenetriaminepentaacetic acid-functionalized SWNTs, labeled with indium-111, into the bloodstream. A rapid clearance rate and no retention of the SWNTs in any of the secondary organs, such as the liver or the spleen, was observed. The SWNTs were excreted as intact nanotubes through the renal excretion route.[168] Another possible solution for visualization of CNT distribution can be the use of gadolinium-labeled CNTs, as produced by Sitharaman et al.[89,90] in an MRI experiment. Blending these labeled CNTs in a degradable bone tissue-engineered construct, followed by implantation in an animal model, gives the opportunity to follow the labeled CNTs over time by MRI (Figure 4.9).

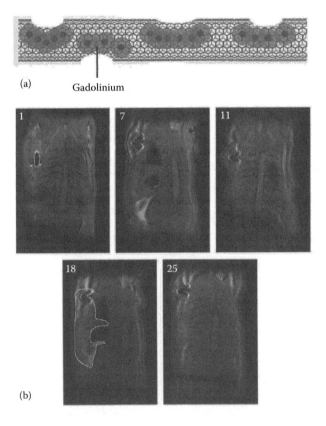

**FIGURE 4.9**
(a) Molecular representation of a functionalized SWNT with gadolinium as contrast agent, and (b) magnetic resonance imaging slices of subcutaneously implanted PLGA scaffold containing such gadolinium-labeled SWNTs on days 1, 7, 11, 18, and 25. Marking on day 1 slide indicates the scaffold and marking on day 18 slide indicates the tissue surrounding the scaffold that has increased intensity due to released SWNTs after degradation of the scaffold.

It can be concluded that there is still a lot of controversy about the use of CNTs. More research into the biological interactions between the body and CNTs is an absolute necessity before application in bone-substituting materials as such can be considered. However, with increased knowledge on minimizing or completely eliminating the toxicity of this material, it might be possible to take advantage of the unique characteristics of CNTs for tissue engineering applications.

## 4.5 Summary

From this overview, it can be concluded that nanomaterials can play an important role in future (bone) tissue engineering applications. Already, many positive reports on nanoceramics, nanofibers, and CNTs exist. The materials have the ability to improve biocompatibility, mechanical, and electrical properties of bone tissue engineering constructs. These constructs can even be further modified by incorporation of biological agents. On the other hand, toxicological issues associated with the nanoscale size of these materials might have a negative effect, which is most evident for CNTs. Therefore, extensive research on each new application of nanomaterials is required.

## References

1. Abrams GA, Bentley E, Nealey PF, and Murphy CJ. Electron microscopy of the canine corneal basement membranes. *Cells Tissues Organs* 2002;170:251–7.
2. Abrams GA, Goodman SL, Nealey PF, Franco M, and Murphy CJ. Nanoscale topography of the basement membrane underlying the corneal epithelium of the rhesus macaque. *Cell Tissue Res.* 2000;299:39–46.
3. Chew SY, Wen Y, Dzenis Y, and Leong KW. The role of electrospinning in the emerging field of nanomedicine. *Curr. Pharm. Des.* 2006;12:4751–70.
4. Ferraz MP, Monteiro FJ, and Manuel CM. Hydroxyapatite nanoparticles: A review of preparation methodologies. *J. Appl. Biomater. Biomech.* 2004;2:74–80.
5. Jarcho M, Kay JF, Gumaer KI, Doremus RH, and Drobeck HP. Tissue, cellular and subcellular events at a bone–ceramic hydroxylapatite interface. *J. Bioeng.* 1977;1:79–92.
6. Tsai SW, Hsu FY, and Chen PL. Beads of collagen-nanohydroxyapatite composites prepared by a biomimetic process and the effects of their surface texture on cellular behavior in MG63 osteoblast-like cells. *Acta Biomater.* 2008;4:1332–41.
7. Webster TJ, Ergun C, Doremus RH, Siegel RW, and Bizios R. Enhanced functions of osteoblasts on nanophase ceramics. *Biomaterials* 2000;21:1803–10.
8. Webster TJ, Ergun C, Doremus RH, Siegel RW, and Bizios R. Specific proteins mediate enhanced osteoblast adhesion on nanophase ceramics. *J. Biomed. Mater. Res.* 2000;51:475–83.

9. Webster TJ, Siegel RW, and Bizios R. Enhanced surface and mechanical properties of nanophase ceramics to achieve orthopaedic/dental implant efficacy. *Bioceramics* 2000;192–5:321–4.

10. Wu LQ and Payne GF. Biofabrication: Using biological materials and biocatalysts to construct nanostructured assemblies. *Trends Biotechnol.* 2004;22:593–9.

11. Barrere F, Layrolle P, van Blitterswijk CA, and de Groot K. Biomimetic coatings on titanium: A crystal growth study of octacalcium phosphate. *J. Mater. Sci. Mater. Med.* 2001;12:529–34.

12. Barrere F, van der Valk CM, Dalmeijer RAJ, van Blitterswijk CA, de Groot K, and Layrolle P. *In vitro* and *in vivo* degradation of biomimetic octacalcium phosphate and carbonate apatite coatings on titanium implants. *J. Biomed. Mater. Res. A* 2003;64A:378–87.

13. Christenson EM, Anseth KS, van den Beucken LJJP et al. Nanobiomaterial applications in orthopedics. *J. Orthop. Res.* 2007;25:11–22.

14. Dalton JE and Cook SD. *In vivo* mechanical and histological characteristics of Ha-coated implants vary with coating vendor. *J. Biomed. Mater. Res.* 1995;29:239–45.

15. Bouyer E, Gitzhofer F, and Boulos MI. Morphological study of hydroxyapatite nanocrystal suspension. *J. Mater. Sci. Mater. Med.* 2000;11:523–31.

16. Kumar R, Prakash KH, Cheang P, and Khor KA. Temperature driven morphological changes of chemically precipitated hydroxyapatite nanoparticles. *Langmuir* 2004;20:5196–200.

17. Janackovic D, Petrovic-Prelevic I, Kostic-Gvozdenovic L, Petrovic R, Jokanovic V, and Uskokovivc D. Influence of synthesis parameters on the particle sizes of nanostructured calcium-hydroxyapatite. *Bioceramics* 2000;192–1:203–6.

18. Manuel CM, Ferraz MP, and Monteiro FJ. Synthesis of hydroxyapatite and tricalcium phosphate nanoparticles preliminary studies. *Bioceramics 15* 2003;240–2:555–8.

19. Gross KA, Chai CS, Kannangara GSK, Ben Nissan B, and Hanley L. Thin hydroxyapatite coatings via sol–gel synthesis. *J. Mater. Sci. Mater. Med.* 1998;9:839–43.

20. Masuda Y, Matubara K, and Sakka S. Synthesis of hydroxyapatite from metal alkoxides through sol–gel technique. *Nippon Seramikkusu Kyokai Gakujutsu Ronbunshi-J. Ceram. Soc. Jpn.* 1990;98:1255–66.

21. Jillavenkatesa A and Condrate RA. Sol–gel processing of hydroxyapatite. *J. Mater. Sci.* 1998;33:4111–9.

22. Liu YL, Layrolle P, de Bruijn J, Van Blitterswijk C, and de Groot K. Biomimetic coprecipitation of calcium phosphate and bovine serum albumin on titanium alloy. *J. Biomed. Mater. Res.* 2001;57:327–35.

23. Sundaram J, Durance TD, and Wang R. Porous scaffold of gelatin-starch with nanohydroxyapatite composite processed via novel microwave vacuum drying. *Acta Biomater.* 2008;4:932–42.

24. Kong L, Ao Q, Wang A et al. Preparation and characterization of a multilayer biomimetic scaffold for bone tissue engineering. *J. Biomater. Appl.* 2007;22:223–39.

25. Du C, Cui FZ, Feng QL, Zhu XD, and de Groot K. Tissue response to nanohydroxyapatite/collagen composite implants in marrow cavity. *J. Biomed. Mater. Res.* 1998;42:540–8.

26. Liu L, Liu J, Wang M et al. Preparation and characterization of nano-hydroxyapatite/silk fibroin porous scaffolds. *J. Biomater. Sci. Polym. Ed.* 2008;19:325–38.

27. Huang YX, Ren J, Chen C, Ren TB, and Zhou XY. Preparation and properties of poly(lactide-co-glycolide) (PLGA)/nano-hydroxyapatite (NHA) scaffolds by thermally induced phase separation and rabbit MSCs culture on scaffolds. *J. Biomater. Appl.* 2008;22:409–32.

28. Ren J, Zhao P, Ren TB, Gu SY, and Pan KF. Poly (D,L-lactide)/nano-hydroxyapatite composite scaffolds for bone tissue engineering and biocompatibility evaluation. *J. Mater. Sci. Mater. Med.* 2008;19:1075–82.

29. Wang H, Li Y, Zuo Y, Li J, Ma S, and Cheng L. Biocompatibility and osteogenesis of biomimetic nano-hydroxyapatite/polyamide composite scaffolds for bone tissue engineering. *Biomaterials* 2007;28:3338–48.

30. Heo SJ, Kim SE, Wei J et al. *In vitro* and animal study of novel nano-HA/PCL composite scaffolds fabricated by layer manufacturing process. *Tissue Eng. A* 2008;5:977–89.

31. Arts JJC, Verdonschot N, Schreurs BW, and Buma P. The use of a bioresorbable nano-crystalline hydroxyapatite paste in acetabular bone impaction grafting. *Biomaterials* 2006;27:1110–8.

32. Kokubo T, Kim HM, and Kawashita M. Novel bioactive materials with different mechanical properties. *Biomaterials* 2003;24:2161–75.

33. Kokubo T, Miyaji F, Kim HM, and Nakamura T. Spontaneous formation of bonelike apatite layer on chemically treated titanium metals. *J. Am. Ceram. Soc.* 1996;79:1127–9.

34. Li P, Nakanishi K, Kokubo T, and de Groot K. Induction and morphology of hydroxyapatite, precipitated from metastable simulated body fluids on sol–gel prepared silica. *Biomaterials* 1993;14:963–8.

35. Tas AC. Synthesis of biomimetic Ca-hydroxyapatite powders at 37 degrees C in synthetic body fluids. *Biomaterials* 2000;21:1429–38.

36. Liu DM, Troczynski T, and Tseng WJ. Water-based sol–gel synthesis of hydroxyapatite: Process development. *Biomaterials* 2001;22:1721–30.

37. Stigter M, de Groot K, and Layrolle P. Incorporation of tobramycin into biomimetic hydroxyapatite coating on titanium. *Biomaterials* 2002;23:4143–53.

38. Wen HB, de Wijn JR, van Blitterswijk CA, and de Groot K. Incorporation of bovine serum albumin in calcium phosphate coating on titanium. *J. Biomed. Mater. Res.* 1999;46:245–52.

39. Shirkhanzadeh M. Direct formation of nanophase hydroxyapatite on cathodically polarized electrodes. *J. Mater. Sci. Mater. Med.* 1998;9:67–72.

40. Jaworek A and Sobczyk AT. Electrospraying route to nanotechnology: An overview. *J. Electrostat.* 2008;66:197–219.

41. Leeuwenburgh S, Wolke J, Schoonman J, and Jansen J. Electrostatic spray deposition (ESD) of calcium phosphate coatings. *J. Biomed. Mater. Res. A* 2003;66A:330–4.

42. Moerman R, Frank J, Marijnissen JCM, Schalkhammer TGM, and van Dedem GWK. Miniaturized electrospraying as a technique for the production of microarrays of reproducible micrometer-sized protein spots. *Anal. Chem.* 2001;73:2183–9.

43. Moerman R, Knoll J, Apetrei C, van den Doel LR, and van Dedem GWK. Quantitative analysis in nanoliter wells by prefilling of wells using electrospray deposition followed by sample introduction with a coverslip method. *Anal. Chem.* 2005;77:225–31.

44. Thundat T, Warmack RJ, Allison DP, and Ferrell TL. Electrostatic spraying of DNA molecules for investigation by scanning tunneling microscopy. *Ultramicroscopy* 1992;42:1083–7.
45. Uematsu I, Matsumoto H, Morota K et al. Surface morphology and biological activity of protein thin films produced by electrospray deposition. *J. Colloid Interface Sci.* 2004;269:336–40.
46. Huang J, Jayasinghe SN, Best SM, Edirisinghe MJ, Brooks RA, and Bonfield W. Electrospraying of a nano-hydroxyapatite suspension. *J. Mater. Sci.* 2004;39:1029–32.
47. Teo WE, He W, and Ramakrishna S. Electrospun scaffold tailored for tissue-specific extracellular matrix. *Biotechnol. J.* 2006;1:918–29.
48. Murugan R and Ramakrishna S. Nano-featured scaffolds for tissue engineering: A review of spinning methodologies. *Tissue Eng.* 2006;12:435–47.
49. Vasita R and Katti DS. Nanofibers and their applications in tissue engineering. *Int. J. Nanomed.* 2006;1:15–30.
50. Fennessey SF and Farris RJ. Electrospinning: Mechanical behavior of twisted and drawn polyacrylonitrile nanofiber. *Abstr. Pap. Am. Chem. Soc.* 2004;228:U507.
51. Kim K, Yu M, Zong XH et al. Control of degradation rate and hydrophilicity in electrospun non-woven poly(D,L-lactide) nanofiber scaffolds for biomedical applications. *Biomaterials* 2003;24:4977–85.
52. Loscertales IG, Barrero A, Marquez M, Spretz R, Velarde-Ortiz R, and Larsen G. Electrically forced coaxial nanojets for one-step hollow nanofiber design. *J. Am. Chem. Soc.* 2004;126:5376–7.
53. Smith LA and Ma PX. Nano-fibrous scaffolds for tissue engineering. *Colloids Surf. B Biointerfaces* 2004;39:125–31.
54. Dzenis Y. Spinning continuous fibers for nanotechnology. *Science* 2004;304: 1917–9.
55. Li M, Mondrinos MJ, Gandhi MR, Ko FK, Weiss AS, and Lelkes PI. Electrospun protein fibers as matrices for tissue engineering. *Biomaterials* 2005;26:5999–6008.
56. Matthews JA, Wnek GE, Simpson DG, and Bowlin GL. Electrospinning of collagen nanofibers. *Biomacromolecules* 2002;3:232–8.
57. Huang L, Nagapudi K, Apkarian RP, and Chaikof EL. Engineered collagen–PEO nanofibers and fabrics. *J. Biomater. Sci. Polym. Ed.* 2001;12:979–93.
58. Li MY, Guo Y, Wei Y, MacDiarmid AG, and Lelkes PI. Electrospinning polyaniline-contained gelatin nanofibers for tissue engineering applications. *Biomaterials* 2006;27:2705–15.
59. Li WJ, Laurencin CT, Caterson EJ, Tuan RS, and Ko FK. Electrospun nanofibrous structure: A novel scaffold for tissue engineering. *J. Biomed. Mater. Res.* 2002;60:613–21.
60. Shin HJ, Lee CH, Cho IH et al. Electrospun PLGA nanofiber scaffolds for articular cartilage reconstruction: Mechanical stability, degradation and cellular responses under mechanical stimulation *in vitro*. *J. Biomater. Sci. Polym. Ed.* 2006;17:103–19.
61. Yoshimoto H, Shin YM, Terai H, and Vacanti JP. A biodegradable nanofiber scaffold by electrospinning and its potential for bone tissue engineering. *Biomaterials* 2003;24:2077–82.
62. He W, Ma ZW, Yong T, Teo WE, and Ramakrishna S. Fabrication of collagen-coated biodegradable polymer nanofiber mesh and its potential for endothelial cells growth. *Biomaterials* 2005;26:7606–15.

63. Fertala A, Han WB, and Ko FK. Mapping critical sites in collagen II for rational design of gene-engineered proteins for cell-supporting materials. *J. Biomed. Mater. Res.* 2001;57:48–58.

64. Zhong SP, Teo WE, Zhu X, Beuerman R, Ramakrishna S, and Yung LYL. Formation of collagen-glycosaminoglycan blended nanofibrous scaffolds and their biological properties. *Biomacromolecules* 2005;6:2998–3004.

65. Chew SY, Wen J, Yim EKF, and Leong KW. Sustained release of proteins from electrospun biodegradable fibers. *Biomacromolecules* 2005;6:2017–24.

66. Zeng J, Aigner A, Czubayko F, Kissel T, Wendorff JH, and Greiner A. Poly(vinyl alcohol) nanofibers by electrospinning as a protein delivery system and the retardation of enzyme release by additional polymer coatings. *Biomacromolecules* 2005;6:1484–8.

67. Jiang HL, Fang DF, Hsiao BJ, Chu BJ, and Chen WL. Preparation and characterization of ibuprofen-loaded poly(lactide-co-glycolide)/poly(ethylene glycol)-g-chitosan electrospun membranes. *J. Biomater. Sci. Polym. Ed.* 2004;15:279–96.

68. Katti DS, Robinson KW, Ko FK, and Laurencin CT. Bioresorbable nanofiber-based systems for wound healing and drug delivery: Optimization of fabrication parameters. *J. Biomed. Mater. Res. B Appl. Biomater.* 2004;70B:286–96.

69. Kenawy ER, Bowlin GL, Mansfield K et al. Release of tetracycline hydrochloride from electrospun polymers. *Abstr. Pap. Am. Chem. Soc.* 2002;223:C115.

70. Kim K, Luu YK, Chang C et al. Incorporation and controlled release of a hydrophilic antibiotic using poly(lactide-co-glycolide)-based electrospun nanofibrous scaffolds. *J. Control. Release* 2004;98:47–56.

71. Verreck G, Chun I, Peeters J, Rosenblatt J, and Brewster ME. Preparation and characterization of nanofibers containing amorphous drug dispersions generated by electrostatic spinning. *Pharm. Res.* 2003;20:810–7.

72. Zeng J, Xu X, Chen X et al. Biodegradable electrospun fibers for drug delivery. *J. Control. Release* 2003;92:227–31.

73. Zong XH, Kim K, Fang DF, Ran SF, Hsiao BS, and Chu B. Structure and process relationship of electrospun bioabsorbable nanofiber membranes. *Polymer* 2002;43:4403–12.

74. Larrondo L and Manley RSJ. Electrostatic fiber spinning from polymer melts. 1. Experimental-observations on fiber formation and properties. *J. Polym. Sci. B Polym. Phys.* 1981;19:909–20.

75. Larrondo L and Manley RSJ. Electrostatic fiber spinning from polymer melts. 2. Examination of the flow field in an electrically driven jet. *J. Polym. Sci. B Polym. Phys.* 1981;19:921–32.

76. Larrondo L and Manley RSJ. Electrostatic fiber spinning from polymer melts. 3. Electrostatic deformation of a pendant drop of polymer melt. *J. Polym. Sci. B Polym. Phys.* 1981;19:933–40.

77. Li CM, Vepari C, Jin HJ, Kim HJ, and Kaplan DL. Electrospun silk-BMP-2 scaffolds for bone tissue engineering. *Biomaterials* 2006;27:3115–24.

78. Foldvari M and Bagonluri M. Carbon nanotubes as functional excipients for nanomedicines: II. Drug delivery and biocompatibility issues. *Nanomedicine* 2008;4:183–200.

79. Kagan VE, Bayir H, and Shvedova AA. Nanomedicine and nanotoxicology: Two sides of the same coin. *Nanomedicine* 2005;1:313–6.

80. Ajayan PM, Schadler LS, Giannaris C, and Rubio A. Single-walled carbon nano-tube-polymer composites: Strength and weakness. *Adv. Mater.* 2000;12:750–3.
81. Calvert P. Nanotube composites—A recipe for strength. *Nature* 1999;399:210–1.
82. Shi XF, Hudson JL, Spicer PP, Tour JM, Krishnamoorti R, and Mikos AG. Injectable nanocomposites of single-walled carbon nanotubes and biodegrad-able polymers for bone tissue engineering. *Biomacromolecules* 2006;7:2237–42.
83. Abarrategi A, Gutierrez MC, Moreno-Vicente C et al. Multiwall carbon nano-tube scaffolds for tissue engineering purposes. *Biomaterials* 2008;29:94–102.
84. Wang W, Watari F, Omori M et al. Mechanical properties and biological behav-ior of carbon nanotube/polycarbosilane composites for implant materials. *J. Biomed. Mater. Res. B Appl. Biomater.* 2007;82B:223–30.
85. Helland A, Wick P, Koehler A, Schmid K, and Som C. Reviewing the environ-mental and human health knowledge base of carbon nanotubes. *Cien. Saude Colet.* 2008;13:441–52.
86. Terrones M and Terrones H. The carbon nanocosmos: Novel materials for the twenty-first century. *Philos. Trans. R. Soc. Lond. A Math. Phys. Eng. Sci.* 2003;361:2789–806.
87. Vajtai R, Wei BQ, and Ajayan PM. Controlled growth of carbon nanotubes. *Philos. Trans. R. Soc. Lond. A Math. Phys. Eng. Sci.* 2004;362:2143–60.
88. Shi XF, Hudson JL, Spicer PP, Tour JM, Krishnamoorti R, and Mikos AG. Rheological behaviour and mechanical characterization of injectable poly(propylene fumarate)/single-walled carbon nanotube composites for bone tissue engineering. *Nanotechnology* 2005;16:S531–8.
89. Sitharaman B, Tran LA, Pham QP et al. Gadofullerenes as nanoscale magnetic labels for cellular MRI. *Contrast Media Mol. Imaging* 2007;2:139–46.
90. Sitharaman B and Wilson LJ. Gadonanotubes as new high-performance MRI contrast agents. *Int. J. Nanomed.* 2006;1:291–5.
91. Sitharaman B, Zakharian TY, Saraf A et al. Water-soluble fullerene (C60) deriva-tives as nonviral gene-delivery vectors. *Mol. Pharm.* 2008;5:567–78.
92. Iijima S. Helical microtubules of graphitic carbon. *Nature* 1991;354:56–8.
93. Bethune DS, Kiang CH, Devries MS et al. Cobalt-catalyzed growth of carbon nanotubes with single-atomic-layer walls. *Nature* 1993;363:605–7.
94. Ebbesen TW and Ajayan PM. Large-scale synthesis of carbon nanotubes. *Nature* 1992;358:220–2.
95. Iijima S. Growth of carbon nanotubes. *Mater. Sci. Eng. B Solid State Mater. Adv. Technol.* 1993;19:172–80.
96. Dresselhaus MS, Dresselhaus G, and Eklund PC. Fullerenes. *J. Mater. Res.* 1993;8:2054–97.
97. Harris PJF. New perspectives on the structure of graphitic carbons. *Crit. Rev. Solid State Mater. Sci.* 2005;30:235–53.
98. Terrones M, Hsu WK, Kroto HW, and Walton DRM. Nanotubes: A revolution in materials science and electronics. *Fullerenes Relat. Struct.* 1999;199:189–234.
99. Maser WK, Munoz E, Benito AM et al. Production of high-density single-walled nanotube material by a simple laser-ablation method. *Chem. Phys. Lett.* 1998;292:587–93.
100. Eklund PC, Pradhan BK, Kim UJ et al. Large-scale production of single-walled carbon nanotubes using ultrafast pulses from a free electron laser. *Nano Lett.* 2002;2:561–6.
101. Baker RTK. Catalytic growth of carbon filaments. *Carbon* 1989;27:315–23.

102. Amelinckx S, Zhang XB, Bernaerts D, Zhang XF, Ivanov V, and Nagy JB. A formation mechanism for catalytically grown helix-shaped graphite nanotubes. *Science* 1994;265:635–9.
103. Nikolaev P. Gas-phase production of single-walled carbon nanotubes from carbon monoxide: A review of the HiPco process. *J. Nanosci. Nanotechnol.* 2004;4:307–16.
104. Webster TJ and Ejiofor JU. Increased osteoblast adhesion on nanophase metals: Ti, Ti6Al4V, and CoCrMo. *Biomaterials* 2004;25:4731–9.
105. de Oliveira PT and Nanci A. Nanotexturing of titanium-based surfaces upregulates expression of bone sialoprotein and osteopontin by cultured osteogenic cells. *Biomaterials* 2004;25:403–13.
106. Elias KL, Price RL, and Webster TJ. Enhanced functions of osteoblasts on nanometer diameter carbon fibers. *Biomaterials* 2002;23:3279–87.
107. Kay S, Thapa A, Haberstroh KM, and Webster TJ. Nanostructured polymer/nanophase ceramic composites enhance osteoblast and chondrocyte adhesion. *Tissue Eng.* 2002;8:753–61.
108. Webster TJ, Siegel RW, and Bizios R. Design and evaluation of nanophase alumina for orthopaedic/dental applications. *Nanostruct. Mater.* 1999;12:983–6.
109. Webster TJ, Siegel RW, and Bizios R. Osteoblast adhesion on nanophase ceramics. *Biomaterials* 1999;20:1221–7.
110. Du C, Cui FZ, Zhu XD, and de Groot K. Three-dimensional nano-HAp/collagen matrix loading with osteogenic cells in organ culture. *J. Biomed. Mater. Res.* 1999;44:407–15.
111. Zhu XL, Eibl O, Scheideler L, and Geis-Gerstorfer J. Characterization of nano hydroxyapatite/collagen surfaces and cellular behaviors. *J. Biomed. Mater. Res. A* 2006;79A:114–27.
112. Herten M, Rothamel D, Schwarz F, Friesen K, Koegler G, and Becker J. Surface- and nonsurface-dependent *in vitro* effects of bone substitutes on cell viability. *Clin. Oral Investig.* 2008;2:149–55.
113. Laschke MW, Witt K, Pohlemann T, and Menger MD. Injectable nanocrystalline hydroxyapatite paste for bone substitution: *In vivo* analysis of biocompatibility and vascularization. *J. Biomed. Mater. Res. B Appl. Biomater.* 2007;82:494–505.
114. Busenlechner D, Tangl S, Mair B et al. Simultaneous *in vivo* comparison of bone substitutes in a guided bone regeneration model. *Biomaterials* 2008;29:3195–200.
115. Rothamel D, Schwarz F, Herten M et al. Dimensional ridge alterations following socket preservation using a nanocrystalline oxyapatite paste. A histomorphometrical study in dogs. *Int. J. Oral Maxillofac. Surg.* 2008;37:741–7.
116. Meirelles L, Albrektsson T, Kjellin P et al. Bone reaction to nano hydroxyapatite modified titanium implants placed in a gap-healing model. *J. Biomed. Mater. Res. A* 2008;87A:624–31.
117. Shields KJ, Beckman MJ, Bowlin GL, and Wayne JS. Mechanical properties and cellular proliferation of electrospun collagen type II. *Tissue Eng.* 2004;10:1510–7.
118. Zhang Y, Venugopal JR, El Turki A, Ramakrishna S, Su B, and Lim CT. Electrospun biomimetic nanocomposite nanofibers of hydroxyapatite/chitosan for bone tissue engineering. *Biomaterials* 2008;29:4314–22.
119. Zhang YZ, Ouyang HW, Lim CT, Ramakrishna S, and Huang ZM. Electrospinning of gelatin fibers and gelatin/PCL composite fibrous scaffolds. *J. Biomed. Mater. Res. B Appl. Biomater.* 2005;72B:156–65.

120. Hu J, Liu XH, and Ma PX. Induction of osteoblast differentiation phenotype on poly(L-lactic acid) nanofibrous matrix. *Biomaterials* 2008;29:3815–21.
121. Leong MF, Rasheed MZ, Lim TC, and Chian KS. *In vitro* cell infiltration and *in vivo* cell infiltration and vascularization in a fibrous, highly porous poly(D,L-lactide) scaffold fabricated by cryogenic electrospinning technique. *J. Biomed. Mater. Res. A* 2008;1:231–40.
122. Simonet M, Schneider OD, Neuenschwander P, and Stark WJ. Ultraporous 3D polymer meshes by low-temperature electrospinning: Use of ice crystals as a removable void template. *Polym. Eng. Sci.* 2007;47:2020–6.
123. Kim HW, Lee HH, and Chun GS. Bioactivity and osteoblast responses of novel biomedical nanocomposites of bioactive glass nanofiber filled poly(lactic acid). *J. Biomed. Mater. Res. A* 2008;85A:651–63.
124. Schneider OD, Loher S, Brunner TJ et al. Cotton wool-like nanocomposite biomaterials prepared by electrospinning: *In vitro* bioactivity and osteogenic differentiation of human mesenchymal stem cells. *J. Biomed. Mater. Res. B Appl. Biomater.* 2008;84B:350–62.
125. Fujihara K, Kotaki M, and Ramakrishna S. Guided bone regeneration membrane made of polycaprolactone/calcium carbonate composite nano-fibers. *Biomaterials* 2005;26:4139–47.
126. Wutticharoenmongkol P, Sanchavanakit N, Pavasant P, and Supaphol P. Preparation and characterization of novel bone scaffolds based on electrospun polycaprolactone fibers filled with nanoparticles. *Macromol. Biosci.* 2006;6:70–7.
127. Kim KH, Jeong L, Park HN et al. Biological efficacy of silk fibroin nanofiber membranes for guided bone regeneration. *J. Biotechnol.* 2005;120:327–39.
128. Fu Y, Nie H, Ho M, Wang C, Huang H, and Wang C. Optimized bone regeneration based on sustained release from 3D scaffold. *Calcif. Tissue Int.* 2008;82:S64–5.
129. Shin M, Yoshimoto H, and Vacanti JP. *In vivo* bone tissue engineering using mesenchymal stem cells on a novel electrospun nanofibrous scaffold. *Tissue Eng.* 2004;10:33–41.
130. Piskin E, Isoglu IA, Bolgen N et al. *In vivo* performance of simvastatin-loaded electrospun spiral-wound polycaprolactone scaffolds in reconstruction of cranial bone defects in the rat model. *J. Biomed. Mater. Res. A* 2008;4:1137–51.
131. Colvin VL. The potential environmental impact of engineered nanomaterials. *Nat. Biotechnol.* 2003;21:1166–70.
132. Kipen HM and Laskin DL. Smaller is not always better: Nanotechnology yields nanotoxicology. *Am. J. Physiol. Lung Cell. Mol. Physiol.* 2005;289:L696–7.
133. Maynard AD, Baron PA, Foley M, Shvedova AA, Kisin ER, and Castranova V. Exposure to carbon nanotube material: Aerosol release during the handling of unrefined single-walled carbon nanotube material. *J. Toxicol. Environ. Health A* 2004;67:87–107.
134. Oberdorster E, Zhu SQ, Blickley TM, McClellan-Green P, and Haasch ML. Ecotoxicology of carbon-based engineered nanoparticles: Effects of fullerene (C-60) on aquatic organisms. *Carbon* 2006;44:1112–20.
135. Oberdorster G, Oberdorster E, and Oberdorster J. Nanotoxicology: An emerging discipline evolving from studies of ultrafine particles. *Environ. Health Perspect.* 2005;113:823–39.
136. Shvedova AA, Castranova V, Kisin ER et al. Exposure to carbon nanotube material: Assessment of nanotube cytotoxicity using human keratinocyte cells. *J. Toxicol. Environ. Health A* 2003;66:1909–26.

137. Monteiro-Riviere NA, Nemanich RJ, Inman AO, Wang YYY, and Riviere JE. Multi-walled carbon nanotube interactions with human epidermal keratinocytes. *Toxicol. Lett.* 2005;155:377–84.
138. Ding L, Stilwell J, Zhang T et al. Molecular characterization of the cytotoxic mechanism of multiwall carbon nanotubes and nano-onions on human skin fibroblast. *Nano Lett.* 2005;5:2448–64.
139. Soto KF, Carrasco A, Powell TG, Garza KM, and Murr LE. Comparative *in vitro* cytotoxicity assessment of some manufactured nanoparticulate materials characterized by transmission electron microscopy. *J. Nanopart. Res.* 2005;7:145–69.
140. Cui D, Tian F, Ozkan CS, Wang M, and Gao H. Effect of single wall carbon nanotubes on human HEK293 cells. *Toxicol. Lett.* 2005;155:73–85.
141. Manna SK, Sarkar S, Barr J et al. Single-walled carbon nanotube induces oxidative stress and activates nuclear transcription factor-kappa B in human keratinocytes. *Nano Lett.* 2005;5:1676–84.
142. Pulskamp K, Diabate S, and Krug HF. Carbon nanotubes show no sign of acute toxicity but induce intracellular reactive oxygen species in dependence on contaminants. *Toxicol. Lett.* 2007;168:58–74.
143. Raja PMV, Connolley J, Ganesan GP et al. Impact of carbon nanotube exposure, dosage and aggregation on smooth muscle cells. *Toxicol. Lett.* 2007;169:51–63.
144. Wick P, Manser P, Limbach LK et al. The degree and kind of agglomeration affect carbon nanotube cytotoxicity. *Toxicol. Lett.* 2007;168:121–31.
145. Carrero-Sanchez JC, Elias AL, Mancilla R et al. Biocompatibility and toxicological studies of carbon nanotubes doped with nitrogen. *Nano Lett.* 2006;6:1609–16.
146. Hu H, Ni YC, Montana V, Haddon RC, and Parpura V. Chemically functionalized carbon nanotubes as substrates for neuronal growth. *Nano Lett.* 2004;4:507–11.
147. Nimmagadda A, Thurston K, Nollert MU, and McFetridge PSF. Chemical modification of SWNT alters *in vitro* cell–SWNT interactions. *J. Biomed. Mater. Res. A* 2006;76A:614-25.
148. Zanello LP, Zhao B, Hu H, and Haddon RC. Bone cell proliferation on carbon nanotubes. *Nano Lett.* 2006;6:562–7.
149. Sayes CM, Liang F, Hudson JL et al. Functionalization density dependence of single-walled carbon nanotubes cytotoxicity *in vitro*. *Toxicol. Lett.* 2006;161:135–42.
150. Jia G, Wang HF, Yan L et al. Cytotoxicity of carbon nanomaterials: Single-wall nanotube, multi-wall nanotube, and fullerene. *Environ. Sci. Technol.* 2005;39:1378–83.
151. Muller J, Huaux F, Moreau N et al. Respiratory toxicity of multi-wall carbon nanotubes. *Toxicol. Appl. Pharmacol.* 2005;207:221–31.
152. Cherukuri P, Bachilo SM, Litovsky SH, and Weisman RB. Near-infrared fluorescence microscopy of single-walled carbon nanotubes in phagocytic cells. *J. Am. Chem. Soc.* 2004;126:15638–9.
153. Shi XF, Sitharaman B, Pham QP et al. Fabrication of porous ultra-short single-walled carbon nanotube nanocomposite scaffolds for bone tissue engineering. *Biomaterials* 2007;28:4078–90.
154. Kam NWS, Jessop TC, Wender PA, and Dai HJ. Nanotube molecular transporters: Internalization of carbon nanotube–protein conjugates into mammalian cells. *J. Am. Chem. Soc.* 2004;126:6850–1.
155. Bottini M, Bruckner S, Nika K et al. Multi-walled carbon nanotubes induce T lymphocyte apoptosis. *Toxicol. Lett.* 2006;160:121–6.

156. Grubek-Jaworska H, Nejman P, Czuminska K et al. Preliminary results on the pathogenic effects of intratracheal exposure to one-dimensional nanocarbons. *Carbon* 2006;44:1057–63.
157. Huczko A and Lange H. Carbon nanotubes: Experimental evidence for a null risk of skin irritation and allergy. *Fullerene Sci. Technol.* 2001;9:247–50.
158. Wang HF, Wang J, Deng XY et al. Biodistribution of carbon single-wall carbon nanotubes in mice. *J. Nanosci. Nanotechnol.* 2004;4:1019–24.
159. Warheit DB, Laurence BR, Reed KL, Roach DH, Reynolds GAM, and Webb TR. Comparative pulmonary toxicity assessment of single-wall carbon nanotubes in rats. *Toxicol. Sci.* 2004;77:117–25.
160. Lam CW, James JT, McCluskey R, and Hunter RL. Pulmonary toxicity of single-wall carbon nanotubes in mice 7 and 90 days after intratracheal instillation. *Toxicol. Sci.* 2004;77:126–34.
161. Li JG, Li WX, Xu JY et al. Comparative study of pathological lesions induced by multiwalled carbon nanotubes in lungs of mice by intratracheal instillation and inhalation. *Environ. Toxicol.* 2007;22:415–21.
162. Shvedova AA, Kisin ER, Mercer R et al. Unusual inflammatory and fibrogenic pulmonary responses to single-walled carbon nanotubes in mice. *Am. J. Physiol. Lung Cell. Mol. Physiol.* 2005;289:L698–708.
163. Nel A, Xia T, Madler L, and Li N. Toxic potential of materials at the nanolevel. *Science* 2006;311:622–7.
164. Radomski A, Jurasz P, Alonso-Escolano D et al. Nanoparticle-induced platelet aggregation and vascular thrombosis. *Br. J. Pharmacol.* 2005;146:882–93.
165. Sitharaman B, Shi X, Walboomers XF et al. *In vivo* biocompatibility of ultra-short single-walled carbon nanotube/biodegradable polymer nanocomposites for bone tissue engineering. *Bone* 2008;43:362–70.
166. Kreyling WG, Semmler M, Erbe F et al. Translocation of ultrafine insoluble iridium particles from lung epithelium to extrapulmonary organs is size dependent but very low. *J. Toxicol. Environ. Health A* 2002;65:1513–30.
167. Geiser M, Rothen-Rutishauser B, Kapp N et al. Ultrafine particles cross cellular membranes by nonphagocytic mechanisms in lungs and in cultured cells. *Environ. Health Perspect.* 2005;113:1555–60.
168. Singh R, Pantarotto D, Lacerda L et al. Tissue biodistribution and blood clearance rates of intravenously administered carbon nanotube radiotracers. *Proc. Natl. Acad. Sci. U.S.A.* 2006;103:3357–62.

# Section III

# Nanotechnology and Agrofood and Water

# 5

## Nanotechnologies in Agrofood and Water

**Frans W. H. Kampers**

## CONTENTS

Food is a material that has a structural hierarchy, from the macrolevel where we enjoy its macroscopic properties, all the way down to the molecular and supramolecular levels where the nutritional and structural properties find their origin. Food can therefore be seen as a natural nanomaterial. Changing the characteristics of a foodstuff, to create new functionality, therefore usually requires changing the material at the nanolevel. In the past, mankind has used very crude methods to achieve this, such as cooking, mixing, and pressing, or letting other organisms do the job, for example, in the case of fermentation and other biological conversions. With the advent of nanotechnologies, man has started to develop the ability to act at the nanolevel directly and to interfere with the nanotechnology that nature through evolution has devised and optimized. We now have the first basic abilities to modify specific biochemical processes and to create new functions or properties, and science is rapidly developing more. Nanotechnology is an enabling technology that will provide us with tools to do business at the nanolevel, although at this point in time it is still in its infancy. The result will be that new and improved food products will be developed that will benefit the individual consumer, the society as a whole, and the environment (Moraru et al. 2003). However, as with all new technologies, there are also drawbacks and risks to be taken into account. These have to weigh up against the benefits; otherwise, the public will not accept the applications of this technology in something as basic and intimate as food and water, and provide a "license to produce." They will not buy the products, and their economic activity will not be viable. Consumers are very critical with regard to food and water. Although very few food products can still be regarded as unchanged by man, we want to have the illusion that our food and beverages are natural and pristine. Of course, they must also be healthy, tasty, and safe. In our modern society, food must also be convenient, easy and fast to prepare, transportable and storable, and must fit the cultures, lifestyles, and customs of the consumers. Moreover, finally, we are beginning to become aware of our ecological footprint and focus more and more on the sustainability of food production and consumption. Many of these characteristics are in direct contradiction with each other, and technologies need to provide solutions to resolve the conflicts and provide acceptable compromises. In this chapter, we will review most of these aspects and the impact that nanotechnologies can have on them.

## 5.1 Applications of Nanotechnology in Agriculture

If it is to be any good to the consumer, food must be the product of biological processes. In our industrialized society, the primary production of the base materials and products mostly takes place at farms. With the exception of the production of fish, only a very small part of our food supply is taken directly from nature. The reason for this is that the farm is a unit operation that allows optimizing some of the circumstances of the production. Over the centuries, this has evolved to a state where farmers in greenhouses have control over virtually all factors influencing the development of crops. Not only can they push a crop to its maximum potential, they can even control the moment the crop will be ready for harvest. This is, nowadays, common practice in crops such as fruits, vegetables, and flowers. To what extent these possibilities are being exploited with certain crops is not so much a question of biological limitations but more of economic restrictions. Not every crop sufficiently increases in value when costly measures are taken to influence production processes to justify the investment. It is not a question of technological limitations. The opportunities for new technologies to add to the already extensive toolkit of modern farmers therefore lie in improving the economic effectiveness of their deployment.

Preharvest factors that show room for improvement can be grouped into three categories: better monitoring of processes to be able to control the production to a higher extent; optimizing the delivery of production factors such as nutrients and water to the production systems; and developing more efficient methods to limit the influence of quality- and quantity-reducing pests.

### 5.1.1 Process Monitoring

The ability to more accurately monitor processes is fundamental to improved process control and the ability to determine when and what action to take in which circumstances. To be able to monitor processes, it is necessary to measure specific parameters that provide information on these processes. With the advent of nanotechnologies, some of these parameters can be measured with more accuracy and more specificity. However, the real gain of new technologies is that new parameters come into reach that provide much more information. This is because nanotechnologies work at the molecular and supramolecular levels. They allow the detection and sometimes even the quantification of specific molecules (Lieber 2003).

The human nose (and equivalent organs in other animal species) uses a large number of different receptor molecules (~300–350) that have the ability to bond to certain molecules that come in its vicinity. These receptors, usually very specific proteins, are embedded in the membrane of cells in the nose and cause an amplification process when such a docking event takes place. This process is then detected by a neuron, which communicates the event to the brain. When we smell a specific odor, many of the receptors cause signals of different strengths. Our brain has learnt to interpret the resulting pattern and to link it to, say, a ripe apple. With nanotechnology, it is now possible to attach the same receptor molecules to a silicon surface and to detect the docking event as a small change in the electrical properties of the silicon. By combining many different receptors with information technology to correlate the resulting pattern to specific odors, an electronic nose can be developed (Gardner and Bartlett 2000).

In many biological processes, certain molecules are used for the communication between subprocesses. Well known are the hormones in humans and animals, but also in plants hormones are excreted in specific stages of the development process. However, organisms also produce chemical substances that facilitate communication between individuals (e.g., to attract partners or warn against threats) and species (e.g., to attract pollination agents or repel enemies). Humans usually perceive them as smells and odors. These small volatile molecules until recently could only be measured with expensive scientific instruments that were not suited for measurements under practical circumstances on the farm. Nanotechnologies will allow the development of new principles that not only make them more specific and robust, but also will make it possible to miniaturize them and produce them in large quantities, which will reduce costs.

Of course we are familiar with the smell of ripe fruits. These signaling molecules are produced by plants to attract species that consume the fruits and thus contribute to the distribution and growing conditions of the seeds. The smells change as the fruits ripen. By determining the composition of the smell, the optimal harvesting moment can be determined. Sensors based on nanotechnology can be used in an orchard or a greenhouse to monitor the composition of the smell and signal the farmer to start harvesting when the desired state of ripening has been achieved.

The quantification of volatiles can be used in many more agricultural applications. As explained before, smells are a common means of communication between biological species and they usually come into play when important messages need to be conveyed. The smell of ripe fruits and blooming flowers is a positive example of this, whereas the smell of disease or pest infestation is the opposite. The latter is especially important to detect in the early stages in order to allow small-scale actions for preventing the spread of disease and possibly make it easier to cure individual plants and animals.

Developments in other areas of nanotechnology, such as wireless communication and energy scavenging, in the near future will provide the technology to deploy these kinds of monitoring much more easily. In combination with very large-scale production, these technologies could make it economically possible to employ wireless sensor networks throughout the greenhouse, stable, or even the plot, to monitor growing conditions and/or volatiles and to report back to the farm management system when actions are required. Trials have been conducted to monitor the conditions in potato crops for detecting phytophthora and specific conditions in vineyards (Fonseca 2007). In the future, applications of "smart dust," a military development in which large quantities of sand grain-sized devices monitor troop movements on a battlefield, could be envisioned here.

In animal husbandry applications, the use of RFID (radiofrequency identification) transponders to identify individual animals is already common practice. These transponders are not only small enough to be implanted in the animal's body, but they can also be equipped with sensors to monitor the health and wellbeing of the animal and/or its production status (e.g., heat or pregnancy detection). Sensors in the product flow (e.g., milk) can also be used to monitor the animals and the quality of the product.

The use of chemical sensors to determine the levels of nutrients in the water that is provided to the crops in greenhouses has been common practice for some years (Bergveld 2003). These chemFET sensors benefit from nanotechnology in the sense that they will become more specific, accurate, and inexpensive. These sensors allow more accurate dosing of the nutrients in agreement with the developmental stage of the plants. Moreover, the delivery of the nutrients to plants and animals can also benefit from the developments in nanotechnology, as we will see in the next section.

### 5.1.2 Nutrient Delivery

The primary plant production process on a farm is basically the conversion of $CO_2$, sunlight, water, and nutrients into complex molecules that form the base materials of food and, more and more, raw materials for different industry sectors. The animal production process is not very different in the sense that it also requires water and nutrients, but since it uses the energy content of the plant material in combination with oxygen, it does not require sunlight. The delivery of nutrients to both plants and animals is therefore important and needs to be optimal for optimized production processes. In the animal production system, most nutrients are taken up readily with the food the animal consumes; however, some very specific nutrients require special attention since their availability could be too low in one-sided diets, often occurring in animal husbandry systems where the animals do not have the liberty to find food by their own instincts. In these cases, nutrient delivery systems based on nanotechnology could be used to supply them. Since these systems are very similar to those used in human food applications, these will be discussed in more detail in Section 5.3.

Plants do not have the ability to graze and change their location if certain nutrients at their current location are used up. This means that in farm applications, they are dependent on human intervention to supply the nutrients in the form of fertilizers. Unfortunately, this process is relatively inefficient. Immediately after fertilization, the dose of nutrients could be too high and the plants can develop diseases under unfavorable conditions. If there is too much rain, the nutrients can be washed away into the aqueous environment. Not only are they then lost for the plants for which they were intended, they also cause wild plants and organisms to overdevelop at places where they are undesirable. Delivery systems based on encapsulation of nutrients in clever materials, often structured at the nanolevel to create the desired release function, can create more gradual release of the nutrients in a speed that is compatible with the crop and a rate at which the plants can use it optimally.

### 5.1.3 Crop Protection

Especially in vegetable production, infestations of different organisms can create large damage to the crops. This is, in part, a negative result of the monocultures that are used on farms for efficiency reasons, but therefore are not less undesirable. Normally, when a pest is detected, many plants are already infected and the farmer has no other choice than to apply a strong pesticide over the whole area of the crop. In Section 5.1.1, strategies have been described that in the future will allow early detection of pests. When the pest is detected at an early stage, measures can be taken locally to eliminate the pest and/ or prevent it from spreading. In some cases, the risk of large-scale damage to the crop by certain pests is very high and the farmer will resort to preventive application of pesticides. Unfortunately, the effectiveness is reduced under unfavorable conditions, such as heavy rain, since the chemicals can be washed off from the plants. Not only do they lose their function for the crop, they can also have negative effects on the soil or the aqueous environment.

Nanotechnologies can be used to produce pesticides that have controlled release mechanisms. By encapsulating the agent in a special encapsulation system that has a shell that can open up under well-defined conditions, the agent will only be released if the conditions for that pest are favorable or through the presence of certain compounds that are associated with the pest. In specific cases, the pest (e.g., certain fungi) produces these compounds themselves and in this way they trigger their own destruction. The shells can also be functionalized to make the system stick to the plants more effectively, thus reducing the amount that is washed off before it could be effective.

Although weeds are less of a threat to crops, their presence is also undesirable because they can limit the development of the crop because they compete for certain resources such as light, water, and nutrients. Especially when the crop is still small, its development can be seriously restricted, which results in crop loss at harvest. Although herbicides are applied in a much narrower and better-defined time window, these substances can also benefit from the concepts mentioned above for pesticides.

### 5.1.4 Other Applications

Since nanotechnologies are enabling technologies that can be applied in many different areas, many other applications can be envisioned in agriculture (Pérez-de-Luque and Rubiales 2009). Here are some examples.

In greenhouse applications, nanotechnology is used to improve the light transmission of a greenhouse deck, either by modifying the reflection properties of the deck material or by changing the spectrum of the light transmitted. Self-cleaning surfaces, based on the lotus effect in which a microstructure and a nanostructure are combined to create superhydrophobic behavior, or on catalysis of nanoparticles of $TiO_2$ in combination with light to break down organic molecules, are a simple application of nanotechnology in this case to avoid production loss because of dirty glass. Nanotechnology can also be used to make stronger (polymeric) materials to replace glass as a deck material. If the deck can be made lighter, the supporting construction can be lighter, which results in less shadow on the crop and higher yields. It also enables choosing materials predominantly for their spectroscopic properties (which wavelengths they transmit) and less because of their mechanical strength.

## 5.2 Applications in Food Processing and Production

Micro- and nanotechnologies can help improve many of the processes used in the food industry (Kampers 2007, 2009). Since virtually all food materials are derived from biological substances, they consist of a hierarchy of structures starting from the molecular and supramolecular levels through the micro- and mezolevels to the macrolevel where the consumer experiences its specific qualities and texture. To improve on the latter therefore usually means that the underlying structural levels also need to be modified. Traditional processing of foods already makes use of this principle but was largely derived from trial-and-error and best practices that have been handed over from one generation to the next for centuries. They all intervene at the macrolevel but result in structural changes also at the nanolevel. If you cook an egg, you process it at the macroscale; however, it results in conformational changes in the proteins, which provide the desired structural change to give the texture the consumer prefers. With the advent of nanoscience, it is now possible to devise processes that provide much more control at the nanolevel and therefore can result in more accurate structural changes and new functionality. However, we will start the overview of applications in processing and production with the improved measurement technology that will be possible through the use of micro- and nanotechnologies.

### 5.2.1 Process Monitoring

Because food materials are of biological origin, they exhibit large variabilities in structure, composition, and properties. Within one batch, the properties can vary substantially, making it difficult to realize the structural changes everywhere in the same way. Moreover, the physical size of a food product in relation to the macroscopic processing also provides a challenge if precise structural changes are desired. A turkey cooked in an oven can easily be burned on the outside and still raw in the core. Processes in the food industry must be designed in such a way that they are robust for this variability, and centuries of optimization have provided us with a range of processes that can be used successfully. These processes already often use sensors to determine critical parameters. In baking bread, the oven temperature and the time inside the oven are important parameters to monitor, and experience dictates how to use them. However, a baker also uses visual and smell monitoring during the process and intervenes when more accurate control is necessary. Unfortunately, this method is difficult to automate. However, with sensors that mimic the human vision and olfactory systems, new opportunities could arise.

One of the areas of research in micro- and nanotechnologies is directed toward the development of an electronic nose (Gardner and Bartlett 2000). The human olfactory system employs 300–350 different receptors located in the membrane of certain cells in the nose that generate different signal patterns when different smells are perceived. The brain has learned to interpret these patterns, to recognize them and connect them to circumstances in our direct environment, for example, making the observation that someone recently baked bread. These receptors are based on the principle that a small volatile molecule present in the atmosphere near the receptor can dock to the receptor because it fits with respect to shape and charge distributions. The docking results in a shift of charges in the receptor, which in turn gives rise to a conformational change in the receptor molecule. These changes trigger a cascade of effects in the cell that eventually causes a neuron to fire and the brain to become aware of the docking event.

By linking these receptors to a semiconductor surface, it is also possible to detect the charge shifts in the receptor when docking takes place through a small change in the impedance of the semiconductor. By combining different receptors on a large number of patches on the semiconductor, it is in principle, possible to create a device that is sensitive to a number of selected volatiles. As always, it is much less easy to develop this principle in practice. The problems encountered include the conformational changes of the proteins when they are taken out of their usual working environment, that is, embedded in the cell membrane, and covalently bond them to a hard surface.

In practical applications, the sensors of course need not detect all substances the human nose can detect. They probably will be targeted at molecules that are relevant in the process for which they are intended. In fact these molecules could be different from the ones the human nose is sensitive for. At first instance, receptors from other species, such as dogs or insects, could probably be used; however, later on, when nanoscience leads to new receptor architectures that are suitable for ligands that no species has receptors for, or which are more suitable for the detection of specific ligands in combination with the unfavorable conditions of the silicon-based detection systems, completely new, artificial receptor molecules could also be implemented.

The electronic nose is just one example of new sensor principles that come within reach through the application of micro- and nanotechnologies. Many of them are based on the same principle of mimicking biological processes. Although they are usually not as good as their biological counterparts, they do outperform more traditional sensors in sensitivity, specificity, and accuracy.

Electronic noses are still under development. It will require some major breakthroughs regarding aspects such as the conformational changes these molecules exhibit when taken out of their normal operating environment, the orientation of the receptors away from the surface that they are bound to, fine tuning the affinity between ligand and receptor to prevent the ligand from becoming permanently bound to the receptor (which would make the sensor a one-time-use device) or to prevent the occurrence of too little binding, etc.

## 5.2.2 Process Innovation and Optimization

The ability to create very well-defined structures in silicon and silicon-like or silicon-based materials—that are developed on the basis of the processes from microelectronics in microtechnology—has enabled new concepts in the processing of food materials. Since the possibilities in this field are virtually limitless, there are many opportunities for the food industry to improve on important processes. Here, three examples will be given: separation and fractionation, emulsification, and low-volume/high-value microproduction of specific chemical components.

Cees van Rijn (2004) has made an extensive description of the possibilities of microtechnology devices in separation technology. With the lithography processes developed for the microelectronics industry, it is possible to make very well-defined structures with high precision. It has been demonstrated that it is possible to make a very thin SiN membrane with holes having the same size and shape, which can be used to sieve out certain components from fluid food substances. In this way, yeast cells can be cleared from beer, but also bacteria from milk, resulting in pasteurized milk without heating treatment. There are obvious advantages to this process with respect to product quality, cost, and sustainability. Having full control over the shape of the holes, uniformity in the size of the holes, and thinness of the membrane are prerequisites for this process. On the basis of the same principle, it is also in theory possible to separate a complex mixture into its individual components. If applied to milk, it would be feasible to fractionate milk into proteins, casein micelles, fat, and bacteria. Although no new products are created, just by fractionating milk, a lot of value is added to the components that are now available to different processes.

Derived from the same technology as the microsieves, it is also possible to innovate the emulsion process (Joscelyne and Trägårdh 2000). Traditionally, an emulsion, for example, oil in water (mayonnaise), is created by applying high shear forces (stirring) on a mixture of two components and some surface-active additives. The result are droplets from one component in the continuous phase of the other component. A large variety of droplet sizes are created in this way. With membrane emulsification, the discontinuous phase (in mayonnaise, the oil) is pressed through the same well-defined holes as described above. They then form droplets in the continuous phase, which flows over it. Since all the holes are of the same size, all droplets are also equally sized, forming a monodisperse emulsion. The advantage of a monodisperse emulsion is that the stability is higher. However, now that micro- and nanotechnologies allow control over these kinds of processes at the nanolevel, it is also possible to devise new products such as double emulsions. In a double emulsion, the inside of the discontinuous phase in its turn also contains a discontinuous component. In the example of mayonnaise, the oil droplets could have a core of water again. Since this would replace a lot of the oil in mayonnaise with water, it would result in a real low-calorie mayonnaise but with full fat taste and mouth feel, thus not diminishing consumer satisfaction.

If only small volumes of very expensive chemicals are needed, a micro-reactor may be the thing to go for (Ehrfeld et al. 2000). In a microreactor, very small channels of the order of magnitude of micrometers are used to bring certain chemicals in contact with each other. Microfluidics, and with increasing miniaturization often also nanofluidics, is the science that has provided us with the understanding of the remarkable behavior of fluids in small channels, and has allowed us to redesign processes to make use of this behavior. One of the aspects of fluids in microchannels is that they flow lamellar, which means that two fluids in one channel do not mix spontaneously. This means that it can be controlled when and where they mix, as well as the exact conditions in which the chemical reaction takes place. Moreover, in a thin channel, the interaction of the flowing component and the wall is very intricate and since the wall often plays a role in the reactions that take place, this means that this role is enhanced. It also means that the energy exchange with the wall is much better, resulting in a high control of parameters such as the reaction temperature. This is extremely important since temperature variations often give rise to other chemical reactions taking place that produce unwanted side products. Small channels mean that very little reagent is in play, which in turn means that reactions that previously cannot be done safely on a large scale now become feasible.

Of course, one of the biggest drawbacks is that this way of doing chemistry only yields very small amounts of products. If these products have a high value and/or only very little is needed for the application in mind, this is not a problem. However, usually, more is needed. In traditional chemical process development, small-scale laboratory production is scaled up to pilot plant production and next to industrial scale production. Usually these scaling steps pose a very big risk for the company since laboratory production in general is not a guarantee for good large-scale production. In fact, in many cases, scaling has been the bottleneck that kills a new product. With microreactor production, this need not be the case since the proof-of-concept at the laboratory in a microreactor scales linearly toward larger production volumes, simply by putting more microreactors in parallel. If the reaction performs well in one microreactor, it will also do well in a thousand similar microreactors, yielding a thousand times more products. Of course, if still larger production volumes are required, a redesign of the microreactor for mass parallelization would be wise from an economic point of view.

## 5.3 Opportunities for Food Product Development

The biggest opportunities that applications of nanotechnologies have to offer to the food industry and to the consumers lie in the development of new products. Food is a material with a structural hierarchy from the macroscopic level where we experience its benefits, such as taste, smell, and texture, through the meso- and microlevels, all the way down to the nanolevel. It is therefore not surprising that a technology that allows the industry to modify the materials at the nanolevel will provide new opportunities for new products and modifications to specific characteristics of existing products. Although virtually all processing that is being done to food products, including cooking at home, modifies structural elements at the nanolevel, nanotechnology now enables to do that with a precision not encountered before. Boiling an egg, for instance, modifies the structure of the proteins, causing the textural changes that allow the egg to be sliced. This is a macroscopic process, and all components of the egg are affected by the treatment. Nanotechnology would allow, for instance, to modify only specific proteins or change the structure of the proteins in a defined way. Although this may seem not to be very useful in the case of an egg, it will prove to be very useful in other foodstuffs.

### 5.3.1 Texture Modification

Production of sufficient high-quality (protein-rich) food will be a global challenge for the next decades. Emerging and rapidly developing economies combine large populations with steeply rising standards of living. These populations will develop a demand for more protein, preferably of animal source. Unfortunately, the traditional way of producing animal protein, through animal husbandry and the meat industry, is highly inefficient. To be able to fulfill the higher demand for proteins, it will be necessary to find new ways to convert plant protein directly in a product that sufficiently mimics the properties of meat to be acceptable as a meat replacement. Meat, especially the high-quality kind, is made up of muscle tissue. Muscle has a structural hierarchy with fascicles, fibers, and fibrils. This hierarchy is also the basis of the structure of meat. When new products are being developed that in future have the potential to fulfill the demands of consumers, it is necessary to recreate the structural hierarchy. This requires the ability to first create a nanostructure of protein fibrils to build upon toward the higher structural levels. With the addition of nanotechnology to the toolbox of the food technologist, these abilities come into reach (Manski et al. 2007).

Because it is now possible to modify and control the texture all the way down to the nanolevel, it is possible to create totally new sensations for the consumer. In part, these new sensations could comprise the texture of foods, which is the experience of structure in the mouth of the consumer (Wilkinson et al. 2000). In fact, the recreation of the structural hierarchy to create meat from nonanimal sources is the ultimate texture engineering. However, texture modification could also be less ambitious. Some food products are too soft or hard for the taste of specific consumer groups. By modifying the structure at the nanolevel, for example, by manipulating the extent and the type of cross linking of protein fibrils, the texture of the food product can be tailored to the tastes of these consumers.

## 5.3.2 Encapsulation and (Targeted) Delivery

In the same way as has been mentioned in Sections 5.1.2 and 5.1.3, encapsulation mechanisms allow the delivery of specific nutrients where they are most effective. Using self-assembly mechanisms, a structure can be created that can contain specific nutrients. Depending on the type of substance on the inside and outside, oily or watery, these structures are called either vesicles or micelles. In fact, these structures have been used in the food industry for a very long time, and also natural components of certain food products are part of these categories of structures. Nanotechnology allows modifying the wall of these structures to create new functionality, for example, to release of the contents of the structure when a specific trigger is present. Triggers can be a change in pH; however, the presence of certain enzymes, present only at the desired location in the gastrointestinal tract, could also be used to release the nutrients. This is called targeted release and can be very effective in the delivery of nutrients necessary to maintain good health (Weiss et al. 2006).

At the same time, these concepts can be used to encapsulate food components that would spoil the desired characteristics of food products. Certain ingredients are considered to be beneficial to health but have a bad taste. When simply added to a food product in the normal way, this would spoil the taste of the product, which, of course, is unacceptable. Certain peptides that taste bitter and omega-3 fatty acids that can give a "fishy taste," are examples of this effect. By encapsulating these ingredients in a vesicle or micelle, the ingredient can be released beyond the mouth region so as to circumvent the experience of the taste.

Another reason to encapsulate a food ingredient is to make it more bio-available. Encapsulation can maintain the dispersion of the material, which increases the surface area and enables a faster exchange of molecules to the phase in which the molecules are taken up by the organ of interest.

Finally, encapsulation is used to protect certain ingredients from the processing conditions or to prevent them from being destroyed by other molecules in the food product. Some combinations of nutrients are essential for the desired biological effect, but can also react with each other before consumption, effectively destroying the beneficial effect. Vitamin A and iron are examples of such a problem. With nanotechnology, new structures can be engineered that keep the nutrients in separate compartments and prevent premature reactions. These concepts will make fortification of popular products possible, thus helping certain groups in society to maintain their health.

## 5.4 Improving Shelf Life and Quality Assurance of Food Products

Because food predominantly is made of biological materials, it is extremely perishable and the quality of the products rapidly deteriorates without proper actions to protect it from outside influences and internal processes. Man has learned to employ a variety of techniques to slow down the deterioration process, of which packaging, cooling, and chemical protection through salt, sugar, or alcohol are the most commonly used. Unfortunately, these strategies are less and less popular since they reduce the freshness of the food. Consumers have a strong tendency to prefer fresh or mildly preserved products. The result is that, at the moment, in the industrialized societies of the Western world, about 30% to 40% of all the foods that are being produced end up as waste, without being eaten by the consumers for whom they were intended. In view of the ever-growing world population and the food scarcity in large parts of the world, this is a highly undesirable situation.

### 5.4.1 Barrier Properties

Many of the quality deterioration processes are driven by oxygen, either through direct oxidation of the product or components of the product, or because the organisms responsible for spoilage, such as bacteria or fungi, need oxygen to function and propagate. Therefore, reducing the amount of oxygen in the atmosphere of the product is an effective way of slowing down the spoilage processes. Maintaining the oxygen-deprived atmosphere obviously requires packaging that is tight for oxygen. Glass or metals are effective barriers against oxygen and have been used extensively in the past. Unfortunately, they have specific disadvantages and consumers more and more prefer other packaging materials, which are, however, invariably less effective as a barrier against oxygen. Together with the demand for low-weight, which means thin, and often transparent packaging—because consumers want to be able to inspect the product inside the package—this makes it virtually impossible to fulfill the oxygen barrier requirements. Here, nanotechnologies can come to the rescue.

In nanocomposite materials, nanosized clay platelets are incorporated into the matrix of the polymer packaging material (Rhim and Ng 2007). These platelets increase the diffusion path length of oxygen, effectively improving the barrier properties of the material (Sorrentino et al. 2007). Because the particles are nanosized, they do not scatter visible light and therefore do not interfere with the transparency of the original material. Other strategies make use of very specific nanosized layers on top of the packaging material to reduce the oxygen permeability. In some applications, oxygen scavenger molecules are included in the packaging concept to catch oxygen getting into the package (Brody 2006). Which of these strategies is used strongly depends on the product to be protected, the packaging concept, and price.

### 5.4.2 Antimicrobial Activity

For some products, deprivation of oxygen is not an option and microbial activity is difficult to stop. However, here, nanotechnologies can help by enabling antimicrobial activity in or on the packaging material (Cha and Chinnan 2004). It is well known that nanosilver particles, already widely used in wound dressings and textiles, work as antimicrobial agents. By incorporating nanosilver particles into the matrix of the packaging material, microbes that come in contact with these materials are killed. This effect reduces the microbial pressure on the food product inside, effectively prolonging its shelf life. Unfortunately, nanosilver is a persistent nanoparticle that can exert its action even after its intended use, making it a potential environmental hazard. Nanothick layers of polymer brushes that have positively charged atoms incorporated in them have the same effect, but are much better attached to the packaging material and will be destroyed when incinerated or will degrade when discarded, although this might take some time.

### 5.4.3 Monitoring Quality Deterioration

Even after effective packaging or other measures, there are only very few food products that can be stored for a very long time. This means that processes that are responsible for quality deterioration are only slowed but not stopped. (Some of these processes are actually desirable and by maturing the product, its quality can be improved. However, these processes are beyond the scope of this chapter.) Having information on the quality and safety of the product is very important to the consumer. Until now, the quality of a product is assessed based on the storage time, sell-by date, or consume-by date. This is an indirect method that relies on the manufacturer models of the spoilage process and on the reliability of storage conditions. Especially when the product has to be stored at a low temperature or other conditions that are not maintained easily, there is a chance that this requirement is not fulfilled the entire time the product in storage. In these cases, the quality may not be in agreement with the sell-by or consume-by date, and consumption of the product could cause health problems. A better system is based on the product of time and storage temperature, which is used by Onvu (www.onvu.com). The food industry has done a tremendous job in controlling large parts of the chain that is necessary to bring the product from primary production to the consumer's plate, resulting in a very high level of food safety in industrialized countries. Unfortunately, there are still parts of the chain that cannot be controlled. Especially, storage by the consumer is highly unreliable and can cause serious problems.

To overcome this problem, it would be better to have a direct indication of the quality of the product inside a package. Spoilage processes often have characteristic volatiles as by-products. As a matter of fact, we become aware of these volatiles when we perceive that a product smells "off." Unfortunately, our nose is not very sensitive and we can only use this method on an open package and if the concentration of the volatiles is diluted in the ambient atmosphere. This means that we can only rely on this method of quality assessment in very specific cases. With nanotechnology, it is possible to create devices that are much more sensitive to the specific volatile molecules associated with the spoilage process of the product packaged. Moreover, by including them in the packaging concept, they can monitor the atmosphere inside the packaging where the concentration of these molecules will be highest.

The detection of the presence of (too high concentrations of) the volatiles can be done through a chemical reaction resulting in a color change or other visible signals. This can be effective for the individual consumer but is difficult to incorporate in a more complex logistical system that optimizes storage times, delivery distance, and optimal consumer quality. Such a computerized system needs sensors that can be read electronically. These sensors can be combined with RFID systems to communicate wirelessly with the logistic system outside. With such a concept, it would also be possible to assess the quality of the product at the checkout counter and maybe automatically give a price reduction on the basis of the remaining storage time. In the further future, such devices would also be able to communicate with home appliances, such as refrigerators, to signal that consumption is required before the product is spoiled.

Quality sensing devices based on nanotechnologies and incorporated in the packaging concept will, in most cases, need to be disposable. Not only does this limit the possibilities from an environmental point of view, it also necessitates a production method that makes them very cheap. With nanotechnologies, which usually have economic advantages when produced in large quantities, and especially when advances in other fields of nanotechnology research make it possible to print these types of electronic circuitry on packaging materials, these concepts will become viable (www.polyapply.org).

### 5.4.4 Detection of Spoilage Organisms

Raw materials for food and primary food products are always infected with certain bacteria and other organisms. These organisms after harvest start to propagate and eventually spoil the product. The amount of spoilage organisms in combination with storage conditions and models for the spoilage processes can be used to accurately predict quality deterioration of the product and therefore allows logistical decisions about where to market the specific, usually fresh product. Unfortunately, it requires extensive laboratories, qualified personnel, and especially time for the determination of the amount

of spoilage organisms. Time is something that is scarce in the fresh produce business. Fast, cheap, and easy-to-use diagnostic tests that can quantify certain spoilage organisms in a sample of the fresh product would very
much help the fresh markets. These tests can be developed with micro- and
nanotechnologies. Depending on the organisms to be determined, different
types of diagnostic kits can be developed. Needless to say, these applications
greatly benefit from developments in the medical diagnostic field.

In the previous section, the aim was to quantify the spoilage organisms.
However, there are also organisms, such as campylobacter, in the meat industry that are not allowed at all. In this case, a yes/no test is called for. Although
this seems an easier task than to quantify organisms, there are some specific
difficulties surrounding these determinations. One of the more important
problems is related to the regulatory framework that is designed to assure
food safety in these products. Regulation prescribes that not one organism
is allowed in a 25 g sample of the product. A 25 g sample obviously does not
agree with tests based on micro- and nanotechnology principles since they
work with very small amounts of material. Sample pretreatment and amplification of the substance to be detected need to be done to increase the sensitivity and to make the translation from milligrams or micrograms to 25 g. An
alternative could be that nanotechnology tests are used as a prescreening of
the official tests and allow internal decisions within the fresh food production company. Another alternative would be that regulations are changed to
accommodate new test strategies. However, this will only be initiated after
the effectiveness of these tests is proven, and this is a lengthy procedure.

## 5.5  Applications in Water

Water is abundant on Earth. However, the problem is that most of it contains
unwanted substances. Only a very small part of all the water on the planet
is sweet, and even that water can easily be polluted owing to the unwanted
effects of different economic activities such as agricultural and chemical production. Unfortunately, virtually all land-dwelling biological organisms and
many of the species that live in water rely on the availability of sweet water
of sufficient quality. Providing enough clean, sweet water to all humans, animals, and plants is one of the major problems mankind faces in the coming
decades. There are two routes in which nanotechnology can help solve this
problem: purification and filtration.

### 5.5.1  Filtration

To get rid of larger components in water by filtration is a simple method.
With microtechnology, very accurate and reproducible holes can be created

in extremely thin membranes of, for example, silicon nitride. These micro-sieves can be used to filter bacteria from milk or yeast cells from beer, and for other food applications, but can also be employed in water cleaning (van Rijn 2004). Infected water is a very big problem in less developed countries with a high death toll, especially among young children (WHO 2002). Sieving out bacteria from water would greatly reduce this risk. Unfortunately, this can only be done effectively with high-technology equipment, and therefore expensive membranes from microtechnology, because it requires the combi-nation of high porosity to achieve sufficient throughput and a narrow pore size distribution to prevent the passage of some bacteria through larger holes and into the clean water stream. High-volume production of these mem-branes would make such an application also available to poor economies but it would probably require extensive subsidization from developed countries to reach an economically viable scale.

By reducing the size of the holes in the sieve, we automatically enter the realm of nanofiltration and the possibility to start separating smaller biologi-cal organisms, such as viruses, or even larger molecules from water. However, this principle can also be achieved with certain materials that by nature are only permeable for very small molecules. Semipermeable membranes are often employed in biology to maintain a certain pressure on structures: tur-gor. This principle, although in a small scale, is also used in military applica-tions to extract potable water from a dirty water source. A bag partly made of a semipermeable membrane containing a sugar solution through osmosis extracts water from the dirty water source. After some time, the bag contains clean, though sweetened, water. With nanotechnology, this principle can be improved by replacing sugar with magnetic nanoparticles. Because of their small size, they create a high concentration solution on the inside of the bag but because of their magnetic properties they can easily be extracted from the water inside the bag before consumption.

Microsieves, but especially nanosieves, have a high surface area that comes in contact with the water to be sieved. This surface can be exploited to attach enzymes or other substances that can convert certain unwanted molecules to more desirable ones. These catalytic properties are also used in combination with nanoparticles, as we will see below.

### 5.5.2 Remediation

Many of the polluting substances are higher-level organic molecules that are by-products of industrial activity, or that come into the aqueous environment after their useful lifetime. Not only do they threaten the life of the organ-isms living in this environment, they are also a problem in water purification installations. These installations in part rely on microorganisms to do some part of the cleaning process. Nanoparticles can help break down these sub-stances. It has been known already for a long time that some metallic com-pounds strongly speed up certain chemical reactions without being used by the reaction themselves. This is widely used in the chemical industry. The catalytic effect takes place at the surface of the metal. Molecules bond to the atoms of the metal and can dissociate, providing opportunities for other molecules or molecule fragments to bond to these fragments and form new molecules. Looking for the right catalysts in combination with the appropriate reaction conditions is an ongoing topic in chemical research. Since these processes take place at the surface, a larger surface area makes the process more efficient. Smaller particles have a larger surface-to-volume ratio and are therefore more effective catalysts. Especially since some catalysts, such as platinum or rhodium, are very expensive metals, a high surface-to-volume ratio can make a process economically viable for the chemical industry. Making small metal particles and maintaining the dispersion of these particles under reaction conditions has been one of the more important research goals for many decades and can be regarded as "nanotechnology avant la lettre."

Usually catalysis is used to create high-order chemical molecules. However, the dissociation of the molecules at the surface of the metal can also be used to make them react to smaller molecules, eventually ending up as biocompatible molecules and water. This principle is used in some of the remediation concepts for polluted sites. Of course, also in this case, a high surface-to-volume ratio makes the process more efficient and therefore nanoparticles are also employed. Depending on the kind of pollution, the soil, and geological circumstances, different strategies are used. Sometimes the catalytic nanoparticles are injected into the soil and sometimes the water is extracted and allowed to flow through a purification installation. If nanoparticles are entered into the soil, not only should they not be more polluting themselves, the reaction conditions cannot be controlled and will be very mild. In purification installations, these limitations are absent, but they can only be employed if the pollution can be extracted from the ground.

Another method of catalytic breakdown of more complex organic molecules is the use of titanium dioxide nanoparticles or layers in combination with light, preferably of small wavelengths (ultraviolet). This principle is also used in small-scale water purification in aquaria. Coatings of titanium dioxide are used in self-cleaning surfaces of glass but are also employed on street surfaces to break down organic by-products of traffic before they enter the aqueous environment, effectively reducing the pressure on sewage cleaning installations.

## 5.6 Discussion

From the above, it has become clear that nanotechnology will have many applications in agriculture, food, and water. This is not surprising since it is a very broad enabling technology. Most of the applications will be highly beneficial to individual users, the society, and the planet, but they can also have negative side effects (Gerloff et al. 2009; Borm and Berube 2008). These potential hazards attract a lot of attention at the moment, both from the government side and from the different societal concern groups (Seaton et al. 2009). As with all hazards, there is a lot of emotion involved in the discussions and there is very little room for the objective evaluation of real risks. Although this is usually characteristic of new technologies, it is especially true in the case of nanotechnologies since they are not very well known to the public and require some knowledge of scientific principles to be assessed. Moreover, it is not very easy to obtain objective information from the normal sources since the press is also not often objective and balanced in its coverage of the subject. Bad news and hazards sell more newspapers than positive reports. As a consequence, most people, even well-educated persons, at the moment have a limited understanding of nanotechnologies and predominantly associate it with nanoparticles. As a matter of fact, if nanotechnology is discussed, the actual discussion is about nanoparticles and the risks associated with them (Brayner 2008). Hardly anybody understands that nanotechnologies are much broader and that nanoparticles are just a first, very crude application of them. Compared with the advent of electricity in the beginning of the previous century, with nanotechnology mankind is really at a very early stage. In analogy with electricity, the applications at the moment can be compared with resistors, coils, and capacitors. We are still far away from the development of a radio, let alone computers and telecom networks. If we look at our great example, biology and the molecular processes that are the basis of all forms of life, we can get some idea of what the potential of nanotechnologies can be. The future holds many promises with regard to nanotechnologies. Which of these promises will actually be developed and in the end will benefit mankind will largely be determined by the acceptance of the application of the technology.

### 5.6.1 Consumer Acceptance

The biggest issue associated with applications of nanotechnologies in food and water is the acceptance of the technology by the consumer. Nanotechnologies generally are regarded as unnatural and risky, whereas consumers want food to be natural and safe (Siegrist et al. 2009). To get consumers to accept the technology, the benefits must be clear and the individual consumer must be able to make his of her own risk/benefit evaluation. Unfortunately, there is very little understanding with the general public about nanotechnologies. Moreover, people have difficulty distinguishing between hazard and risk. They mistake hazards in circumstances they have difficulty to oversee, for example, an application of a complex technology, with risks that they are exposed to. However, since risk is the combination of hazard and exposure, risks of potentially hazardous situations are often negligible. Lions are extremely dangerous animals but pose no risk to a visitor of a zoo since the exposure is low. Finally, mankind has difficulty in objectively assessing low-chance events and systematically underestimates high-risk situations. That is why people buy tickets to lotteries and have no difficulty in getting into a car to get from A to B.

Projected on applications of nanotechnologies in food (and agriculture) and water, the distorted assessment results in a strong focus on possible adverse health effects of nanotechnologies. Since these negative effects are virtually exclusively associated with nanoparticles, the focus is strongly on these products of nanotechnologies, suppressing the benefits of other applications from the equation. To make a good risk assessment and from that an objective risk/benefit evaluation requires communication and education of the general public. For the time being, it probably requires that consumers be informed about the use of nanotechnologies in individual products. This will enable informed consumers to decide whether they want to accept the (perceived) risks of nanoproducts in favor of the associated benefits.

Apart from extensive communication by both academia and the industry on the products, the technologies used, and the benefits and risks involved, consumer acceptance also requires regulation of products that employ hazardous nanoparticles. Good governance, including enforcement of well-devised regulation by high-level, objective bodies will build trust with consumers since they can rely on this governance to make the risk assessments that, because of the complexity of the technologies and their applications, is difficult for most of them (Grobe 2008). Because of the intimate and emotional relationship that most people have with the food they eat, this especially holds true for these kinds of products. Only if a trust base can be created with large parts of the society can we expect to get a license to produce nanotechnology-enabled food products.

### 5.6.2 Nanotechnology and the Environment

As described in Section 5.5.2, the environment can benefit from applications of nanotechnology of new concepts of polluted soil remediation. However, it can also be damaged by nanoparticles. In this case, nanotechnology is really a two-edged sword (Colvin 2003). The risks of nanoparticles for the environment are also concerns of the general public in different applications of nanotechnologies and affect the acceptance of some of the applications. Although, also in this case, the confusion between nanotechnologies in the broad sense and nanoparticles plays a role, the lack of knowledge of the long-term effects of persistent nanoparticles does give some justification of the concerns. Science has only a limited understanding of the effects of certain types of nanoparticles on the environment (Wijnhoven et al. 2009). This type of research is currently starting to be initiated. Until demonstrated that it is safe, it seems prudent to apply the precautionary principle and refrain from large-scale applications of persistent nanoparticles.

Applications in agriculture, food, and water are often large-scale applications. Fortunately, as has been shown above, they largely do not involve persistent nanoparticles. Applications in food aim at bioavailability, which is contradictory to persistent. However, it cannot be excluded that in the future, other applications with a more persistent nature will be developed. However, even in the applications described above, caution is prudent. Herbicides and pesticides employed in agriculture to make them more effective can also be more effective when they end up in the environment, and antimicrobial particles such as nanosilver do not stop being antimicrobial after their primary application in packaging materials. Since these packaging materials are designed to be discarded, such an application can be large scale and the exposure to these kinds of particles could be extensive, creating a serious risk if the particles are sufficiently hazardous. One thing seems clear: more research into the effects of persistent nanoparticles is necessary.

## Bibliography

Bergveld, P. 2003. Thirty years of ISFETOLOGY: What happened in the past 30 years and what may happen in the next 30 years? *Sens. Actuators B Chem.*, vol. 88, no. 1, pp. 1–20.

Borm, P.J.A. and D. Berube. 2008. A tale of opportunities, uncertainties, and risks. *Nano Today*, vol. 3, nos. 1–2, pp. 56–59.

Brayner, R. 2008. The toxicological impact of nanoparticles. *Nano Today*, vol. 3, nos. 1–2, pp. 48–55.

Brody, A.L. 2006. Nano and food packaging technologies converge. *Food Technol.*, vol. 60, no. 3, pp. 92–94.

Cha, D.S. and M.S. Chinnan. Biopolymer-based antimicrobial packaging: A review. *Crit. Rev. Food Sci. Nutr.*, vol. 44, no. 4, pp. 223–237.

Colvin, V. 2003. The potential environmental impact of engineered nanomaterials. *Nat. Biotechnol.*, vol. 21, no. 10, pp. 1166–1170.

Ehrfeld, W., V. Hessel and H. Löwe. 2000. *Microreactors: New Technology for Modern Chemistry.* Vch Verlagsgesellschaft Mbh.

Fonseca, L., C. Cane and B. Mazzolai. 2007. Application of micro and nanotechnologies to food safety and quality monitoring. *Meas. Control*, vol. 40, no. 4, pp. 116–119.

Gardner, J.W. and P.N. Bartlett. 2000. Electronic noses. Principles and applications. *Meas. Sci. Technol.*, vol. 11, no. 7, p. 1087.

Gerloff, K., C. Albrecht, A.W. Boots, I. Förster and R.P.F. Schins. 2009. Cytotoxicity and oxidative DNA damage by nanoparticles in human intestinal Caco-2 cells. *Nanotoxicology*, vol. 3, no. 4, pp. 355–364.

Grobe, A., O. Renn and A. Jaeger. 2008. Report No. ISBN 978-2-9700631-4-8.

Joscelyne, S.M. and G. Trägårdh. 2000. Membrane emulsification—A literature review. *J. Memb. Sci.*, vol. 169, no. 1, pp. 107–117.

Kampers, F. 2007. Micro- and nanotechnologies for food and nutrition. *Food Sci. Technol. (London)*, vol. 21, no. 1, pp. 20–24.

Kampers, F.W.H. 2009. Opportunities for bionanotechnology in food and the food industry. In *Bionanotechnology, Global Prospects*, D.E. Reisner (ed.), pp. 79–90. Boca Raton: CRC Press, Taylor & Francis Group.

Lieber, C. 2003. Nanoscale science and technology: Building a big future from small things. *MRS Bull.*, vol. 28, no. 7, pp. 486–491.

Manski, J.M., A.J. van der Goot and R.M. Boom. 2007. Formation of fibrous materials from dense calcium caseinate dispersions. *Biomacromolecules*, vol. 8, no. 4, pp. 1271–1279.

Moraru, C., C. Panchapakesan, Q. Huang, P. Takhistov, S. Liu and J. Kokini. 2003. Nanotechnology: A new frontier in food science. *Food Technol. (Chicago)*, vol. 57, no. 12, pp. 24–29.

Pérez-de-Luque, A. and D. Rubiales. 2009. Nanotechnology for parasitic plant control. *Pest Manag. Sci.*, vol. 65, no. 5, pp. 540–545.

Rhim, J.W. and P.K.W. Ng. 2007. Natural biopolymer-based nanocomposite films for packaging applications. *Crit. Rev. Food Sci. Nutr.*, vol. 47, no. 4, pp. 411–433.

Seaton, A., L. Tran, R. Aitken and K. Donaldson. 2009. Nanoparticles, human health hazard and regulation. *J. R. Soc. Interface*, vol. 7, (Suppl 1), pp. S119–S129.

Siegrist, M., N. Stampfli and H. Kastenholz. 2009. Acceptance of nanotechnology foods: A conjoint study examining consumers' willingness to buy. *Br. Food J.*, vol. 111, nos. 6–7, pp. 660–668.

Sorrentino, A., G. Gorrasi and V. Vittoria. 2007. Potential perspectives of bio-nanocomposites for food packaging applications. *Trends Food Sci. Technol.*, vol. 18, no. 2, pp. 84–95.

van Rijn, C.J.M. 2004. *Nano and Micro Engineered Membrane Technology*, 1st ed. Amsterdam: Elsevier.

Weiss, J., P. Takhistov and D.J. McClements. 2006. Functional materials in food nanotechnology. *J. Food Sci.*, vol. 71, no. 9, pp. R107–R116.

WHO. 2002. *Global Strategy for Food Safety: Safer Food for Better Health*. Geneva: World Health Organization.

Wijnhoven, S.W.P., W.J.G.M. Peijnenburg, C.A. Herberts, W.I. Hagens, A.G. Oomen, E.H.W. Heugens, and B. Roszek et al. 2009. Nano-silver—A review of available data and knowledge gaps in human and environmental risk assessment. *Nanotoxicology*, vol. 3, no. 2, pp. 109–138.

Wilkinson, C., G. Dijksterhuis and M. Minekus. 2000. From food structure to texture. *Trends Food Sci. Technol.*, vol. 11, no. 12, pp. 442–450.

# 6

## Nanofoods: Environmental, Health, and Socioeconomic Risks or the Achilles' Heel of Nanotechnologies?

**Simon Beaudoin, Louise Vandelac, and Christian Papilloud**

### CONTENTS

### 6.1 Introduction

After more than 20 years of laboratory and research and development (R&D) work, advances in the nanotechnology field permeate almost all research areas in live and material sciences (e.g., chemistry, physics, biology, medicine, engineering). They are widely commercialized owing to substantial help from public authorities, themselves banking heavily on the competitive advantages touted by the industry (Roco 2005). Since early 2000, more than 60 countries in the world show strong activities in this field. The major league players, including the United States, China, South Korea, the European Union, Russia, and Japan (PCAST 2012), accelerate their strategic development plans in the hope of better market shares (EEB 2009). The rise of nanotechnologies can also be clearly observed through the multiplication of specialized and vernacular publications (from a little more than 30,000 in 1998 to more than 100,000 in 2009; cf. ObservatoryNANO 2011), as well as the increasing annual rate of patent submissions (+34.5% between 2000 and 2008; cf. Dang et al. 2010).

Economic predictions regarding the exponential growth of the nanotechnology market can be factored into the skyrocketing popularity of the field. According to the consulting firm Cientifica (2011), whose work notably includes the nanotechnology field, the governments around the world would have invested through the past 11 years more than 67.5 billion US dollars in research funds. This amount could reach 100 billion US dollars by 2014. Currently, public authorities would be investing about 10 billion US dollars per year in R&D (Cientifica 2011; ObservatoryNANO 2012), a sum that could increase by 20% in the coming 3 years (Cientifica 2011). Including corporate research and private funding, which have outspent public investments since the middle of the 2000s, Cientifica estimates that global investment for 2015 could reach up to about a quarter of a trillion US dollars.

Even if these projections vary considerably from report to report, it should be noted that the global economic importance of this field is punctuated by impressive developments. It is not surprising to find a convergence of large multinational companies, along with a certain number of startups on the fringes. As Cientifica underlines, "The picture in 2007 is one still dominated by a large, raw-material-based industry, the nanomaterials being produced by the global chemical industry and dominated by large multinationals while more recent start-ups attempt to find higher value niche markets" (Cientifica 2007). According to Foladori and Invernizzi (2007), "there is [also] an ongoing centralization process in companies that produce nanomaterials, reducing small firms and concentrating production in large multinational chemical corporations."

This convergence effect can be observed in every sector of nanotechnologies, markedly in nanofoods. While representing only 10% of the available nanoproducts, nanofoods is already considered a growing market in the field of "nano-enabled" products with a relatively high estimated market share (cf. HKC 2007; Cientifica 2007; Scrinis and Lyons 2007), and a lot of the biggest worldwide food industries are involved [e.g., Atria (Kraft Foods), Associated British Food, Ajinomoto, BASF, Bayer, Cadbury Schweppes, Campbell's Soup, Cargill, DuPont Food Industry Solutions, General Mills, Glaxo-SmithKline, Goodman Fielder, Group Dannone, John Lust Group Plc, H.J. Heinz, Hershey Foods, La Doria, Maruha, McCain Foods, Mars, Inc., Nestlé, Northern Foods, Nichirei, Nippon Suisan Kaisha, PepsiCo, Sara Lee, Syngenta, Unilever, United Foods] (FOE Australia 2008). At the same time, nanofoods are also a precarious area, notably because of the controversial exposure of the public to these products (PEN 2011), which remains not addressed within a broader and controlled framework involving not only scientists and industries but also policy makers, stakeholders, and civilian representatives (Papilloud 2010).

## 6.2 Nanofood Sector

Nanofoods find their origins in technologies developed for parallel fields such as pharmaceutical, medical, and cosmetic (FAO/WHO 2009). They are generally understood as the use of nanotechnology techniques or tools during cultivation, production, processing, or packaging of food (Joseph and Morisson 2006; Chaudhry et al. 2010); hence, nanotechnologies are integrated throughout the food chain production (Table 6.1).

The number of nanofood applications on the consumer market varies widely depending on the source, going from approximately 100 (PEN 2011), to 300 (HKC 2007), or even as much as 150 to 600 (FOE Australia 2008). A close examination of nanosilver applications alone outputs 565 nanosilver products or product ranges among 441 companies within all application sectors, not specifically nanofood products and cookware, but disregarding medicinal colloidal silver. Most of these applications were sourced in Southeast Asia; more specifically, 36% originated from China and 38% from South Korea (Berge 2012).

Yet, the lack of reliable data certainly leads to an underestimation of nanofood products integrated into the food chain. It is worth noting that there are no common definitions or national inventories (House of Lords 2010a), no mandatory labeling of foods that incorporate nanotechnologies (FOE Australia 2008), and that the principal companies involved are reluctant to disclose any information pertaining to their nanoproducts or divulge any research information (Chun 2009).

In this context, it also becomes difficult to know the exact number of companies, their involvement in research, and/or current usage of nanotechnologies in food applications. Some data from 2006 estimated this number to be between 200 (ISFT 2006) and 400 (Cientifica Ltd. 2006 in Chaudhry et al. 2010). They are mostly large multinationals in the food and beverage sector, who invest massively in R&D (FOE Australia 2008; Kuzma and VerHage 2006), but do so covertly (Benoit Browaeys 2009), sometimes erasing from their websites any nanotechnology-related information or advances they make in the field,* while the impact from start-ups and research centers varies considerably as they are often bought out and absorbed by multinationals (see Scrinis and Lyons 2007).

Thus, it is difficult to evaluate the breadth of the nanofood sector, its real economic importance, its outcome in terms of products and economic growth, the diversity of their uses, and the value of their related patents within the industry—in short, the overall social and economic benefits and short ends of nanofoods. Despite a thorough review of the scientific literature, of (inter-)national reports, and gray literature, there are very few credible information, which often are incomplete, so that the global picture of the field remains quite shady.

---

* At the start of the 2000s, Kraft Foods put together a consortium called "Nanotek"; it involved 15 universities and research laboratories around the world. However, shortly following the wave of uncertainties concerning nanofoods and the industry reticence in publicly sharing their activities, Kraft Foods yielded the Nanotek consortium to its partner, Philipp Morris USA (Altria owner), which changed its name to "Interdisciplinary Network of Emerging Science and Technologies" (INEST), thereafter erasing all traces and references to nanotechnologies, a dubious transparency operation (Berdot 2007; House of Lords 2010a).

**TABLE 6.1**

Sectors, Applications, and Functions Developed in Nanofood Field

| Sector/Application | Function |
|---|---|
| *Agriculture* | |
| Nanobiotechnology | New transgenesis techniques |
| Synthetic DNA | Creation of new life forms based on the conception of new nucleotides |
| Germination | Improvement of germination rates following nanoparticle application |
| Nanofertilizers and nanopesticides | "Protection" and controlled release of active substances |
| Nanocaptors | Fields and herds dubbed "intelligent" |
| Nanofluidic | Treatment and analysis of biological material such as DNA, proteins, or sperm cells in minute quantities |
| Nanomedicine | New delivery systems for pharmaceutical substances for veterinary treatment |
| Nanoculture | Transgenic plants engineered for soil mineral extraction |
| Nanofilters | Treatment of wastewater as well as soil and agricultural waste |
| *Food Transformation* | |
| Nanocaptors | Contamination detection and quality analysis |
| Nanostructured food | Improvement of taste, color, flavor, texture, consistency, etc. |
| Biocide surfaces | Integration of silver nanoparticles (and others) for their antimicrobial properties |
| *Nanopackaging* | |
| Improved nanopackaging | Improvement of mechanical properties (rigidity, strength, flexibility, durability) and barrier properties (temperature, humidity, light, oxygen and other gasses) |
| Active nanopackaging | Intelligent systems where an intentional substance transfer between the packaging and the contents actively improves or maintains product quality with the goal of prolonging shelf life, improving or maintaining organoleptic properties; two types: absorbers and releasers |
| Biocidal nanopackaging | Reduction or prevention of microbial growth enabled by nanoparticle presence |
| Intelligent nanopackaging | Inclusion of nanometric captors capable of measuring certain transport and storage conditions of food |
| Biodegradable or edible nanopackaging | Packaging made from polymers and natural nanocomposites |

*(continued)*

**TABLE 6.1 (Continued)**

Sectors, Applications, and Functions Developed in Nanofood Field

| Sector/Application | Function |
| --- | --- |
| *Consumption* | |
| Nanoceuticals | Increase in absorption and bioavailability of nutrients, health supplements, nutraceuticals (e.g., cooking oil), and active ingredients |
| Surfaces biocides | Prevention or reduction of microbial growth |

*Source:* ETC Group, *Down on the Farm: The Impact of Nano-Scale Technologies on Food and Agriculture.* Ottawa: ETC Group, 68 p., 2004; Joseph, T. and M. Morrison, *Nanoforum Report: Nanotechnology in Agriculture and Food.* (Glasgow, UK): European Nanotechnology Gateway, 14 p., 2006; Chaudhry, Q. et al., *Food Addit. Contam. Part A Chem. Anal. Control. Expo. Risk Assess.*, 25, 241, 2008; Chaudhry, Q., R. Watkins and L. Castle, Nanotechnologies in the food arena: new opportunities, new questions, new concerns. In *Nanotechnologies in Food*, Q. Chaudhry, L. Castle and R. Watkins (eds.), Cambridge: RSC Nanoscience and Nanotechnology, no. 14, pp. 1–17, 2010, Reproduced by permission of The Royal Society of Chemistry; FOE (Friends of the Earth) Australia, *Out of the Laboratory and on to Our Plates: Nanotechnology in Food and Agriculture.* Cam Walker (Melbourne): FOE Australia, 62 p., 2008; Imran, M. et al., *Crit. Rev. Food Sci. Nutr.*, 50, 799, 2010; Smolander, M. and Q. Chaudhry, Nanotechnologies in food packaging. In *Nanotechnologies in Food*, Q. Chaudhry, L. Castle and R. Watkins (eds.), pp. 86–101. Cambridge: RSC Nanoscience and Nanotechnology, no. 14, 2010, Reproduced by permission of The Royal Society of Chemistry; CEST (Commission de L'éthique en Science et en Technologie), *Enjeux Ethiques des Nanotechnologies dans le Secteur Agroalimentaire: Supplément 2011 à L'avis Éthique et Nanotechnologies: Se Donner les Moyens D'agir.* Quebec: Government of Quebec, 72 p., 2011.

## 6.3 Nanofood Public Policies

This situation reflects the transnational lack of a consensus regarding the definition of nanotechnologies at large, as well as their peculiar applications, the proper definition of related product categories, and their boundaries. In the area of nanofoods, this is particularly critical since product categories and composition constantly evolve. This is not unrelated to the fact that no government has imposed any mandatory disclosure on nanotechnologies, all sectors mingled, which would enable the tracking and inventory of the products circulating in the country.

Furthermore, North American and European regulatory frameworks contain numerous gaps, permitting for the majority of applications or nanocomposites to enter their markets freely, without prior control (see Maniet 2010, 2011, 2012). This stems in part from the fact that nanoparticles are generally considered to be existing substances (United States and Canada) or the close equivalent to existing macrosized substances (European Union). Additionally, the quantity thresholds required to demand the production of toxicological or ecotoxicological data are inadequate. The entirety of the work required to establish adequate governance, and the burden of proof of nanomaterial toxicity, rests on the shoulders of administrations often under unrealistic deadlines, without the considerable means in terms of budget, manpower, and equipment such an endeavor would require (ibid).

In addition to these gaps in the regulatory framework, the United States as well as other countries, use another exemption measure called GRAS (Generally Recognized As Safe), which stipulates that "substances can be marketed without FDA's approval or even its knowledge because such substances are generally recognized among qualified experts as having been shown, through scientific procedures or experience based on common use, to be safe" (GAO 2010). These substances are "hundreds of spices and artificial flavors, emulsifiers and binders, vitamins and minerals, and preservatives— to enhance a food's taste, texture, nutritional content, or shelf life" (ibid). Despite the latest regulatory developments,* in the case of nanomaterials, they "may escape pre-market review on the basis that they fit within certain exceptions to the definition of 'food additive' in the FFDCA [Federal Food, Drug, and Cosmetic Act]" (Duvall 2012).

This avoidance measure called GRAS, which served as the cornerstone for the large-scale distribution of genetically modified organisms (GMOs), also based on substantial equivalence (SRC 2001), in the fields and on plates all over the Americas without any labeling, is a commercial postulate devoid of any scientific foundation. According to this marketing assumption, transgenic products, nanoproducts, or any product resulting from such fabrication processes, are sufficiently different to require patents but not sufficiently different to require a rigorous and complete social and scientific assessment.

If this portrait does paint a complex picture of the field of nanotechnologies, it also bears witness to the mechanisms that continue to "produce ignorance," which, while rooted in certain founding concepts of existing regulatory frameworks, are also caused by the weaknesses in the budgets dedicated to risk analysis.† As an indicator, the risk analysis budgets for the National Nanotechnology Initiative in the United States have gone from 2.8% to 5.1% of the total budgets in 2006 and 2010 (Sargent 2011). It is therefore unsurprising that despite the downpour of money invested in this field, large portions of the impact analyses for nanotechnologies are still missing and that public policy regarding impact prevention is absent.

Notwithstanding the important hurdles that public authorities must tackle, a number of national and international agencies as well as nongovernmental organizations have attempted to identify the various commercialized

---

* "In the specific instance of nanotechnology, a food substance manufactured for the purpose of creating very small particle sizes with new functional properties likely would not be covered by an existing GRAS determination for a related food substance manufactured without using nanotechnology" (FDA 2012).
† This concept of "ignorance production" is borrowed from the lawyer and politician Corinne Lepage, Eurodeputy and member of the Committee on the Environment, Public Health and Food Safety at the European Parliament.

products, patented or still in development, and some potential impacts of these products. A few attempts have been made for drafting a range of models aimed at the evaluation and framing of nanotechnologies (FAO/WHO 2009; CEST 2011; Scott and Chen 2003; EFSA 2009, 2011; Robinson and Morrison 2009; AFSSA 2009; House of Lords 2010a, 2010b; FSA 2008; FSAI 2008; FASFC et al. 2010; FOE 2008; ETC Group 2004; Kuzma and VerHage 2006).

It is the case notably in the United States (FDA 2012), in Europe (EFSA 2011), and in the United Kingdom (United Kingdom Government 2010), where this work has begun, not in anticipation of potential impacts but in response to alerts, petitions, appeals for moratoriums, and even a lawsuit by organizations of civil society and other agencies (ETC Group 2004; VivAgora; FOE 2008; CTA et al. 2006, 2008, 2011; Foladori and Invernizzi 2007; House of Lords 2010a, 2010b). Some regulatory frameworks have also been suggested for the framing of biocide products containing, among other components, nanosilver particles intended to eliminate pathogens (EPA 2011; FDA 2011; European Parliament 2012). It appears, however, that no new legislation specifically designed for nanotechnologies or nanofoods has seen the light of day. One of the major obstacles to creating this legislation could lie in our inability to accurately measure the breadth of the suspected risks. Nonetheless, because the food and beverage sector has seen its fair share of massive scandals in the last 20 years, public sensibility concerning food has been sharpened and quickened by growing suspicion. This, coupled to the absence of any framework permitting sound scientific evaluation, compromises advances in the fields of nanofoods and nanotechnologies in general.

## 6.4 Nanofood Scientific and Social Assessment

Some argue that current risk analysis studies, almost all based on the risk evaluation paradigm initially proposed in 1983 by the National Research Council (NRC) to evaluate traditional chemicals, would be applicable to nanotechnologies as a whole (OECD 2012; Oberdörster et al. 2005), including nanofoods (AFSSA 2009; EFSA 2009, 2011; EFSA 2011; FSAI 2008). However, "it has also been pointed out that the current testing methodologies would need certain adaptations in view of the special features of ENMs [engineered nanomaterials]" (Chaudhry et al. 2011).

To palliate for the inadequacies of this risk assessment model, based on tests developed to estimate risks for macrometer-sized substances, many suggest allowing for alternative dosimetric parameters as opposed to keeping with the traditional weight or concentration parameters used for conventional substances [agglomeration/aggregation, water solubility, crystalline phase, dustiness, crystallite size, representative transmission electron microscopy picture(s), particle size distribution, specific surface area, zeta potential (surface charge), surface chemistry, photocatalytic activity, pour density, porosity, octanol–water partition coefficient, redox potential, radical formation potential (OECD 2012)]. However, many authors and organizations argue that the quantitative assessment of nanorisks is impossible (Bensaude-Vincent 2009; IRSST 2008; Aitken et al. 2009; AFSSET 2010) because of the lack of data to complete the process and the lack of understanding of phenomena occurring at the nanometric scale, which cause difficulties in all aspects of risk analysis, notably at the risk evaluation stage. It is true that the bulk of funds dedicated to research in the field are allocated to development and that financial support for the analysis of the impacts and issues is minute in comparison, so much so that it becomes difficult to conclude with any precision on the nature, types, and levels of risks. The absence of independent, in-depth, and contradictory expertise should be noted (e.g., lifespan exposure studies on animals), as well as the failure to take into account the many impacts and issues that may arise within the complex socioeconomic, political, cultural, and ecological spheres (e.g., nanopesticides and bees), such studies should be requisitioned in the broader structure of scientific and social assessment of nanotechnologies.

In light of some of the major hurdles only just exposed here, proceeding with rigorous risk analysis demands the development of new models for apprehending the impacts associated with nanofood applications. A broader net must be cast, one that takes into account the socioeconomic factors, as well as the impacts of current methods of evaluation and commercialization on public health and environment, as opposed to evaluating one specific nanofood application at a time.

## 6.5 Nanofood's Potential Impacts

Generally speaking, the presence of synthetic nanoparticles (intentionally created) in foods; in food manipulation and preparation; and in their accidental or voluntary discarding into air, soil, and water, present certain risks. These "nano"-related risks are bound to evolve during the life cycle stages of the products that contain them (Williams et al. 2010), indeed through the whole of the food chain (Holbrook et al. 2008; Bouldin et al. 2008; Zhu et al. 2010; Judy et al. 2011; Cedervall et al. 2012), and this must be taken into account in order to protect workers in this field as well as the general population and more globally biodiversity (CEST 2006). Toxicological data has indicated, for many years already, that certain nanoparticles can cross natural biological barriers such as the skin, the blood–brain barrier, the lungs, the intestines, and the placental barrier (Oberdörster et al. 2005). In animals, many toxic effects have been demonstrated for certain nanoparticles at multiple organ levels (heart, lungs, kidneys, reproductive system) as well as some genotoxicity and cytotoxicity (IRSST 2008).

An increase in scientific studies dedicated to health risks following oral exposure to nanosized substances has been observed in the last few years (Card and Magnuson 2009). Some studies have demonstrated that oral administration of metal nanoparticles, often used in nanofoods, present higher-risk factors than larger-sized particles (notably in terms of translocation in the gastrointestinal tract and distribution to various organs and tissues) (Chaudhry 2010). Other studies highlight the fact that many *in vivo* research is for acute exposition (Card et al. 2010) and that dietary matrices, because of their vast complexity, would generate some difficulties in analyzing the results (Bouwmeester et al. 2009).

"There are only a limited number of published oral toxicity studies on some classes of ENMs, with those on solid particulates largely limited to insoluble metals and metal oxides. The quality of many of these studies is questionable, severely limiting the use of this information for risk assessment purposes (EFSA 2009). Common limitations include use of a single size of ENM, poorly characterized ENM, administration of ENMs at unrealistically high doses, study of only a narrow range of biological parameters, or omission of an appropriate larger particle of the same composition and a soluble form of the parent material as comparators to allow distinction between the effects of particle sizes and those of release of particle surface material into solution (Oberdörster et al. 2007). This leads to the conclusion that the current state of knowledge does not permit reliable prediction of the toxicological characteristics of any given ENM from data on other ENMs or from a consideration of the characteristics of the ENM itself. The capacity to predict computationally (e.g., using QSAR) the toxicological properties of conventional materials, however, although considerably greater than for ENMs, is nonetheless limited and of variable reliability" (FAO/WHO 2009).

Given the presence of nanofood products in the market, exposition to nanoparticles via food supplies is very likely, especially considering that "Exposure to nanomaterials in the human food chain may occur not only through intentional uses in food manufacturing, but also via uses in agricultural production and carry over from use in other industries" (Magnuson et al. 2011).

## 6.6 Conclusion

Keeping in mind the importance of public investments in the development of nanotechnologies, it is paradoxical to see that these same public authorities (1) have established no regulatory, legal or assessment framework in line with the potential impacts of these productions or able to limit or prevent its risks; (2) no analytical framework permitting the understanding of global social, environmental, and health issues; (3) nor the appreciation of cascading effects stemming from the accelerated industrial concentration brought about by these patented nanos.

In fact, it is possible to wonder if this lack of framework is not related to a will to facilitate market access in order to get a quicker return on investment, which could be coupled to the diverse forms of public support aimed at invigorating this innovating sector. This phenomenon was observed with GMOs where scientific assessment framework as well as costs and delays in approval were much lower than that of pesticides in general, despite the principal characteristics of marketed GMOs being pesticide function (Séralini and Vélot 2011).

It is possible to surmise that devices facilitating the production of ignorance (Kleinman and Suryanarayanan 2012) were established, making some of the tools and analytical systems used by scientists and public authorities alike, inexact or even inoperative. As previously stated, the GRAS (generally recognized as safe) notion, similar to that of "substantial equivalence" in the case of GMOs, is a political and economic postulate that enables the bypass of any scientific assessment of nanotechnologies, as well as any strategic evaluations regarding the soundness and pertinence of certain orientations in development.

In the field of nanotechnologies, more specifically in a sector as sensitive as food supply, the rush to get products on the market without any prior definitions, measurement standards, assessment frameworks, approval devices, postmarketing follow-ups, or even mandatory disclosure is troubling at best. The powerful implication of public authorities in nanofood, in the name of their economic mission, coupled to an effective lack of consideration and funding for their social, health, and environmental missions, could effectively lead to a loss of confidence from the public in regard to nanofood and potentially even other nanoproducts.

The nanofood sector condenses a vast array of complex issues at the crossroads of many systems representations of science, but also of democracy and ethics. It is at the junction of a veritable transformation of the agrifood cycle and tends to amplify productivist orientations, which are more and more contested in light of their economic concentration effects on global land and seed appropriation, on the widening socioeconomic gaps and their effects on food security, and on more global ecological considerations, from erosion to biodiversity to soil degradation and diffuse pollution.

Concerning the representations of science, development of nanofoods perfectly illustrates a certain self-legitimating discourse in science, which attempts to label as antiscience speech any question or criticism, even when these discussions bear on the necessity for increased scientific requirements in terms of rigor and independent counterexpertise. In a field such as food nanotechnology, at the junction of nanotechnological innovation and the complexity of the digestive system, it has become impossible to remain confined in a model of a "system of scientists doing research (...) in which expert researchers choose problems to work on, based on their expectation that the results will be interesting and useful in some way" (Easterbrook 2012). Not only does such a field require a very high level of interdisciplinary integration, but the products often result from a commercial market niche rather than sound scientific understanding.

In such system thinking, "Questions about whether certain kinds of research are ethical, or who might yield the benefits from this research lie outside the boundary of this system, and so are not considered" (ibid) or at least not as heavily as they should. What is more is that this scientific discourse, despite only covering certain aspects of the problem, effectively contributes in reassuring the public. The possibility of critical distance between a researcher and his object is then lessened. Worst in such system, "science is seen as a neutral pursuit of knowledge, and therefore, attempts to disrupt experiments must be 'anti-knowledge', or 'anti-science'" (ibid). However, in application sectors like nanotechnologies, pressing marketing requirements precede the bulk of the work that needs to be done in order to understand the nature and potential impacts of the product. Although obviously, "People who operate within this system tend to frame the discussion in terms of an attack" (ibid), it is widely recognized that not one scientist can claim to be able to establish on his own, the appropriate usage that should be reserved for a specific technology according to their environmental, social, health, and economic externalities. This is the case for silver nanoparticles used in socks, underwear, and washing machines (Benn and Westerhoff 2008), despite the fact that these types of nanoparticles are already found in fish environments and some effects are beginning to be measured. The nanosilver antiseptic bandages for burn victims are not put into question here, but rather the massive distribution and usage of such products, their ubiquity, and when the effects of contamination are already observed in the environment.

Aside from the importance of questioning the scientific paradigms at work in the development of nanotechnologies, notably in the nanofood sector, it is important to bring to light the increased industrial concentration effects generated by these sociotechnical innovations and their multiple socioeconomic, political, and cultural impacts (employment, working conditions, consumption patterns associated with their diffusion, land and food control, etc.) on the agrifood systems at a global scale; this constitutes a blind spot in many published texts concerning the nanofood sector.

In centering solely on the analysis of potential impacts on health and the environment, as if they represented the Alpha and Omega of social acceptability, it is clear that the evaluation premises and the insufficient budget allowance, which oscillate between 2% and 6% of the investments in the field, condemns us to decades of marginal and obsolete research in comparison with these speedy developments fuelled by the market and the states (Papilloud 2010; Laurent 2010). If it took, since the end of the 1960s, more than 50 years of research to begin shedding light on the importance of endocrine-disrupting effects associated with a number of pesticides and chemical synthetic products and which contribute substantially to the chronic disease epidemic, such as cancer, how is it that we can hope to achieve these kinds of results in much more complex fields such as GMOs, and moreover nanotechnology, while the inexistence of labeling laws impede even a summary knowledge of its distribution?

In terms of public policy, nanotechnologies, just as GMOs, were not only authorized but widely encouraged by public authorities, based on a discourse taken on by public relations firms and some key actors within the public apparatus (Roco 2005), a discourse according to which these technologies would revolutionize all aspects of industrial production, so much so that any state dominating these fields would also dominate international competition.

Moreover, questions regarding potential health and environmental impacts cannot drive out the importance of including within the impact analyses, evaluation and homologation strategy, the essential premises that are the very soundness and pertinence of these innovations, in light notably, of the "precaution principle." Inasmuch as the dissemination of these "nano" applications in the food chain stems from political and economical orientations on innovation, driven by the competitiveness of the main economic powers in concert with large multinational agrifood and agrichemical companies, this examination postfact should also inspect market mechanisms that seem to be driving toward a new "nanotechnological" determinism. Furthermore, insofar as they demand large investments, nanofood developments should be examined at a macroscopic scale, highlighting the impacts of an increasing industrial concentration and the integration of these products throughout the production and marketing systems, which may come with the weakening or even the disappearance of small and medium producers and distributors altogether, and this comes with expected impacts on food security and working conditions in the sector.

In order to circumvent the outright rejection of large areas of applications for nanotechnologies, is it not essential to tackle the surfacing issues, sometimes even the soundness of commercial orientations, all the while stressing the necessity to establish social and scientific assessment procedures in order to avoid letting the market alone decide of an "anything and everything nano" and in finally, to avoid nanofoods becoming the Achilles' heel of the vast field of nanotechnologies.

---

## Acknowledgments

The research for this chapter was funded by the Social Sciences and Humanities Research Council of Canada and by Quebec's Ne³LS network funds. We must also thank Aleck Guess, master student at the Institute of Environmental Sciences, working on nano public policies, for the translation of this chapter.

# Bibliography

AFSSA (Agence Française de Sécurité Sanitaire des Aliments). 2009. *Nanotechnologies et Nanoparticules dans L'alimentation Humaine et Animale*, AFFSA: Maisons-Alfort (Val-de-Marne), 27 p.

AFSSET (Agence Française de Sécurité Sanitaire de L'environnement et du Travail). 2010. *Évaluation des Risques Liés aux Nanomatériaux pour la Population Générale et pour L'environnement*. Paris: Saisine n°2008/005, Rapport D'expertise Collective. Comité d'Experts Spécialisés «Agents physiques, nouvelles technologies et grands aménagements», Groupe de Travail "Nanomatériaux—Exposition du consommateur et de l'environnement," March, 207 p.

Aitken, R.J., S.M. Hankin, B. Ross, C.L. Tran, V. Stone, T.F. Fernandes, and K. Donaldson et al. 2009. *EMERGNANO: A Review of Completed and Near Completed Environment, Health and Safety Research on Nanomaterials and Nanotechnology*. Institute of Occupational Medicine (IOM), SAFENANO, Edinburgh, 189 p.

Benn, T.M. and P. Westerhoff. 2008. Nanoparticle silver released into water from commercially available sock fabrics. *Environ. Sci. Technol.*, vol. 42, pp. 4133–4139.

Benoit Browaeys, D. 2009. *Le Meilleur des Nanomondes*. Buchel Chastel, Paris, 276 p.

Bensaude-Vincent, B. 2009. *Les Vertige de la Technoscience: Façonner le Monde Atome par Atome*. Paris: La Découverte, 224 p.

Berdot, C. 2007. *Après les OGM, les Nanotechnologies Entrent dans la Chaîne Alimentaire!* ATTAC 06. Online. http://www.local.attac.org/attac06/spip.php?article141 (6-08-2009).

Berge, M. 2012. *Le Développement du Nano-Argent: Entre Représentations Hygiénistes et Déterminisme Technologique*. Montreal, Master in Environmental Sciences, University of Quebec at Montreal [September 2012].

Bouldin, J.L., T.M. Ingle, A. Sengupta, R. Alexander, R.E. Hannigan and R.A. Buchanan. 2008. Aqueous toxicity and food chain transfer of Quantum DotsTM in freshwater algae and *Ceriodaphnia dubia*. *Environ. Toxicol. Chem.*, vol. 27, no 9, pp. 1958–1963.

Bouwmeester, H., S. Dekkers, M.Y. Noordam, W.I. Hagens, A.S. Bulder, C. de Heer, S.E. ten Voorde, S.W. Wijnhoven, H.J. Marvin and A.J. Sips. 2009. Review of health safety aspects of nanotechnologies in food production. *Regul. Toxicol. Pharmacol.*, vol. 53, no 1, pp. 52–62.

Card, J.W. and B.A. Magnuson. 2009. Proposed minimum characterization parameters for studies on food and food-related nanomaterials. *J. Food Sci.*, vol. 74, no 8, pp. vi–vii.

Card J.W. and Magnuson, B.A. 2010. A method to assess the quality of studies that examine the toxicity of engineered nanomaterials. *Intl J Toxicol*, vol. 29, no 4, pp. 402–410.

Cedervall, T., L.-A. Hansson, M. Lard, B. Frohm and S. Linse. 2012. Food chain transport of nanoparticles affects behaviour and fat metabolism in fish. *PLoS ONE*, vol. 7, no 2. http://www.plosone.org/article/info%3Adoi%2F10.1371%2Fjournal.pone.0032254

CEST (Commission de L'éthique de la Science et de la Technologie). 2006. *Éthique et Nanotechnologies: Se Donner les Moyens D'agir*. Quebec: Government of Quebec, 121 p.

CEST (Commission de L'éthique en Science et en Technologie). 2011. *Enjeux Ethiques des Nanotechnologies dans le Secteur Agroalimentaire: Supplément 2011 à L'avis Éthique et Nanotechnologies: Se Donner les Moyens D'agir.* Quebec: Government of Quebec, 72 p.

Chaudhry, Q. 2010. Food Applications of Nanotechnologies: An Overview of Potential Benefits and Risks. In *Nanotechnology in the Food Chain: Opportunities and Risks,* A Huyghebaert, X. Van Huffel and G. Houins, pp. 27–36. Brussels (24 novembre).

Chaudhry, Q., H. Bouwmeester and R.F. Hertel. 2011. The current risk assessment paradigm in relation to the regulation of nanotechnologies. In *International Handbook on Regulating Nanotechnologies,* G.A. Hodge, D.M. Bowman and A.D. Maynard (eds.), Cheltenham (UK): Edward Elgar Pub, pp. 124–143.

Chaudhry, Q., M. Scotter, J. Blackburn, B. Ross, A. Boxall, L. Castle, R. Aitken and R. Watkins. 2008. Applications and implications of nanotechnologies for the food sector. *Food Addit. Contam. Part A Chem. Anal. Control. Expo. Risk Assess.,* vol. 25, no. 3, pp. 241–258.

Chaudhry, Q., R. Watkins and L. Castle. 2010. Nanotechnologies in the food arena: new opportunities, new questions, new concerns. In *Nanotechnologies in Food,* Q. Chaudhry, L. Castle and R. Watkins (eds.), Cambridge: RSC Nanoscience and Nanotechnology, no. 14, Royal Society of Chemistry Publishing, pp. 1–17.

Chun, A.L. 2009. Will the public swallow nanofood? *Nat. Nanotechnol.,* vol. 4, no 12, pp. 790–791.

Cientifica. 2007. *Half way to the trillion-dollar market? A critical review of the diffusion of nanotechnologies.* London: Cientifica Ltd.

Cientifica. 2011. *Global Funding of Nanotechnologies and Its Impact.* London: Cientifica Ltd, 7 p.

CTA (International Center for Technology Assessment), Friend of the Earth, The Action Group on Erosion, Technology and Concentration, The Center for Environmental Health, Food and Water Watch and The Institute for Agriculture and Trade Policy. 2011. *Complaint for Declaration and Injunctive Relief.* San Francisco (CA): United States District Court for the Northern District of California, December 21, 23 p.

CTA (The International Center for Technology Assessment) et al. 2006. *Petition Requesting FDA Amend Its Regulations for Products Composed of Engineered Nanoparticles Generally and Sunscreen Drug Products Composed of Engineered Nanoparticles Specifically.* Rockville (MD): Dockets Management Branch, Food and Drug Administration, Department of Health and Human Services, May 16, 79 p.

CTA (The International Center for Technology Assessment) et al. 2008. *Petition for Rulemaking Requesting EPA Regulate Nano-Silver Products as Pesticides.* Washington (DC)/Arlington (VA): Office of Pesticide Programs, Environmental Protection Agency, May 1, 116 p.

Dang, Y., Y. Zhang, L. Fan, H. Chen and M.C. Roco. 2010. Trends in worldwide nanotechnology patent applications: 1991 to 2008. *J. Nanopart. Res.,* vol. 12, no 3, pp. 687–706.

Duvall, M.N. (ed.). 2012. *FDA Regulation of Nanotechnology.* Washington (DC): Beveridge & Diamond, P.C., 135 p.

Easterbrook, S. 2012. *Systems Thinking and Genetically Modified Food.* Online. http://www.easterbrook.ca/steve/?p = 2905 (25-05-2012)

EEB (European Environmental Bureau). 2009. *EEB Position Paper on Nanotechnologies and Nanomaterials: Small Scale, Big Promises, Divisive Messages.* Brussels: EEB, 12 p.

EFSA (European Food Safety Authority) Scientific Committee. 2009. The potential risks arising from nanoscience and nanotechnologies on food and feed safety. *EFSA J.*, vol. 7, no. 3, 39 p.

EFSA (European Food Safety Authority) Scientific Committee. 2011. Scientific opinion on guidance on the risk assessment of the application of nanoscience and nano-technologies in the food and feed chain. *EFSA J.*, vol. 9, no. 5, 36 p.

EPA (Environmental Protection Agency). 2011. Pesticides; policies concerning prod-ucts containing nanoscale materials; opportunity for public comment. *Fed. Reg.* [*June 17, Proposed Rules; Docket ID: EPA-HQ-OPP-2010-0197*], vol. 76, no 117, pp. 35383–35395.

ETC Group. 2004. *Down on the Farm: The Impact of Nano-Scale Technologies on Food and Agriculture*. Ottawa: ETC Group, 68 p.

European Parliament. 2012. Nano-biocides regulated. *Nanoforum*. Online. http:// www.nanoforum.org/nf06~modul~showmore~folder~99999~scc~news~ scid~4270~.html?action = longview& (2-05-2012)

FAO/WHO (Food and Agriculture Organization of the United Nations/World Health Organization). 2009. *FAO/WHO Expert Meeting on the Application of Nanotechnologies in the Food and Agriculture Sectors: Potential Food Safety Implications. Meeting Report*. Rome, 104 p.

FASFC (Belgian Federal Agency for the Safety of the Food Chain) in collaboration with DG SANCO of the European Commission and the EFSA (European Food Safety Agency). 2010. Nanotechnology in the food chain: opportunities and risks. In *International Symposium (24 November)*, A. Huyghebaert, X. Van Huffel and G. Houins (eds.), Organised by the FASFC in the Framework of the Belgian EU Presidency.

FDA (Food and Drug Administration). 2012. *Guidance for Industry: Assessing the Effects of Significant Manufacturing Process Changes, Including Emerging Technologies, on the Safety and Regulatory Status of Food Ingredients and Food Contact Substances, Including Food Ingredients that Are Color Additives. Draft Guidance*. Washington (DC): US Department of Health and Human Services, Food and Drug Administration, Center for Food Safety and Applied Nutrition, April, 26 p.

FDA (Food and Drugs Administration). 2011. *Considering Whether an FDA-Regulated Product Involves the Application of Nanotechnology Guidance for Industry: Draft Guidance*. Washington (DC): US Department of Health and Human Services, Food and Drug Administration, Office of the Commissioner.

FOE (Friends of the Earth) Australia. 2008. *Out of the Laboratory and on to Our Plates: Nanotechnology in Food and Agriculture*. Cam Walker (Melbourne): FOE Australia, 62 p.

Foladori, G. and N. Invernizzi. 2007. *Agriculture and Food Workers Challenge Nanotechnologies*. Montevideo (Uruguay): Regional Latinoamericana de la Unión Internacional de Trabajadores de la Alimentación, Agrícolas, Hoteles, Restaurantes, Tabaco y Afines (Rel-UITA), March.

FSA (Food Standards Agency). 2008. *Report of FSA Regulatory Review: A Review of Potential Implications of Nanotechnologies for Regulations and Risk Assessment in Relation to Food*. London: FSA, 28 p.

FSAI (Food Safety Authority of Ireland). 2008. *The Relevance for Food Safety Applications of Nanotechnology in the Food and Feed Industries*. Dublin: FSAI, 82 p.

GAO (United States Government Accountability Office). 2010. *Food Safety: FDA Should Strengthen Its Oversight of Food Ingredients Determined to Be Generally Recognized as Safe (GRAS)*. Washington (DC): Report to Congressional Requesters, February, 69 p.

HKC (Helmut Kaiser Consultancy). 2007. *Strong Increase in Nanofood and Molecular Food Markets in 2007 Worldwide*. Online. http://www.hkc22.com/ Nanofoodconference.html (17-10-2008)

Holbrook, R.D., K.E. Murphy, J.B. Morrow and K.D. Cole. 2008. Trophic transfer of nanoparticles in a simplified invertebrate food web. *Nat. Nanotechnol.*, vol. 3, no. 6, pp. 352–355.

House of Lords. 2010a. *Nanotechnologies and Food. Volume I: Report*. London: The Stationery Office Limited. Science and Technology Committee, 1st Report of Session 2009-10, 112 p.

House of Lords. 2010b. *Nanotechnologies and Food. Volume II: Evidence*. London: The Stationery Office Limited. Science and Technology Committee, 1st Report of Session 2009-10, 372 p.

IFST (Institute of Food Science and Technology). 2006. *Information Statement: Nanotechnology*. Cambridge: IFST, 22 p.

Imran, M., A.M. Revol-Junelles, A. Martyn, E.A. Tehrany, M. Jacquot, M. Linder and S. Desobry. 2010. Active food packaging evolution: Transformation from micro-to nanotechnology. *Crit. Rev. Food Sci. Nutr.*, vol. 50, no. 9, pp. 799–821.

IRSST (Institut de recherche Robert-Sauvé en santé et en sécurité du travail), C. Ostiguy, B. Soucy, G. Lapointe, C. Woods and L. Ménard. 2008. *Les Effets sur la Santé Reliés aux Nanoparticules*. Montreal: IRSST, report R-558, 112 p.

Joseph, T. and M. Morrison. 2006. *Nanoforum Report: Nanotechnology in Agriculture and Food*. (Glasgow, UK): European Nanotechnology Gateway, 14 p.

Judy, J.D., J.M. Unrine and P.M. Bertsch. 2011. Evidence for biomagnification of gold nanoparticles within a terrestrial food chain. *Environ. Sci. Technol.*, vol. 45, pp. 776–781.

Kleinman, D.L. and S. Suryanarayanan. 2012. Dying bees and the social production of ignorance. *Sci. Technol. Human Values*, pp. 1–26. http://sth.sagepub.com/ content/early/2012/04/27/0162243912442575

Kuzma, J. and P. VerHage. 2006. *Nanotechnology in Agriculture and Food Production: Anticipated applications*. Washington (DC): Project on Emerging Nanotechnologies, 41 p.

Laurent, B. 2010. *Les Politiques des Nanotechnologies: Pour un Traitement Démocratique d'une Acience Emergente*. Paris: Charles Léopold Mayer, 243 p.

Magnuson, B., T.S. Jonaitis and J.W. Card. 2011. A brief review of the occurrence, use, and safety of food-related nanomaterials. *J. Food Sci.*, vol. 76, no. 6, pp. R126–R133.

Maniet, F. 2010. *L'encadrement Juridique des Nanotechnologies au Canada et dans L'Union Européenne*. Montreal, Master in Environmental Sciences, University of Quebec at Montreal, 236 p.

Maniet, F. 2011. *L'encadrement des Nanotechnologies: Réflexions de Droit Comparé. 79ᵉ Congrès de L'Association Francophone pour le Savoir* (Acfas) (Sherbrooke, May 9–13, 2011), *Colloque Technosciences, Environnement, Santé, Risques, Gouvernance et Société*. Organisé par l'Institut des sciences de l'environnement, le GRETESS

(Gouvernance, Risques, Environnement, Technosciences, Santé et Société) (UQÀM) et Pôle Risques de la Maison de la recherche en sciences humaines de l'Université de Caen Basse-Normandie.

Maniet, F. 2012. *Nanotechnologies et Produits de Consommation: Quels Risques? Quels Encadrements?* Cowansville (Can.): Yvon Blais, Thomson Reuters, 296 p.

NRC (National Research Council of the National Academies). 1983. *Risk Assessment in the Federal Government: Managing the Process.* Washington (DC): National Academies Press.

Oberdörster, G., E. Oberdörster and J. Oberdörster. 2005. Nanotoxicology: An emerging discipline evolving from studies of ultrafine particles. *Environ. Health Perspect.,* vol. 113, no. 7, pp. 823–839.

Oberdörster, G., V. Stone and K. Donaldson. 2007. Toxicology of nanoparticles: A historical perspective. *Nanotoxicol,* vol. 1, no 1, pp. 2–25.

ObservatoryNano. 2011. *ObservatoryNANO Factsheets.* Online. http://www.observatorynano.eu/project/catalogue/F/(7-05-2012)

ObservatoryNano. 2012. *Public Funding of Nanotechnology.* Online. http://www.observatorynano.eu/project/document/1835/(7-05-2012).

OECD (Organisation for Economic Co-operation and Development). 2012. *Important Issues on Risk Assessment of Manufactured Nanomaterials.* Paris: Series on the Safety of Manufactured Nanomatérials, no. 33, 57 p.

Papilloud, C. 2010. *Gouverner L'infiniment Petit.* Paris: L'Harmattan, 161 p.

PCAST (President's Council of Advisors on Science and Technology). 2012. *Report to the President and Congress on the Fourth Assessment of the National Nanotechnology Initiative.* Washington (DC), 46 p.

PEN (Project on Emerging Nanotechnologies). 2011. *Inventories.* Online. http://www.nanotechproject.org/inventories/(12-06-2011)

Robinson, D.K.R. and M.J. Morrison. 2009. *Nanotechnology Developments for the Agrifood Sector.* Report of the ObservatoryNANO, European Commission, 46 p.

Roco, M.C. 2005. International perspective on government nanotechnology funding in 2005. *J. Nanopart. Res.,* vol. 7, no. 6, pp. 707–712.

Sargent Jr., J.F. 2011. *Nanotechnology and Environmental, Health, and Safety: Issues for Consideration.* Congressional Research Service, CRS Report for Congress, Prepared for Members and Committees of Congress, 37 p.

Scott, N.R. and H. Chen. 2003. *Nanoscale Science and Engineering for Agriculture and Food Systems.* Washington (DC): A Report Submitted to Cooperative State Research, Education and Extension Service, The United States Department of Agriculture. National Planning Workshop (November 18–19, 2002), 63 p.

Scrinis, G. and K. Lyons. 2007. The emerging nano-corporate paradigm: Nanotechnology and the transformation of nature, food and agri-food systems. *Int. J. Sociol. Food Agric.,* vol. 15, no. 2, pp. 22–44.

Séralini, É. and C. Vélot. 2011. Les OGM agricoles aujourd'hui: Que sont-ils et participent-ils à la faim dans le monde? *Écol. Politique,* no. 43, pp. 23–34.

Smolander, M. and Q. Chaudhry. 2010. Nanotechnologies in food packaging. In *Nanotechnologies in Food,* Q. Chaudhry, L. Castle and R. Watkins (eds.), pp. 86–101. Cambridge: RSC Nanoscience and Nanotechnology, no. 14, Royal Society of Chemistry Publishing.

SRC (Société Royale du Canada). 2001. *Éléments de Précaution: Recommendations pour la Réglementation de la Biotechnologie Alimentaire au Canada.* Royal Society of Canada, Ottawa, 269 p.

United Kingdom Government, Secretary of State for Health by Command of Her Majesty. 2010. *Government Response to the Lord's Science and Technology Select Committee Report into Nanotechnologies and Food.* Crown, London, 18 p.

VivAgora. Online. http://www.vivagora.fr/

Williams, R.A., K.M. Kulinowski, R. White and G. Louis. 2010. Risk characterization for nanotechnology. *Risk Anal.*, vol. 30, no. 11, pp. 1671–1679.

Zhu, X., J. Wang, X. Zhang, Y. Chang and Y. Chen. 2010. Trophic transfer of TiO$_2$ nanoparticles from daphnia to zebrafish in a simplified freshwater food chain. *Chemosphere*, vol. 79, no. 9, pp. 928–933.

# Section IV

# Bionanotechnology and the Environment

# 7

# Benefits of Nanotechnology for the Environment

Danail Hristozov

## CONTENTS

## 7.1 Introduction

Maintaining and improving the quality of soil, water, and air resources represent some of the greatest challenges standing before our society today. Pollution from a variety of sources, such as oil and chemical spills, pesticide and fertilizer runoff, abandoned industrial and mining sites, as well as airborne gaseous contaminants and particulate matter (PM) from car exhaust, seriously affects the environment and threatens the health of human populations. Enormous amounts of carbon dioxide ($CO_2$) are released daily into the atmosphere from combustion of fossil fuels and warm it up irreversibly. The world's climate system is an integral part of the complex of life-supporting processes. Climate and weather have always had a powerful impact on human health and wellbeing.

"In the light of these enormous and complex challenges, it is perhaps ironic that one prospective solution is diminutive in size but immensely powerful in capacity" [1]. Nanotechnology holds promise to provide solutions to some environmental problems and contribute to environmental sustainability. Masciagnoli and Zhang [1] divided the benefits of nanotechnology for the environment into three categories: sensing and detection (environmental monitoring), remediation and treatment, and pollution prevention. Some other important benefits were identified at the European Nanoforum Joint Workshop in 2007, and they include energy and material conservation [2]. The latter benefits, however, will not be discussed in this chapter since the conservation of energy and materials do not directly contribute to the preservation of human health.

## 7.2  Environmental Pollution, Human Health, and Nanotechnology

"Pollution" is the introduction of contaminants into the environment, which causes instability, disorder, harm, or discomfort to ecosystems [3]. Pollution has many forms, but most often it is expressed as chemical substances, biological agents, noise, heat, or light. Environmental pollution has always had negative effects on human health, which can greatly vary in their kind or magnitude in accordance with the types of pollutants involved and the extent of the human exposure to them.

Air pollution can cause severe health problems and even death in both human and animal populations. Ozone, for instance, can result in respiratory and cardiovascular diseases, throat inflammation, chest pains, and congestion [4]. PM induces respiratory problems, reduced lung function, chest pain, and asthmatic responses [5]. Exposure to volatile organic compounds (VOCs) causes skin irritation and nausea, and increases the risk of cancer [6]. Short-term exposures to high levels of sulfur dioxide ($SO_2$) can be life threatening. Long-term exposure to persistent levels of $SO_2$ can lead to respiratory problems, such as lung inflammation and asthma hypersensitivity [7].

Many sources of water are now contaminated with heavy metals (e.g., mercury, cadmium, arsenic, lead, chromium), persistent organic pollutants

(POPs), and nutrients (e.g., nitrogen and phosphorus), which have the capacity to cause adverse health effects. Runoff from agriculture contains pesticides, such as dichlorodiphenyltrichloroethane (DDT), chlordane, and atrazine, that can heavily contaminate water bodies and enter the drinking water sources. Pesticides can cause both endocrine and reproductive health damages, and long-term exposure to some of them is carcinogenic [8]. Inadequately treated municipal sewage can carry microbial pathogens, causing the spread of diseases such as diarrhea or cholera. Domestic wastewater, agricultural runoff, and industrial effluents contain phosphorus and nitrogen, which can lead to eutrophication in surface waters, significantly reducing their quality. The excessive use of fertilizers causes nitrate contamination of groundwater, which can spread to drinking water sources and cause oxygen deficiency in organ tissues, followed by a dangerous condition called methemoglobinemia [9]. Many of the synthetic compounds in use today are found in the aquatic environment and accumulate in the food chain. POPs are extremely harmful for ecosystems and for human health: they can easily accumulate in animals, plants, and especially in aquatic organisms and thus enter the human food chain. Overexposure to most POPs can lead to severe acute effects, while at lower exposure levels long-term effects, such as endocrine disruption, reproductive and immune dysfunction, neurobehavioral and developmental disorders, and cancer can occur [10]. Oil spills can cause skin irritations and rashes. Lead and other heavy metals have been shown to induce neurological problems, while chemical and radioactive substances in water can cause cancer and birth defects.

A substantial portion of the global pollution, responsible for the health effects, listed above is generated as a result of industrial production processes. Although it is largely recognized that the current production paradigm is environmentally unsustainable, following an increasing linear trend of resource consumption and overcontamination, society has always been reluctant to face this issue and find a long-term solution. To preserve the environment, keeping it clean for future generations, radical changes are necessary in both the way society consumes and the way industry produces, as the right balance has to be found. It was recognized that the majority of people are not willing to change their consumer patterns and since in the context of the free market economy it is the consumer behavior that shapes the industrial policies, it becomes evident that if society stays passive, then it is the industry that should find a way to produce sustainably. Today, industry creates goods mostly by shaping matter in a top–down approach, relying on energy-intensive production processes, generating substantial amounts of waste. The total opposite of this would be a bottom–up approach, based on product design using molecular building blocks, precisely positioned through well-controlled, low-energy processes, barely creating any waste. It is exactly what manufacturing on the nanoscale has promised: an alternative that may fundamentally shift the current production practices to a more sustainable paradigm.

To protect the health of their citizens, many nations have enacted legislation for pollution control. Some important examples are the European (EU) Directive 96/61/EC, the United States (US) Clean Air and Clean Water Acts, and the Japanese Chemical Substances Control Law. Pollution control largely relies on monitoring to obtain data about the occurrence and concentrations of contaminants in the environment. Environmental monitoring data are traditionally produced using analytical techniques such as mass spectrometry, gas chromatography, and infrared spectrometry, but it was recognized that those conventional methods do not adequately reflect the dynamic behavior of environmental contaminants since they use large static devices, often fixed to the ground, which cannot be easily reassembled and applied at different spatial scales. Nanotechnology holds promise for substantial contribution to pollution control through the development and application of more sensitive environmental monitoring technologies, suitable to apply anywhere and able to provide real-time measurements.

Excessive environmental pollution should not be allowed, but once present, it should be removed by means of remediation. A variety of techniques for environmental remediation exist today (e.g., surfactant enhanced aquifer remediation, pump and treat, solidification and stabilization, *in situ* oxidation, soil vapor extraction) and being applicable to a vast array of contaminants, they all share the major disadvantage of being too costly. Nanotechnology has promised to contribute to environmental quality through the development and application of more effective and cheaper treatment and remediation technologies.

The following sections aim to provide a broad overview of the benefits of nanotechnology for the environments in the areas of environmental sensing and detection, remediation, and treatment, which have direct implications for human health. In addition, the chapter seeks to discuss these benefits in the context of the risks surrounding the production and large-scale commercialization of nano-enabled products.

## 7.3 Nanotechnology and Environmental Monitoring

Environmental monitoring is defined as "…gathering, assessing and reporting environmental information, obtained through continuous or periodic sampling, observation and analysis of both natural variation or changes, and anthropogenic pressures and their effects on humans and the environment…" [11]. It provides important information about the concentrations of pollutants in the environment, which is essential for their human and eco-logical exposure and risk assessment and regulation.

## 7.3.1 Air Monitoring Systems

Analytical methods, such as mass spectrometry, gas chromatography, chemi-luminescence, and infrared spectrometry are capable of precise air compo-sition analyses; however, they are time consuming, relatively expensive, and difficult to use in the field. The enormous pollution complexity and its intensive dynamics required the application of new, more flexible, and cost-effective systems, operating at higher spatial resolutions. This demand determined the development of the solid-state gas sensors (SGSs), which are able to analyze air samples faster and less expensive than their conventional alternatives [12].

SGSs consist of one or more oxides of the transition metals (e.g., tin, alu-minum, zinc, cobalt, tungsten). These materials are processed into paste, which is then used to construct bead-type sensors. Another type is the film-chip sensors, which are fabricated as the metal oxides are vacuum deposited onto silica chips [13]. Nowadays, nanoparticles (NPs) and thin films of metal oxides (<100 nm thick) are used to construct the sensors. This offers consider-able advantages over the standard technology, increasing the sensitivity and reducing the response time of the devices.

The SGSs operate in a simple fashion. As ambient gas molecules are cap-tured within the sensor, the metal oxide causes the gas to dissociate into charged ions or complexes, and electron transfer takes place [14]. This effect changes the electrical conductivity of the semiconducting material in accor-dance with the composition of the surrounding air. A pair of very thin elec-trodes is attached to the metal oxide to measure the changes in conductivity and report them as signals [14]. SGSs typically produce strong signals, as their strength depends on the gas concentrations and the size of the particles used to build the semiconductor [15].

Currently, nanostructured metal oxides are the main types of materi-als used to fabricate gas sensors. That is why the devices are often called "conductimetric nanosensors." The reason to employ nanomaterials in the SGSs is that they have very high surface-area-to-volume ratios (sa/vol) [16], which allows that more ambient gas molecules are adsorbed on the material interface [16]. The higher gas concentrations invoke stronger changes in con-ductivity of the semiconductors and stronger electrical signals, respectively, which increases the sensitivity of the devices [16].

Today, metal oxides, shaped as nanowires, nanobelts, and nanocombs, are tested for use in SGSs. The results show that these morphologies sig-nificantly increase the effective surface area of the semiconducting material [16] and they may be integrated into the next generation of SGSs, which will emerge on the market in the next 3 to 5 years.

An important benefit of nanotechnology for air monitoring is that it decreases the size of the SGS devices considerably, making them compact enough to be fitted anywhere. They can be integrated into flexible, mobile monitoring systems, which can be easily reconfigured and applied on different spatial scales, providing reliable, real-time air quality data. If the sensors are connected in an intelligent sensor network equipped with a GPS (global positioning system), data can be transmitted from remote locations to a central service site, modeled using GIS (geographic information system) software and published on the Internet [17].

### 7.3.2 Water Monitoring Systems

When the European Water Framework Directive was implemented in 2000, new regulations for water monitoring of organic substances were imposed and measurements had to be done down to microgram per liter ($\mu g$ $L^{-1}$) levels. Such accuracy, however, was difficult to achieve with conventional water monitoring technologies, and a necessity for more sensitive systems appeared. Nanotechnology has shown the potential to develop novel biosensor technologies with improved characteristics (i.e., specificity, sensitivity, detection speed, ruggedness, and the ability to handle large volumes). Novel water monitoring technologies use nanostructured biochips to detect a variety of contaminants. A biochip is a small device that has multiple miniaturized test sites (biosensors), arranged as microarrays on a solid substrate [18]. That arrangement allows many tests to be performed simultaneously and thus achieve higher throughput and save time. The sensors can be deposited either on flat passive substrates (e.g., silicon or glass) or on active substrates, consisting of integrated electronics to perform or assist signal transduction [18]. Surface chemistry is used to bind the substrate to the sensor surface.

The Water Framework Directive (known also as Directive 2000/60/EC) is a European directive, which commits all EU member states to achieve good qualitative and quantitative status of all water bodies by 2015 [19]. By means of Directive 2000/60/EC, the EU provides for the management of inland surface waters, groundwater, transitional waters, and coastal waters in order to "prevent and reduce pollution, promote sustainable water use, protect the aquatic environment, improve the status of aquatic ecosystems and mitigate the effects of floods and droughts" [19].

The directive requires the issue of key documents over 6-year planning cycles, as the most important among them are the River Basin Management Plans, which need to be published in 2009, 2015, and 2021 [19].

Immunochemistry* is actively involved in the operation of the biosensor technologies. It involves techniques such as immunoaffinity chromatography† and immunoassay‡ [20]. Sample preparations based on immunoaffinity take advantage of the attraction between an antibody and a specific analyte [20]. By rinsing a water sample over an antibody-treated surface, chemists can isolate particular compounds adhering to the antibody molecules. The isolated compound is then eluted from the immobilized antibody and analyzed, using chromatography or immunoassay techniques [20]. Antibodies can be produced synthetically for a variety of organic pollutants.

An important example of a novel water monitoring nanotechnology, based on an immunoassay technique, is the Automated Water Analyzer Computer Supported System (AWACSS). It was developed by researchers from the Corporate Technology Division of Siemens AG in Erlangen (Germany), in collaboration with the Karlsruhe Water Technology Center and the University of Tübingen [21]. The project was financed by the European Commission (EC) and technically designed by Siemens. AWACSS has the size of a suitcase and it can simultaneously test several samples and send the results to a central server [21]. The system is able, within less than 18 min, to check for 32 different substances, ranging from hormones to pesticides and antibiotics. The device can detect very low concentrations (i.e., <1 $\mu$g L$^{-1}$) [21].

The key component of AWACSS is an array of nanostructured biochips, which can capture molecules of environmental pollutants [21]. The water sample is first mixed with antibodies that are marked with a fluorescent pigment (e.g., Cy5.5, Alexa680, or quantum dots). If the sample contains specific organic molecules, the antibodies attach to them [21]. Then, a pump propels the liquid across the array of small glass biochips, each coated with a layer of captor molecules. These molecules capture the antibodies (as they are bound to the toxins) and the remaining particles are rinsed from the chips [21]. A concentrated light source is used to cause the captured antibodies to glow, making them detectable by an optical sensor [21].

### 7.3.3 Summary and Conclusions

As was shown in previous sections, nanotechnology contributes to the field of environmental monitoring through the development of sensing alternatives with enhanced functionality. The nanostructured SSGs are simple to use, technologically more effective, and cheaper than their conventional counterparts. Current research is focused on the development of a new generation of sensors, incorporating semiconducting nanowires, nanobelts, or

---

* Immunochemistry is a branch of chemistry that involves the study of the reactions and components of the immune system.
† Imunoaffinity chromatography is a column chromatography method using antibody–antigen reactions to purify or detect substances.
‡ An immunoassay is a biochemical test that measures the concentration of a substance in a liquid, using the reaction of an antibody (or antibodies) to its antigen.

nanocombs, which are expected to further improve the detection strength of the devices. Since they are very small, the SSGs can be integrated into mobile monitoring systems, which can be used at different spatial scales, thus allowing more precise illustration of temporal and spatial distributions of the contaminants and the associated human exposure. In addition, the development of micro- and nanofluidic technologies and their convergence with immunochemistry made it possible to design minute biochips, which can analyze water samples for a wide variety of contaminants. Since they are more advanced and less costly than their conventional counterparts, the nano-enhanced sensing technologies will be applied on the large scale in the next 3 to 7 years to contribute to

- Generation of higher-quality data about the human exposure to contaminants
- More precise identification and quantification of exposure sources
- More precise illustration of temporal and spatial exposure trends
- More reliable monitored data to use for human health risk assessment

The provision of high-quality monitoring data can greatly facilitate the analysis of the environmental and human health hazards and risks of exposure to contaminants. This kind of analysis can greatly contribute to a more informed chemical regulation policy and invoke the review of some aspects of the current health and environmental protection programs.

## 7.4  Nanotechnology for Environmental Remediation and Treatment

A major environmental benefit of nanotechnology is the development of remediation and end-of-pipe treatment alternatives. Environmental remediation involves the removal of contaminants from soils, waters, and sediments for the sake of human health and environmental protection [22]. End-of-pipe treatment is the removal of contaminants from emissions, most often through filtration or chemical transformation, before discharge into the environment.

Substances of significant health concern, which need to be removed from the environment, include heavy metals (e.g., arsenic, lead, mercury) and organic compounds (e.g., benzene, chlorinated solvents, creosote, toluene). Novel nano-based remediation and treatment practices have been developed in recent years. Some of the advantages they offer over conventional technologies are better selectivity, higher removal capacity, and lower cost.

## 7.4.1 Remediation Nanotechnologies

### 7.4.1.1 Nanoscale Zero-Valent Iron

Nanoscale zero-valent iron (nZVI) has been widely used for environmental remediation due to its low cost. Its application in packed bed reactors and permeable reactive barriers has been widely reported in the literature. The material has been established as an effective reducing agent for a wide variety of environmental contaminants [24]. A tentative list of these contaminants is given in Table 7.1.

The nZVI particles can remain reactive in soil and water for long periods (>4–8 weeks) [24]. They react rapidly, when applied *in situ*, achieving very fast decontamination rates (trichloroethylene [TCE] reduction of up to 99% in few days after slurry injection) [24]. nZVI is typically mixed with water to form slurry, which can be injected into the contaminated plume. Compared with similar *in situ* methods, nZVI allows remediation at greater depths, which is very important in case the target site is covered by buildings.

In contrast to all benefits, a significant weakness of the nZVI technology is that the hydrophilic behavior of the iron particles allows for the cleanup of aqueous phases only, which excludes the possibility for dense nonaqueous phase liquid (DNAPL) remediation [24].

**TABLE 7.1**

Common Environmental Contaminants that Can Be Transformed by Nanoscale Iron Particles

| Chlorinated Methanes | Trihalomethanes |
|---|---|
| Carbon tetrachloride ($CCl_4$), chloroform ($CHCl_3$), chloromethane ($CH_3Cl$), dichloromethane ($CH_2Cl_2$) | Bromoform ($CHBr_3$), dibromochloromethane ($CHBr_2Cl$), dichlorobromomethane ($CHBrCl_2$) |
| **Chlorinated Benzenes** | **Chlorinated Ethenes** |
| Hexachlorobenzene ($C_6Cl_6$), pentachlorobenzene ($C_6Cl_5$), tetrachlorobenzenes ($C_6Cl_4$), trichlorobenzenes ($C_6H_3Cl_3$), dichlorobenzenes ($C_6H_4Cl_2$), chlorobenzene ($C_6H_5Cl$) | Tetrachloroethene ($C_2Cl_4$), trichloroethene ($C_2HCl_3$), *cis*-dichloroethene ($C_2H_2Cl_2$), *trans*-dichloroethene ($C_2H_2Cl_2$), dichloroethene ($C_2H_2Cl_2$), vinyl chloride ($C_2H_3Cl$) |
| **Pesticides** | **Other Polychlorinated Hydrocarbons** |
| DDT ($C_{14}H_9Cl_5$), lindane ($C_6H_6Cl_6$) | Dioxins, pentachlorophenol ($C_6HCl_5O$), PCBs |
| **Organic Dyes** | **Other Organic Contaminants** |
| Orange II ($C_{16}H_{16}N_2NaO_4S$), chrysoidine ($C_{12}H_{13}ClN_4$), tropaeolin O ($C_{12}H_9N_2NaO_5S$) | *N*-nitrosodimethylamine ($C_4H_{10}N_2O$), TNT ($C_7H_5N_3O_6$) |
| **Heavy Metal Ions** | **Inorganic Anions** |
| Mercury ($Hg^{2+}$), nickel ($Ni^{2+}$), silver ($Ag^+$), cadmium ($Cd^{2+}$) | Dichromate $\left(Cr_2O_7^{2-}\right)$, As $\left(AsO_3^{4-}\right)$, perchlorate ($ClO^{-4}$), nitrate ($NO^{-3}$) |

*Source:* Zhang, W., *J. Nanopar. Res.*, 5, 323, 2003. With permission.

A number of bimetallic systems in which various metals are plated onto nZVI particles have shown the ability to reduce chlorinated organic compounds at rates significantly faster than the nZVI alone [25]. Some combinations available today are Fe/Pt, Fe/Ag, Fe/Ni, Fe/Co, and Fe/Cu [25]. Among them, the palladized iron (Fe/Pd) has the fastest reaction kinetics. Laboratory studies showed that TCE is destroyed twice as fast by Fe/Pd than by nZVI alone [25]. Unfortunately, owing to the high cost of palladium, the *in situ* use of Fe/Pd NPs is infeasible.

As it was shown in this section, nZVI represent a powerful means of groundwater and site remediation. Along with the benefits associated with its utilization, however, scientists are afraid that exposure to the iron NPs can potentially cause environmental and/or health problems.

Most analysts of this issue suggest that the current nZVI-based remediation methods do not appear to pose environmental and human health risks [26–29]. Modeled transport data indicate that NP plumes may travel only slightly faster than most contaminant plumes and as a consequence the human exposure is likely to be minimal [27]. However, there are still many uncertain aspects, for example, the inherent toxicity of the particles, the environmental behavior, and the fate of their transformation by-products. More research is necessary before final conclusions can be drawn about the health risks of nZVI particles.

### 7.4.1.2 Nanoscale Semiconductor Photocatalysts (nSPs)

Semiconductor photocatalysts (SPs) are catalysts built from semiconducting materials (e.g., titanium dioxide [$TiO_2$], zinc oxide, iron oxide, tungsten trioxide), which obtain their activation energy from the light in the UV spectrum [25,30]. It was recognized that building SP materials from NPs greatly enhances their photocatalytic activity. The nanoscale SPs are able to degrade a great variety of inorganic and organic contaminants, which makes them useful for environmental remediation. A tentative list of these contaminants is provided in Table 7.2.

Nanoparticulate $TiO_2$ has been traditionally used in environmental remediation because of its low toxicity, high photoconductivity, high photostability, availability, and low cost [25,30]. Novel technologies and improved processes have enabled the development of a variety of photocatalytic derivatives. Metals such as copper, silver, gold, and platinum have been used to modify the $TiO_2$ particle surfaces and improve their decontamination activity. The combination of $TiO_2$ with copper, for example, results in a "synergistic photocatalytic effect" for the remediation of hexavalent chromium [32]. Coupling the $TiO_2$ NPs with gold or silver results in similar effects [32].

The $TiO_2$-based p–n junction nanotubes represent a novel, fascinating development in the field of nanoscale SPs. The nanotubes contain platinum (in the inside) and $TiO_2$ (on the outside). The $TiO_2$ coating of the tube acts as an oxidizing surface, while the inside of the tube is reductive [33]. The ability

**TABLE 7.2**

Common Environmental Contaminants Transformed by SPs

| Inorganic Contaminants | Organic Contaminants |
|---|---|
| Ammonia ($NH_3$), azide ions $\left(N_3^-\right)$, chromium (Cr) species, copper (Cu), cyanide ions ($CN^-$), gold (Au), halide ions (i.e., fluoride [$F^-$], chloride [$Cl^-$], bromide [$Br^-$], iodide [$I^-$], astatide [$At^-$]), iron (Fe) species, manganese (Mn) species, nitrates $\left(NO_3^-\right)$ and nitrites $\left(NO_2^-\right)$, nitric oxide (NO), ozone ($O_3$), palladium (Pd), silver (Ag) and sulfur (S) species, etc. | Chlorinated aromatics (e.g., chlorophenols, chlorobenzenes, chlorobiphenyls, dichlorodibenzo-*p*-dioxin, chlorodibenzo-*p*-dioxin, 2,4,5-trichlorophenoxyacetic, acid, 2,4-dichlorophenoxyacetic acid), polychlorinated biphenyls (PCBs) ($C_{12}H_{10}$-$xCl_x$), dichlorodiphenyltrichloroethane (DDT) ($C_{14}H_9Cl_{15}$), chlorinated surfactants, chlorinated ethenes (e.g., tetrachloroethene [$C_2Cl_4$], trichloroethene [$C_2HCl_3$], *cis*-dichloroethene [$C_2H_2Cl_2$], *trans*-dichloroethene [$C_2H_2Cl_2$], dichloroethene [$C_2H_2Cl_2$], vinyl chloride [$C_2H_3Cl$]), Nitrogenous compounds (e.g., monuron, nitrotolulene, picoline, piperidene, proline, pyridine, simazine, theophylline, thymine, trietazine, cyclophosphamide, ethylenediaminetetraacetic acid [EDTA]), etc. |

*Source:* Modified after Hoffmann M.R. et al., *Chem. Rev.*, 95, 69, 1995.

of the nanotubes to destroy toluene was tested by Chen et al. [33] and the results showed that they exhibit much higher destruction rates than the non-nanotube material [33].

Along with the benefits associated with the utilization of $TiO_2$ for environmental remediation, it is possible that $TiO_2$ NPs, injected in the underground, can cause environmental problems and/or do harm to human health. Currently, little data regarding the human and environmental exposure to $TiO_2$ NPs, used for environmental remediation, are available and the associated risks are still largely unknown.

Several models describing how $TiO_2$ NPs behave in the environment have been developed thus far, as most of them point out that it is very likely that *in situ* applied $TiO_2$ particles reach surface waters [34,35]. According to Mueller and Nowack [34], among all NPs, $TiO_2$ was of largest environmental concentration in the Swiss surface waters (i.e., 16 µg $L^{-1}$). This was confirmed by Boxall et al. [35], who suggested a nano-$TiO_2$ concentration of 24.5 µg $L^{-1}$ in the British surface waters [35]. From the water, the $TiO_2$ particles can be easily taken up by living organisms and enter the human food chain. Once there, they might potentially cause adverse health effects in the exposed populations. These effects, however, are still largely unexplored. To assess the health risks of exposure to $TiO_2$ NPs, it is essential to investigate their toxicity more deeply.

### 7.4.1.3 Polymeric Nanoparticles

Polymeric NPs are a very broad category of molecules and molecular aggregates suitable for a variety of applications. They have amphiphilic properties, which make them similar to the surfactant micelles. The individual polymer molecules have a hydrophobic and a hydrophilic part and in water they self-assemble and form vesicles with diameters in the nanometer range [36]. Unlike the surfactant micelles, due to the cross-linking of the particle precursor chains, the polymeric NPs are able to maintain stability regardless of precursor chain concentration [36].

The amphiphilic polyurethane (APU) NPs are specifically developed for remedial applications. Researchers have synthesized a number of APU particles using (poly)urethane acrylate anionomer (UAA) and polyethylene glycol–modified urethane acrylate as precursor chains [36]. APU NPs can potentially replace the traditional surfactants that are commonly used to facilitate the remediation of hydrophobic organic contaminants (HOCs).

The HOCs readily sorb to soils or form nonaqueous phase liquids [25,37], which makes it very difficult to remove them from the soil matrix, using pump-and-treat remediation techniques. Because of similar reasons, the conventional pump-and-treat methods have had limited success in removing polynuclear aromatic hydrocarbons (PAHs) from the ground [37]. Surfactants have been shown to significantly enhance the solubility of HOCs and PAHs and improve their recovery rate. However, since they are chemically unstable, the surfactant micelles are easily lost in the process. The cross-linking of polymer chains within UAA particles makes them significantly more stable than surfactant micelles, and having similar desorption capabilities, they may replace them in the near future [36].

### 7.4.1.4 Ferritin-Encapsulated Metal Oxides

Proteins have attracted the attention of researchers for their ability to control the formation of mineral structures. Cage-shaped proteins can function as controlled environments where nanosized materials can be assembled and encapsulated. An example of such a protein is ferritin: a protein able to store iron. Ferritin is composed of 24 polypeptide subunits, which self-assemble into three-dimensional, hollow complexes under certain conditions [38]. The metal ions then become bound to sites in the central cavity. The diameter of the assembled apoferritin (i.e., iron-free ferritin) is about 12 nm, and the inside cavity is approximately 8 nm [25]. Iron molecules can diffuse into the cavity through channels in the protein shell, where iron becomes mineralized and converted to iron oxide (i.e., ferric oxyhydroxide) NPs [38].

The most promising potential benefit of ferritin for remediation is that it can contribute to the photoreduction of contaminants [39]. Despite that normally Fe (III) is able to carry out significant photochemical processes, the Fe (III)-bearing iron oxide quickly becomes photoreduced to Fe (II) and thus deactivated [39]. The ferritin naturally converts Fe (II) to Fe (III) and the protein encapsulation of the iron oxide prevents its conversion back to Fe (II) without inhibiting the rate of decontamination [39].

Kim et al. [39] have demonstrated the ability of ferritin to reduce hexavalent chromium, a dangerous carcinogen, to the chromium trivalent form, which is ubiquitous and less toxic. The researchers also expect to test the new technology on nuclear contaminants [39]. If proven applicable, this technology can be used to remediate groundwater that has been contaminated from the leakage of storage canisters containing nuclear waste [40]. The technology also offers potential remedial capabilities for aromatics and chlorocarbons [25].

### 7.4.1.5 Single-Enzyme Nanoparticles

Enzymes have been proven more effective than synthetic catalysts in many areas of application. However, owing to their chemical instability and relatively short lifetimes, they are considered inappropriate to apply for environmental remediation. A new method of enzyme stabilization has recently been developed, which involves the production of environmentally persistent single enzyme NPs (SENs) [41].

SENs are resistant to extreme conditions such as high/low pH, high contaminant concentration, high salinity, and high/low temperature. They are generally much easier to control than microbial organisms. They need no nutrients to exist and any metabolic by-products or mass transfer limitations, due to cellular transport, are avoided [41].

Specific enzymes are used for the different contaminants. Some examples of enzyme classes appropriate for remediation are the peroxidases, polyphenol oxidases (laccase, tyrosinase), dehalogenases, and organophosphorus hydrolases [42]. The great choice of applicable enzymes implies the possibility for successful remediation of a broad range of organic contaminants in water. Contaminants such as phenols, polyaromatics, dyes, chlorinated compounds, organophosphorus pesticides, and even explosives can be successfully degraded using appropriate enzymes [41].

### 7.4.1.6 Summary and Conclusions

Environmental remediation nanotechnology is still in its infancy, but, rapidly evolving, it holds promise to clean contaminated sites cost-effectively and address challenging site conditions, such as the presence of DNAPL.

The most important example described in this chapter is the nZVI, which has been used in full-scale projects with encouraging success. As a cleanup technology, it has three major advantages: (1) effective for the transformation of a large variety of environmental contaminants, (2) inexpensive, and (3) apparently nontoxic [24].

Similarly to nZVI, nanoparticulate $TiO_2$ has been widely used in environmental remediation because of its low toxicity, high photoconductivity, high photostability, availability, and low cost [25,30]. The $TiO_2$-based p–n junction nanotubes represent a recent innovation in the field of nSPs. They exhibit higher decontamination rates than nonnanotube materials [33], and as their production cost falls they may become the next generation of nSPs.

Ongoing research at the bench- and pilot-scale investigates technologies such as ferritin-encapsulated iron oxides and polymeric and the single-enzyme NPs to determine how to apply their unique characteristics for full-scale remediation. Despite the fact that these technologies deliver no current benefits for the environment, some of them may contribute to environmental remediation at a later stage.

Unfortunately, no quantitative comparison among the costs of application of nano-based remedial tools and their conventional counterparts could be accurately conducted at this time. The reason is that the factors that contribute to the costs of remediation are not only technology specific but also site and contaminant specific, and the remediation cost data in the literature are incomplete. Qualitatively, the vast majority of publications state that nZVI and $TiO_2$ are more cost-effective than their conventional counterparts. Being cheaper and more effective, these technologies will gradually become more widely used and will have significant impact on the future remediation activities.

Despite the dominating predictions that remedial nanotechnologies will deliver significant benefits, there are still many unanswered questions regarding their toxicity. Further research is needed to understand the fate and transport of free NPs in the environment to study their persistence and their potential to bioaccumulate and cause adverse effects in animals and humans.

### 7.4.2 Treatment Nanotechnologies

Nanofiltration is a relatively recent membrane process that holds promise to deliver cost-effective water and air treatment solutions. "Nanofiltration" as a term was coined several years ago to define already used membranes, called at the time "loose reverse osmosis membranes." Other separation processes similar to nanofiltration are the reverse osmosis, ultrafiltration, microfiltration, and particle filtration. The main difference among these processes is the metric scale at which they operate (i.e., the size of particles they are able to retain). Table 7.3 compares the four processes in terms of (1) pore size, (2) materials used to construct the membranes, and (3) type of removed contaminants.

Nanomembranes (NMs) are used not only to remove contaminants from polluted water and air but also for desalination of salty water. There are two types of NMs currently available on the market: nanofilters, using either carbon nanotubes (CNTs) or nanocapillary arrays to mechanically remove impurities, and reactive NMs, where functionalized NPs chemically convert the contaminants into safe by-products.

**TABLE 7.3**

Comparison among Microfiltration, Ultrafiltration, Nanofiltration, and Reverse Osmosis Membrane Processes

|  | **Microfiltration** | **Ultrafiltration** | **Nanofiltration** | **Reverse Osmosis** |
|---|---|---|---|---|
| Pore size | 0.01–1.0 µm | 0.001–0.01 µm | 0.0001–0.001 µm | <0.0001 µm |
| Materials used to construct the membranes | Ceramics, polypropylene, polysulfone, etc. | Ceramics, polysulfone, cellulose acetate, thin film composites | Cellulose acetate, thin film composites | Cellulose acetate, thin film composites |
| Type of contaminants removed | Clay, bacteria, viruses, suspended solids | Proteins, starch, viruses, colloid silica, organics, dyes, fat, etc. | Starch, sugars, pesticides, herbicides, divalent anions, organics, BOD, COD, detergents | Metal cations, acids, sugars, aqueous salts, amino acids, monovalent salts, BOD, COD |

*Source:* Modified after Wagner J., *Membrane Filtration Handbook,* 2nd Ed., Osmonics Inc., 2001. With permission.

### 7.4.2.1 Carbon Nanotube Membranes (CNMs)

Ordered arrays of densely packed, vertically aligned CNTs can be used as membranes to filter out water impurities, while allowing the water to freely flow through the filter. CNMs are able to remove almost all kinds of water contaminants, including bacteria, viruses, and organic contaminants [44]. CMNs are also shown to be effective in desalinating salty water [45]. Table 7.4 compares between the contaminant removal capabilities of CNMs and some alternative water treatment technologies.

Despite the fact that the pores of CNMs are significantly smaller than the pores of other membranes, CNMs have shown the same, or even faster, flow rates. Some CNMs show 10,000 times greater water permeability than some conventional polycarbonate membranes [44]. The reason behind that phenomenon is hidden in the smooth interior of the nanotubes, the walls of which are almost perfectly flat.

CNMs are still relatively expensive but the cost of producing them constantly falls as researchers develop cheaper production methods. It was estimated by Srivastava et al. [45] that CNMs can become much less costly than other filtration membrane technologies (e.g., reverse osmosis, ceramic and polymer filters) [45]. CNM filters are already market competitive in Europe and in the United States but they are still too expensive to apply in developing countries.

**TABLE 7.4**

Comparison among Nanofilters (Including CNMs) and Alternative Water Treatment Technologies in Terms of Contaminant Removal

| Type of Technology | Contaminants Removed | | |
| --- | --- | --- | --- |
| | Inorganic | Organic | Biological |
| *Conventional Treatment Technologies* | | | |
| Coagulation–flocculation | Arsenic, asbestos, cadmium, chromium, selenium | No | Bacteria, fecal coliform, viruses |
| Chemical disinfection | No | No | Bacteria, coliform, fecal coliform, viruses |
| Distillation | All[a] | No | Bacteria, cysts, viruses |
| UV radiation | No | No | Bacteria, spores, coliform, viruses |
| *Nanofiltration Technologies* | | | |
| Carbon nanotube (CNT) membranes | Salts, arsenic, cadmium, mercury, selenium | All[b] | All[c] |
| Nanofibrous filters | Sea salt, arsenic, chromium, lead, radionuclides, etc. | Unspecified | All[c] |
| SAMMS | Arsenic, cadmium, chromium, lead, mercury, radionuclides | Dep. on SAMMS type | Unspecified |

[a] Inorganic contaminants: that is, heavy metals, nitrites, salts, asbestos, radionuclides, calcium, magnesium, and others.

[b] Organic contaminants: that is, pesticides, herbicides, insecticides, industrial effluents, MTBE, PAHS, PCBs, VOCs, and others.

[c] Biological contaminants: that is, bacteria, bacterial spores, *Giardia* and *Cryptosporidium* cysts, coliform, fecal coliform, DNA and RNA, fungi, mold, parasites, protozoa, and viruses.

### 7.4.2.2 Nanomembranes for Carbon Dioxide Removal

Industrial emissions of $CO_2$ contribute to global warming. Around the globe, seasons are shifting, temperatures are climbing, and sea levels are rising. Climate change permanently alters the lands and waters we all depend on for survival. Some expected impacts associated with the greenhouse effect are more heat-related diseases and increased risk of storms, drought, fire, and floods in some regions, which threaten the lives and wellbeing of many people.

Some authors consider the storage $CO_2$ in empty gas fields or aquifers a potential solution to the problem on how to mitigate the effects caused by industrial $CO_2$ emissions [46–49]. In order to store $CO_2$ in the underground, however, it should be captured first. Novel nanostructured membranes might potentially offer an efficient and cost-effective way of separating $CO_2$ from industrial effluents.

The capture and separation of $CO_2$ is a complicated process. Currently, the most widely employed technology involves an absorption process. The flue gasses flow through several baths in which $CO_2$ is bound with amines and chemically removed from the flue gas. This "scrubbing" technology, however, consumes significant amounts of energy and requires expensive, sophisticated installations, which make it very costly. It is expected that the application of NMs for $CO_2$ removal would significantly reduce the costs of infrastructure and operation. Research in the field of $CO_2$ separation NMs is carried out by a number of scientific institutions, as some of it was done in the context of the major European Sixth Framework Programme (FP6) project NANOGLOWA (Nanostructured Membranes against Global Warming).

Until now, several novel NM types have been developed from both polymeric and inorganic materials. Carbon-based membranes, mesoporous oxide membranes, and zeolite membranes are best described in the literature. Polymer membranes are relatively easy to manufacture and are suited for low-temperature applications [50]. It is possible to control the gas permeability and selectivity by just changing the morphology of the monomers building the polymer [50]. Inorganic membranes have much greater thermal and chemical stability than polymeric membranes [51]. Zeolite and silica porous materials can act as molecular sieves, separating gas molecules by their effective size [50]. Since the effective sizes of $CO_2$, nitrogen, hydrogen, and other gases present in fossil fuel conversion systems are very similar, membrane pore spaces must be controlled on a scale comparable to the size differences among these gas molecules [50]. Unfortunately, the gas separation NM technology is still not that developed, although active research continues in this direction.

### 7.4.2.3 Self-Assembled Monolayers on Mesoporous Supports (SAMMS)

The US Pacific Northwest National Laboratory (PNNL) developed the SAMMS. SAMMS are a combination of mesoporous ceramics (with pore diameters between 2 and 50 nm) and self-assembled chemical monolayers. Both the monolayer and the mesoporous support can be functionalized to remove certain contaminants (e.g., mercury, cadmium) [52]. SAMMS exhibit faster adsorption, higher removal capacity, and better selectivity than many other membrane and sorbent technologies (e.g., ion exchange resins, activated alumina filters, ferric oxide filters). The reason behind the rapid kinetics is attributed to the rigid, open pore structure of SAMMS, which leaves all of the binding sites available at all times to bind contaminant molecules [52].

A variety of SAMMS types exist today. The mostly used material is the thiol-SAMMS. Other important materials are the ethylenediamine-, phosphonate-, hydroxypyridone-, and chelate-SAMMS. SAMMS can be assembled into filters and used for the filtration of water and other liquids. SAMMS types for a great variety of contaminants can be designed. Thiol-SAMMS are currently actively used for the removal of mercury from contaminated fluids. The technology is still too expensive for everyday drinking water treatment applications, but its cost is falling.

### 7.4.2.4 Summary and Conclusions

Nanotechnology has led to the development of a variety of end-of-pipe treatment technologies. CNMs have already reached the commercialization phase. They were shown to treat water faster and more effectively than conventional polycarbonate membranes, and since their cost is constantly falling, they may soon become widely used, even in developing countries. In the context of the global water shortage problem, CNMs may deliver significant water treatment benefits.

Some carbon-based, mesoporous oxide and zeolite membranes have been shown to effectively remove $CO_2$ from industrial effluent gases. These technologies are still tested on the bench scale, but they are expected to deliver powerful solutions in near future, which, when applied in industry, will reduce anthropogenic $CO_2$ emissions and impede the positive climate forcing.

## 7.5 Conclusion

Environmental quality and human health are closely related to each other. Controlling the concentrations of contaminants in the environment reduces the probability that humans will be exposed to chemicals that pose hazards to their health. Controlling pollution involves its monitoring and, if the pollution is excessive, its reduction.

Novel nanoengineered technologies provide more sensitive and reliable air and water monitoring solutions. Since they are more advanced than their conventional counterparts, it is likely that they will replace them in the next 3 to 7 years, when the cost of their application falls and they become market competitive. It is likely that high-quality monitored data, which nanosensors can provide for a great range of environmental contaminants, would be of great benefit for the evaluation of their environmental and human health risks. The more precise risk assessment would contribute to more informed chemical regulation policy, and it would likely invoke the review of some of the current environmental and health programs, which might bring about valuable reforms.

Remediation nanotechnologies are different from each other in the way they remove contaminants from the environment. Some of them use chemical conversion mechanisms such as oxidation and reduction, while others act as catalysts. Despite the differences, however, the effective operation of most depends on the effective surface area of their active materials. The large surface areas of NPs make them more effective for the removal of contaminants than their bulk alternatives and are thus preferred for environmental remediation.

Although no quantitative comparison of the costs of nano-based remedial tools and their conventional counterparts could be accurately conducted at this time, the vast majority of published literature qualitatively describe the nZVI and nano-$TiO_2$ as more cost efficient than their traditional alternatives. Being less costly and more effective in terms of operation, these technologies may soon dominate the market, which would ensure their high impact on the future remediation activities.

Nanotechnology has led to the development of a variety of water and gas end-of-pipe treatment technologies. Many of these technologies are still on the bench scale, but some (e.g., CNMs) are already available and competitive on the market. In the context of the global water shortage problem, technologies such as the CNMs are important breakthroughs with the potential to become widely used and, thus, deliver substantial water treatment benefits.

It is expected that in the very near future, NM technology will offer powerful solutions for $CO_2$ separation from flue gases (i.e., highly selective CNT, polymeric, and zeolite membranes). When applied in industry, these technologies may become a valuable ally in the combat against global warming and thus help protect the health and wellbeing of many people all around the globe.

# References

1. Masciagnoli T. and Zhang W.X. Environmental technologies at the nanoscale, *Environ. Sci. Technol.*, 37, 102A–108A, 2003.
2. *Report From the Workshop Organized by Nanoforum and the Institute for Environment and Sustainability, JRC Ispra.* JRC Ispra: Brussels, 2006. Available online: http://www.nanoforum.org/dateien/temp/Nano%20and%20Environment%20work shop%20report.pdf?28082006150510 (accessed December 2, 2009).
3. *"Pollution" Definition from the Merriam-Webster Online Dictionary.* Available online: http://www.merriam-webster.com/dictionary/pollution (accessed December 2, 2009).
4. *Health Effects of Ozone in the General Population.* United States Environmental Protection Agency: Washington, DC, 1999; Available online: http://www.epa.gov/o3healthtraining/population.html (accessed December 2, 2009).
5. *Health and Environmental Effects of Particulate Matter.* United States Environmental Protection Agency: Washington, DC, 1997; Available online: http://www.epa.gov/Region7/programs/artd/air/quality/pmhealth.htm (accessed December 2, 2009).

6. *Volatile Organic Compounds Health Effects Fact Sheet.* Colorado department for Public Health and the Environment (CDPHE): Denver, 2000. Available online: http://www.cdphe.state.co.us/hm/schlage/vocfactsheet.pdf (accessed December 2, 2009).

7. *Public Health Statement: Sulfur Dioxide.* Agency for Toxic Substances and Disease Registry (ATSDR): Atlanta, 1998. Available online: http://www.atsdr.cdc.gov/toxprofiles/tp116-c1-b.pdf (accessed December 2, 2009).

8. *Pesticides: Health and Safety: Human Health Issues.* United States Environmental Protection Agency: Washington, DC, 2009; Available online: http://www.epa.gov/opp00001/health/human.htm (accessed December 2, 2009).

9. *Consumer Factsheet on: Nitrates/Nitrites.* United States Environmental Protection Agency: Washington, DC, 2009; Available online: http://www.epa.gov/OGWDW/contaminants/dw_contamfs/nitrates.html (accessed December 2, 2009).

10. *The POPs Issue and Effects to Human Health.* Environmental Management Bureau-Department of Environment and Natural Resources, Environmental Quality Division: Quezon, Philippines, 2009; Available online: http://www.emb.gov.ph/eeid/pops.htm (accessed December 2, 2009).

11. *Working Group on Environmental Monitoring and Assessment: Environmental Monitoring and Reporting.* United Nations Economic Commission for Europe (UNECE): Geneva, Switzerland, 2008; Available online: http://www.unece.org/env/europe/monitoring/EnvMonRep/ (accessed December 2, 2009).

12. Rickerby D. and Morrison M. Nanotechnology and the environment: A European perspective, *J. Sci. Technol. Adv. Mater.*, 8, 19–24, 2006.

13. Chou J. *Hazardous Gas Monitors: A Practical Guide to Selection, Operation, and Applications*, 1st Ed., McGraw-Hill Professional, New York, 1999, Chap. 1.

14. Capone S. et al. Solid state gas sensors: State of the art and future activities, *J. Optoelectron. Adv. Mater.*, 5, 1335–1348, 2003.

15. Diéguez A. et al. Nanoparticle engineering for gas sensor optimisation: Improved sol–gel fabricated nanocrystalline $SnO_2$ thick film gas sensor for $NO_2$ detection by calcination, catalytic metal introduction and grinding treatments, *Sens. Actuators B*, 60, 125–137, 1999.

16. Rius F., Jiménez-Cadena G., and Riu J. Gas sensors based on nanostructured materials, *Analyst*, 132, 1083–1099, 2007.

17. Dutta J., Pummakarnchana O., and Tripatha, N. Air pollution monitoring and GIS modeling: A new use of nanotechnology based solid state gas sensors, *J. Sci. Technol. Adv. Mater.*, 6, 251–255, 2005.

18. Schena M. *Microarray Biochip Technology*, 1st Ed., Eaton Publishing, Westborough, 2000, Chap. 1.

19. *Directive 2000/60/EC of the European Parliament and of the Council of 23 October 2000 Establishing a Framework for Community Action in the Field of Water Policy.* European Parliament and of the Council of the EU: Brussels, Belgium, 2000; Available online: http://eur-lex.europa.eu/LexUriServ/LexUriServ.do?uri = CONSLEG:2000L0060:20011216:EN:PDF (accessed December 2, 2009).

20. *Immunochemical Analysis of Environmental Samples.* United States Environmental Protection Agency, Environmental Sciences Division: Las Vegas, NV, USA, 1999; Available online: http://www.epa.gov/esd/factsheets/iaes.pdf (accessed December 2, 2009).

21. Proll G. and Gauglitz G. Nanostructured environmental biochemical sensor for water monitoring, presented at Nanotechnology and the Environment workshop, Brussels, Belgium, March 30–31, 2006, 5.

22. *United States Environmental Protection Agency Nanotechnology White Paper.* United States Environmental Protection Agency: Washington, DC, 2007; Available online: http://www.epa.gov/osa/pdfs/nanotech/epa-nanotechnology-whitepaper-0207.pdf (accessed December 2, 2009).

23. *Databases of Innovative Technologies.* United States Environmental Protection Agency: Washington, DC, 2003; Available online: http://www.epa.gov/tio/databases/ (accessed December 2, 2009).

24. Zhang W. Nanoscale iron particles for environmental remediation: An overview, *J. Nanopart. Res.*, 5, 323–332, 2003. With permission.

25. Watlington K. *Emerging Nanotechnologies for Site Remediation and Wastewater Treatment.* North Carolina State University: Raleigh, NC, 2005; Available online: http://www.clu-in.org/download/techdrct/K_Watlington_Nanotech.pdf (accessed December 2, 2009).

26. Tratnyek P. and Johnson R. Nanotechnologies for environmental cleanup, *Nanotoday*, 1, 44–48, 2006.

27. Latif B. *Nanotechnology for Site Remediation: Fate and Transport of Nanoparticles in Soil and Water Systems.* University of Arizona: Tucson, AZ, 2006; Available online: http://www.clu-in.org/download/studentpapers/B_Latif_Nanotechology.pdf (accessed December 2, 2009).

28. Beck B. and Cocoros M. Use of nanoscale zero-valent iron (nZVI) particles for groundwater remediation: A qualitative risk assessment, presented at *22nd Annual International Conference on Soils, Sediments and Water*, Amherst, October 16–19, 2006, 3.

29. Nowack B. Environmental behavior and effects of engineered metal and metal oxide nanoparticles, in *Heavy Metals in the Environment*, Lawrence K. et al., Eds., Taylor & Francis and CRC Press, New York, 2009, Chap. 3.

30. Nagaveni K. et al. Photocatalytic degradation of organic compounds over combustion-synthesized nano-$TiO_2$, *Environ. Sci. Technol.*, 38, 1600–1604, 2004.

31. Hoffmann M.R. et al. Environmental applications of semiconductor photocatalysis, *Chem. Rev.*, 95, 69–96, 1995.

32. Rajeshwar K. et al. Titania-based heterogeneous photocatalysis. Materials, mechanistic issues and implications for environmental remediation, *J. Pure Appl. Chem.*, 73, 1849–1860, 2001.

33. Chen Y. et al. Preparation of a novel $TiO_2$-based p–n junction nanotube photocatalyst, *Environ. Sci. Technol.*, 39, 1201–1208, 2005.

34. Mueller N. and Nowack B. Exposure modeling of engineered nanoparticles in the environment, *Environ. Sci. Technol.*, 42, 4447, 2008.

35. Boxall AB et al. Engineered nanomaterials in soils and water: How do they behave and could they pose a risk to human health? *Nanomedicine*, 2, 919–927, 2007.

36. Tungittiplakorn W. et al. Engineered polymeric nanoparticles for soil remediation, *Environ. Sci. Technol.*, 38, 1605–1610, 2005.

37. Yeom I., Ghosh M., and Cox C. Kinetic aspects of surfactant solubilization of soil-bound polycyclic aromatic hydrocarbons, *Environ. Sci. Technol.*, 30, 1589–1595, 1996.

38. Chasteen N. and Harrison P. Mineralization in ferritin: An efficient means of iron storage, *J. Struct. Biol.*, 126, 182–194, 1999.
39. Kim I. et al. Photochemical reactivity of ferritin for Cr (VI) reduction, *Chem. Mater.*, 14, 4874–4879, 2002.
40. Bonn D. Nanoparticles clean-up, *Front. Ecol. Environ.*, 2, 400, 2004.
41. Kim J. and Grate J. Nano-biotechnology in using enzymes for environmental remediation: Single enzyme nanoparticles, *J. Nanotechnol. Environ.*, 29, 220–225, 2004.
42. Alcalde M. et al. Environmental biocatalysis: From remediation with enzymes to novel green processes, *Trends Biotechnol.*, 24, 283–287, 2006.
43. Wagner J. *Membrane Filtration Handbook*, 2nd Ed., Osmonics Inc., 2001. With permission.
44. *Overview and Comparison of Conventional Water Treatment Technologies and Nanobased Treatment Technologies.* Meridian Institute: Dillon, CO, 2005; Available online: http://www.merid.org/nano/watertechpaper/watertechpaper.pdf (accessed December 2, 2009).
45. Srivastava A. et al. Carbon nanotube filters, *Nat. Mater.*, 3, 610, 2004.
46. Jordan P. et al. Characterizing fault-plume intersection probability for geologic carbon sequestration risk assessment, presented at *Greenhouse Gas Control Technologies (GHGT) Conference*, Washington, DC, November 16–20, 2008, 6.
47. Kvamme B. and Liu S. Reactive transport of $CO_2$ in saline aquifers with implicit geomechanical analysis, *En. Proc.*, 1, 3267–3274, 2009.
48. Nicota J. et al. Pressure perturbations from geologic carbon sequestration: Area-of-review boundaries and borehole leakage driving forces, *Energy Procedia*, 1, 47–54, 2009.
49. Zhang Y. et al. Probability estimation of $CO_2$ leakage through faults at geologic carbon sequestration sites, *Energy Procedia*, 1, 41–46, 2009.
50. Fujioka Y. et al. *Development of Innovative Gas Separation Membranes Through Sub-nanoscale Materials Control.* Research Institute of Innovative Technology for the Earth (RITE): Tokyo, Japan, 2009. Available online: http://gcep.stanford.edu/pdfs/-IUwoO0omIeF6HDYZPqYeg/4.5.2_Fujioka_Web_Public_2009.pdf (accessed December 2, 2009).
51. Kai T., Kazama S., and Fujioka Y. Development of cesium-incorporated carbon membranes for $CO_2$ separation under humid conditions, *J. Memb. Sci.*, 342, 14–21, 2009.
52. *SAMMS Technical Summary.* Pacific Northwest National Laboratory (PNNL): Richland, WA, 2008; Available online: http://samms.pnl.gov/samms.pdf (accessed December 2, 2009).

# Section V

# Nanotoxicology Overview and Problems

# 8

# In Vitro *Study for Nanomaterials*

**Seishiro Hirano and Karim Maghni**

## CONTENTS

## 8.1 Dose Metrics in *In Vitro* Study

Particles are taken up by cells through the process of phagocytosis or endocytosis. Phagocytosis is a major pathway for natural immune-related cells such as macrophages, monocytes, and neutrophils as a host defense mechanism against microorganisms, whereas endocytosis occurs in all types of cells. Phagocytosis of opsonized particles is initiated after cell membrane receptors recognize ligands such as Fcγ and C3bi on the particles. Actin molecules are assembled and the cell membrane extends around the opsonized particle like a zipper closure. On the other hand, endocytosis is initiated by invagination of the cell membranes. In either case, the cell membrane is finally pinched off and the particle is carried inside the cell. In general, particles >1 μm are taken up by phagocytosis and particles <200 nm by endocytosis. The differences between phagocytosis and endocytosis are schematically presented in Figure 8.1. Thus, nanoparticles are more likely taken up by cells via the endocytic pathway unless they are agglomerated [1].

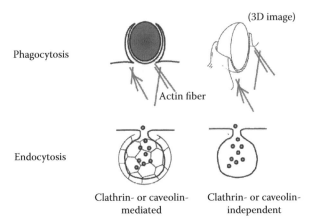

**FIGURE 8.1**
Schematic presentation of phagocytosis and endocytosis. (Adapted from Conner, S.D. and Schmid, S.L., *Nature*, 422, 37, 2003.)

The suspended particles in the culture medium reach the cell monolayer by either diffusional movement or gravitational settling. The time for a particle to travel to the target cell by diffusion is calculated using the following equation:

$$t = \frac{r^2}{2D}, \quad D = \frac{RT}{6N\mu d} \tag{8.1}$$

where
$t$ = average time to reach to the target
$r$ = distance to the target
$D$ = diffusion coefficient (m$^2$ s$^{-1}$)
$R$ = gas constant (8.31 J K-mol$^{-1}$)
$N$ = Avogadoro number (6.02 × 10$^{23}$ mol$^{-1}$)
$\mu$ = viscosity (kg m$^{-1}$ s$^{-1}$)
$d$ = diameter of a particle (m)

On the other hand, gravitational settling is determined by Stoke's law and the time for the particle to settle onto the target cell is expressed by the following equation:

$$t = \frac{r}{v}, \quad v = \frac{2g(\rho_p - \rho_m)d^2}{9\mu} \tag{8.2}$$

where

$v$ = average settling velocity (m s$^{-1}$)
$g$ = gravity acceleration (9.8 m s$^{-2}$)
$\rho_p$ = density of a particle (kg m$^{-3}$)
$\rho_m$ = density of medium (kg m$^{-3}$)

Accordingly, a smaller particle travels in the medium and reaches the target predominantly by diffusional movement and larger and heavier particles settle to the target monolayer by gravitational settling. An image showing how a particle reaches the target cell is shown in Figure 8.2. In general, particles of ca. 50 nm take more time than particles of other sizes to reach the cell monolayer under the usual culture condition because both gravitational settling and diffusional movement are less effective for particles of this size to reach the target cell [2].

A nanoparticle has a large specific surface area and is usually coated with a larger amount of proteins than larger particles are in the culture system. Thus, understanding the particle–protein interaction or the "corona" formation on the nanoparticles is important to investigate the effects of nanoparticles in *in vitro* culture systems. For example, human serum albumin forms a 3.3-nm-thick monolayer on quantum dots and the residential time of albumin on the surface is approximately 100 s [3]. Culture media usually contain biomolecules that are adsorbed on and desorbed from the surface of particles. Thus, the "corona" can be an important determinant for the reactivity of particles with the cells.

Unless nanoparticles are labeled with fluorescence or radioisotopes, quantitative measurement of cellular uptake of nanoparticles is usually difficult. However, as most of nanoparticles are not soluble and refractory, an optical method such as turbidimetry is possible for quantitative measurement of nanoparticles. After lysis of the cells, carbon nanotubes taken up by bronchial epithelial cells were evaluated by turbidimetry (optical density = 640 nm). This simple method enables measurement of <1 µg of multiwalled carbon nanotubes (MWCNTs) per well of a common six-well culture dish [4].

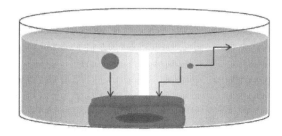

**FIGURE 8.2**
Gravitational settling (left large particle) and diffusional movement (right small particle) to reach to target cell.

## 8.2 Preparation of Nanoparticle Suspension

One of the most serious problems scientists face about *in vitro* nanotoxicology studies is that nanoparticles are not stable in the culture medium and are easily agglomerated. Thus, most of the nanoparticles are usually no longer in the nanosize when they reach the target cells. Nonetheless, the microenvironment where the cell reacts with the agglomerate should be the surface of each nanoparticle, and the total surface area of the agglomerate is almost the same as the sum of the surface area of each single nanoparticle. The cells recognize the outer surface of a particle. Thus, if the particle is porous, the outer surface area of the particle is much smaller than the total surface area measured by the BET (Brunauer-Emmett-Teller) method.

It appears impossible to disperse the particles completely into single particles at concentrations for the practical *in vitro* toxicology experiments (0.1 μg mL$^{-1}$ to 1 mg mL$^{-1}$). To avoid the production of larger agglomerates, *in vitro* toxicologists use different types of detergents. Table 8.1 shows the detergents used in *in vitro* nanotoxicology studies with the rationale to use each detergent. The particle suspension is usually sonicated just before addition to the culture so that the best dispersion is achieved. However, the suspension of nanoparticles is not stable in the culture medium and the particles may start to agglomerate before they reach the target cells. Thus, the cellular response to nanoparticles in the *in vitro* culture system is usually the outcome of complex exposure processes, and the suspended nanoparticles should be characterized when introduced into the culture medium to redefine particle sizes and shapes.

**TABLE 8.1**

Detergents Used in *In Vitro* Nanotoxicology

| Detergent | Type | Rationale |
|---|---|---|
| Serum | Natural | The cells are usually cultured in the presence of 10% fetal bovine serum and the serum may not affect the cells |
| DPPC (dipalmitoylphosphatidylcholine) | Natural | The alveolar surface is covered with surfactant and DPPC is a major component of the lung surfactant |
| Pluronic F68 | Artificial | Nonpyrogenic and "cell culture" type is commercially available |
| Tween 20/80 | Artificial | Nonionic common detergent in biochemistry |
| Humic or fulvic acid | Natural | These are geosolvents and useful for aquatic toxicology (fish, *Daphnia*) |

## 8.3 Cell Type-Based Approach

Various types of cells have been used in *in vitro* nanotoxicology studies depending on the target organ of interest. However, pulmonary cells and macrophages are the most popular among the cell types, probably because the inhalational route is the most probable route of exposure to nanoparticles in industrial and atmospheric environments. The types of cells used in nanotoxicology studies are shown in Table 8.2.

### 8.3.1 Macrophages/Monocytes

Macrophages are phagocytic cells and they engulf a variety of particulate substances efficiently. It is also possible to differentiate monocytic cell lines such as THP-1 and U937 into macrophage-like cells by using a stimulant such as phorbol myristate acetate. Nanomaterials or nanoparticles usually occur as agglomerates, and alveolar macrophages are the primary target cells when nanoparticles are inhaled. It has been shown that polystyrene particles of particle size from 20 to 1000 nm are taken up through a phagocytotic receptor named MARCO (macrophage receptor with collagenous structure). Polystyrene beads of 20 nm were found agglomerated on the plasma membrane and were probably recognized by the cells as larger-sized particles [5]. Carbon and diesel exhaust nanoparticles generate reactive oxygen species (ROS) and cause lipid peroxidation [6–8]. The plasma membrane is seriously damaged when macrophages are exposed to carbon nanotubes [9]. Accordingly, macrophages became necrotic rather than apoptotic after exposure to carbon nanotubes.

**TABLE 8.2**

Cell Types Used in Nanotoxicology Studies Except for Primary Cells

| Cell Type | Cell Name |
| --- | --- |
| Macrophage/monocyte | RAW264.7 (mouse), J774 (mouse), NR8383 (rat), THP-1 (human), U937 (human), HL-60 (human), MonoMac 6 (human) |
| Lung/bronchial cell | A549 (human), SV40-T2 (rat), L2 (rat), Calu-3 (human), BEAS-2B (human) |
| Fibroblast/keratinocyte | NIH-3T3 (mouse), L929 (mouse), HaCaT (human) |
| Endothelial cell, heart/ cardiac cells | HUVEC (human), pulmonary artery cells (human, porcine) |
| Mesothelial cell | MeT-5A (human), MSTO (human) |
| Neural cells | PC12 (rat) |
| Others | Hela (human), germ line cell |

### 8.3.2 Lung and Bronchial Epithelial Cells

The rat lung epithelial cells (L2) appear to be more sensitive to nanoparticles than macrophages [10]. Ultrafine carbon black particles cause oxidative stress–mediated proliferation in endothelial cells [11]. Silicon carbide (SiC) nanoparticles have been shown to cause glutathione depletion and genotoxic effects as examined with the comet assay in A549 human lung epithelial cells, although the cytotoxic effect of SiC nanoparticles was limited [12]. Carbon nanotubes seem to activate nuclear factor-κB, enhance the phosphorylation of MAP kinase pathway components such as p38, and increase the production of proinflammatory cytokines in bronchial epithelial cells [4].

### 8.3.3 Fibroblasts

It was reported that the amount of ceria of various sizes incorporated into human lung fibroblasts largely depended on the particle size and number density, and the surface area was a minor factor [13]. Titanium dioxide nanoparticles increased the number of lysosomes and oxidative stress, and accordingly damaged cytoplasmic organelles and plasma membrane in L929 fibroblasts [14]. Titanium dioxide nanoparticles have also been shown to induce micronuclei and apoptosis in Syrian hamster embryo fibroblasts [15].

### 8.3.4 Endothelial Cell and Heart/Cardiac Cells

Exposure of endothelial cells to aluminum nanoparticles increased both mRNA and protein levels of adhesion molecules such as VCAM-1, ICAM-1, and ELAM-1 [16]. Several lines of evidence suggest that acute exposure to airborne fine particles increases the risk of mortality and morbidity associated with cardiovascular diseases [17]. A gene profiling study using cDNA microarray indicated that exposure to atmospheric nanoparticles upregulated the transcription of genes related to inflammation and clotting, suggesting that those particles may cause adverse cardiovascular health effects [18]. Diesel exhaust nanoparticles and titanium dioxide nanoparticles cause oxidative stress and changes in myofibrillar structure in ventricular cardiomyocytes [19]. Exposure to carbon black nanoparticles also increase the production of proinflammatory cytokines such as IL-6, IL-1β, and TNFα [20], and reduced the expression of connexin 37 and eNOS [21]. Carbon black nanoparticles cause those inflammatory responses in endothelial cells by an ROS-dependent pathway because induction of vascular endothelial growth factors by carbon black nanoparticles was reduced by the antioxidant N-acetylcysteine, a molecule known to increase glutathione levels [22].

### 8.3.5 Neural, Mesothelial, and Other Cells

Mesothelial cells (MSTO) are more sensitive to ferric oxide and cerium oxide nanoparticles than fibroblasts (3T3), while the cytotoxicity of zinc oxide nanoparticles are not different between those two cell types [23]. Unmodified quantum dots increased both extracellular calcium influx and internal calcium release from endoplasmic reticulum and caused cell death in rat primary hippocampal neurons [24]. TiO$_2$ nanoparticles caused intracellular formation of ROS in mouse neuronal and glial cells, whereas exposure to carbon black and superparamagnetic Fe$_2$O$_3$ nanoparticles induced no significant changes in free radical levels [25]. Silver nanoparticles were more cytotoxic than molybdenum nanoparticles, and nanoparticulates were more cytotoxic than the corresponding soluble salts in mouse spermatogonial stem cell line for identical concentrations [26].

## 8.4 Nanomaterial-Based Approach

Nanomaterials are categorized into several groups according to their chemical properties. The most important category is a group of carbon substances such as fullerenes, single-walled carbon nanotubes and MWCNTs, carbon black, and silicon carbide. Other groups of industrial or manufactured nanomaterials are metals such as nanosilver, nanogold, and nanoplatinum; metal oxides such as titanium dioxide, silicon dioxide, and zinc oxide; ceramics such as nanoclay; and organic substances such as dendrimers. Several lines of evidence indicate that the acute toxicity of nanoparticles linearly correlates to the surface area and a classic mass-based dose (mg mL$^{-1}$ or mg cm$^{-2}$) may not be an appropriate metric for nanoparticles [27,28]. It should also be noted that the adverse effects of pure silica zeolites largely depend on the aspect ratio (length vs. width) and the external surface area [27]. It was established that the cytotoxicity of silica particles of different sizes and shapes could be estimated by the following relation:

$$-\ln(1 - y) = ktm \qquad (8.3)$$

where
   $y =$ cell growth inhibition rate ($0 \leq y \leq 1$, $y = 1$, when $m$ has no effect)
   $k =$ constant
   $t =$ time of culture with dusts
   $m =$ dust property (surface area, aspect ratio, radical release, length, etc.)

The high correlation coefficient was obtained in the relation between cytotoxicity and external surface area ($r = 0.953$) or aspect ratio ($r = 0.909$). The aspect ratio is expressed as $(a/\sqrt{bc})$, where $a$, $b$, and $c$ are the three dimensions of a particle and $a$ is the longest side.

An engineered nanoparticle is defined as an intentionally produced particle that has at least one dimension from 1 to 100 nm. However, the toxicological aspects of "nonbulk" materials may emerge from the intrinsic properties such as surface energy and generation of ROS rather than the extrinsic property (size) of nanoparticles [29]. Many toxicological studies suggest that once the toxicological effects are normalized by specific surface area, no significant size-dependent effects would be observed. However, real size-dependent differences are expected in inorganic nanoparticles between <30 nm and >30 nm particles because of "nano-effects" [29].

The theoretical relation between N and S assuming a particle is cuboidal is calculated by Equation 8.4 and the result is shown in Figure 8.3.

$$S = \frac{N^3 - (N-2)^3}{N^3} \qquad (8.4)$$

where
  $S$ = ratio of surface atoms to total atoms
  $N$ = number of atom on one dimension

Thus, the surface of a nanoparticle is exposed to the biological environment very efficiently compared with that of a larger particle.

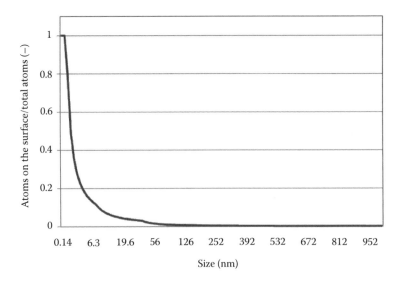

**FIGURE 8.3**
Rate of surface to total iron atoms (atomic diameter = 0.14 nm) assuming that iron particle is cubic.

Of particular interest to nanotoxicologists is the shape of a particle. Asbestos is a fibrous silicate particle that has a high aspect ratio (1:3). The shape of carbon nanotubes is very similar to that of chrysotile asbestos. Although carbon nanotubes are not made of silicates, both asbestos and carbon nanotubes are biopersistent and probably cause similar cellular responses (e.g., for the induction of lung fibrosis).

It has been shown that positively charged nanoparticles are taken up more rapidly via the clathrin-mediated endocytotic pathway than negatively charged nanoparticles [30]. This phenomenon is also proved in the *in vivo* study. When cationic quantum dots were injected into the lung, particles were retained in the lung tissue, while noncationic quantum dots translocated to the extrapulmonary tissues very quickly [31]. The cell surface is negatively charged because of the presence of sialic acid residues of glycoproteins on the plasma membrane, which is the reason why cationic nanoparticles interact quickly and strongly with cells. The trafficking of positively charged polystyrene nanoparticles in rat alveolar epithelial cell monolayers was 20–40 times faster than that of highly negatively charged polystyrene particles [32]. However, the interaction of nanoparticles with red blood cells does not seem to be influenced by the cell surface charge [33]. It should be noted that silica and titanium dioxide particles have negative zeta-potential, while zirconium oxide and cerium oxide particles have positive zeta-potential in pure water. However, the zeta-potential of all those particles shifts to around –18 mV in cell culture medium because of adsorption of proteins [13]. As to metal oxide nanoparticles, solubility was the major factor determining the cytotoxicity of nanoparticles in both mesothelial cells and fibroblasts [23].

## 8.5 Implications and Recommendation for *In Vitro* Study

The *in vitro* study is more appropriate for investigating the "toxicity mechanism" and is not directly linked with "regulation issues." However, once the standard methods are established, the *in vitro* toxicity assay can be used for screening various nanomaterials. As physicochemical characteristics and minor components of nanomaterials vary among industrial nanomaterial products, rapid, reproducible, and accurate screening methods should be developed for the beneficial use of nanomaterials. In this context, the international harmonization research strategy is very important for the standardization of *in vitro* toxicity assay methods of nanomaterials. One of the most difficult issues regarding *in vitro* toxicity assay is to disperse test samples. Especially carbon-based nanomaterials such as carbon nanotubes and fullerene are difficult substances to disperse in culture medium, and the toxicity outcome would be completely different between well-dispersed and agglomerated samples. Biologically inactive and pyrogen-free detergent can be used as long as the stability and characterization of the suspension are documented in detail so that experts can judge the toxicity of the substances and estimate the hazardous level for human health. Of particular interest, the unique physicochemical properties of some nanoparticles (e.g., carbon nanotubes) create interferences with components of some cytotoxic assays, leading to false conclusion on those nanoparticles' potential biosafety [34]. Therefore, several different methods are recommended to be used to validate the *in vitro* nanotoxicity data. Therefore, we also recommend that nanotoxicological studies should include as a first experimental step, the determination of potential interferences of nanoparticles with reagents of cytotoxic assays in a free-cell system.

Which metrics should be appropriate to measure the toxicity of nanoparticles quantitatively is still a matter of argument. The toxicity of nanofibers may be evaluated on the count concentration rather than mass concentration because thin fibers can be more toxic than thick fibers. If nanoparticles are to be dissolved, the mass concentration is more preferable because ionic forms may be more toxic than insoluble forms. If the surface of nanoparticles is highly reactive with biomolecules, the surface area is probably a more proper measure for the toxicity.

## References

1. Conner, S.D. and Schmid, S.L. Regulated portals of entry into the cell. *Nature*, 422, 37–44, 2003.
2. Teeguarden, J.G. et al. Particokinetics *in vitro*: Dosimetry considerations for *in vitro* nanoparticle toxicity assessments. *Toxicol. Sci.*, 95, 300–312, 2007.
3. Rocker, C. et al. A quantitative fluorescence study of protein monolayer formation on colloidal nanoparticles. *Nat. Nanotechnol.*, 4, 577–580, 2009.
4. Hirano, S. et al. Uptake and cytotoxic effects of multi-walled carbon nanotubes in human bronchial epithelial cells. *Toxicol. Appl. Pharmacol.*, 249, 8–15, 2010.
5. Kanno, S., Furuyama, A., and Hirano, S. A murine scavenger receptor MARCO recognizes polystyrene nanoparticles. *Toxicol. Sci.*, 97, 398–406, 2007.
6. Aam, B.B. and Fonnum, F. Carbon black particles increase reactive oxygen species formation in rat alveolar macrophages *in vitro*. *Arch. Toxicol.*, 81, 441–446, 2007.
7. Lundborg, M. et al. Aggregates of ultrafine particles modulate lipid peroxidation and bacterial killing by alveolar macrophages. *Environ. Res.*, 104, 250–257, 2007.
8. Foucaud, L. et al. Measurement of reactive species production by nanoparticles prepared in biologically relevant media. *Toxicol. Lett.*, 174, 1–9, 2007.
9. Hirano, S., Kanno, S., and Furuyama, A. Multi-walled carbon nanotubes injure the plasma membrane of macrophages. *Toxicol. Appl. Pharmacol.*, 232, 244–251, 2008.

10. Sayes, C.M., Reed, K.L., and Warheit, D.B. Assessing toxicity of fine and nanoparticles: Comparing *in vitro* measurements to *in vivo* pulmonary toxicity profiles. *Toxicol. Sci.*, 97, 163–180, 2007.
11. Tamaoki, J. et al. Ultrafine carbon black particles stimulate proliferation of human airway epithelium via EGF receptor-mediated signaling pathway. *Am. J. Physiol. Lung Cell. Mol. Physiol.*, 287, L1127–L1133, 2004.
12. Barillet, S. et al. *In vitro* evaluation of SiC nanoparticles impact on A549 pulmonary cells: Cyto-, genotoxicity and oxidative stress. *Toxicol. Lett.*, 198, 324–330, 2010.
13. Limbach, L.K. et al. Oxide nanoparticle uptake in human lung fibroblasts: Effects of particle size, agglomeration, and diffusion at low concentrations. *Environ. Sci. Technol.*, 39, 9370–9376, 2005.
14. Jin, C.Y. et al. Cytotoxicity of titanium dioxide nanoparticles in mouse fibroblast cells. *Chem. Res. Toxicol.*, 21, 1871–1877, 2008.
15. Rahman, Q. et al. Evidence that ultrafine titanium dioxide induces micronuclei and apoptosis in Syrian hamster embryo fibroblasts. *Environ. Health Perspect.*, 110, 797–800, 2002.
16. Oesterling, E. et al. Alumina nanoparticles induce expression of endothelial cell adhesion molecules. *Toxicol. Lett.*, 178, 160–166, 2008.
17. Dockery, D.W. et al. An association between air pollution and mortality in six U.S. cities. *N. Engl. J. Med.*, 329, 1753–1759, 1993.
18. Karoly, E.D. et al. Up-regulation of tissue factor in human pulmonary artery endothelial cells after ultrafine particle exposure. *Environ. Health Perspect.*, 115, 535–540, 2007.
19. Helfenstein, M. et al. Effects of combustion-derived ultrafine particles and manufactured nanoparticles on heart cells *in vitro*. *Toxicology*, 253, 70–78, 2008.
20. Totlandsdal, A.I. et al. Pro-inflammatory potential of ultrafine particles in mono- and co-cultures of primary cardiac cells. *Toxicology*, 247, 23–32, 2008.
21. Yamawaki, H. and Iwai, N. Mechanisms underlying nano-sized air-pollution-mediated progression of atherosclerosis: Carbon black causes cytotoxic injury / inflammation and inhibits cell growth in vascular endothelial cells. *Circ. J.*, 70, 129–140, 2006.
22. Chang, C.C. et al. The induction of vascular endothelial growth factor by ultra-fine carbon black contributes to the increase of alveolar-capillary permeability. *Environ. Health Perspect.*, 113, 454–460, 2005.
23. Brunner, T.J. et al. *In vitro* cytotoxicity of oxide nanoparticles: Comparison to asbestos, silica, and the effect of particle solubility. *Environ. Sci. Technol.*, 40, 4374–4381, 2006.
24. Tang, M. et al. Unmodified CdSe quantum dots induce elevation of cytoplasmic calcium levels and impairment of functional properties of sodium channels in rat primary cultured hippocampal neurons. *Environ. Health Perspect.*, 116, 915–922, 2008.
25. Gramowski, A. et al. Nanoparticles induce changes of the electrical activity of neuronal networks on microelectrode array neurochips. *Environ. Health Perspect.*, 118, 1363–1369, 2010.
26. Braydich-Stolle, L. et al. *In vitro* cytotoxicity of nanoparticles in mammalian germline stem cells. *Toxicol. Sci.*, 88, 412–419, 2005.

27. Fenoglio, I. et al. Pure-silica zeolites (Porosils) as model solids for the evaluation of the physicochemical features determining silica toxicity to macrophages. *Chem. Res. Toxicol.*, 13, 489–500, 2000.
28. Oberdorster, G., Oberdorster, E., and Oberdorster, J. Nanotoxicology: An emerging discipline evolving from studies of ultrafine particles. *Environ. Health Perspect.*, 113, 823–839, 2005.
29. Auffan, M. et al. Towards a definition of inorganic nanoparticles from an environmental, health and safety perspective. *Nat. Nanotechnol.*, 4, 634–641, 2009.
30. Harush-Frenkel, O. et al. Targeting of nanoparticles to the clathrin-mediated endocytic pathway. *Biochem. Biophys. Res. Commun.*, 353, 26–32, 2007.
31. Choi, H.S. et al. Rapid translocation of nanoparticles from the lung airspaces to the body. *Nat. Biotechnol.*, 28, 1300–1303, 2010.
32. Yacobi, N.R. et al. Polystyrene nanoparticle trafficking across alveolar epithelium. *Nanomedicine*, 4, 139–145, 2008.
33. Rothen-Rutishauser, B.M. et al. Interaction of fine particles and nanoparticles with red blood cells visualized with advanced microscopic techniques. *Environ. Sci. Technol.*, 40, 4353–4359, 2006.
34. Wörle-Knirsch, J.M., Pulskamp, K., and Krug, H.F. Oops they did it again! Carbon nanotubes hoax scientists in viability assays. *Nano Lett.*, 6, 1261–1268, 2006.

# 9

# Toxicokinetics and Interaction of Nanoparticles with Biological Matrices

**Claude Emond**

## CONTENTS

## 9.1 Introduction

Toxicological studies provide information on the defined disease mechanisms, based on dose–response relations and related to the nanoparticle (NP) characteristics that influence toxicity, including the size, surface area, chemistry or reactivity, solubility, and shape. Toxicology studies aim to determine the biological plausibility of health effects from NPs and to identify cascades of mechanisms that are causal for the gradual transition from the physiological status toward pathophysiological alterations, and eventually chronic diseases. Until recently, all toxicological experiments focusing on NPs described the external exposure or the *in vitro* characterization [1]. Techniques for measuring NPs in various biological and chemical matrices are also outlined [2]. The toxicology field is currently well positioned to understand the biological relevance between NPs and biological issues. Nanotoxicokinetics is a branch of toxicology and a new area in which this field evaluates NPs at the local and systemic levels. Nanotoxicokinetics is focused on understanding and predicting what is going to happen to the xenobiotics in the biota. Typically, we segment nanotoxicokinetics into four different steps, namely absorption, distribution, metabolism, and excretion (ADME). In the past, we did not imagine that particles might affect tissues at the systemic level. The nanotoxicology field is also considering the interaction between insoluble NPs and biological systems (e.g., body fluids, proteins, and cells).

We recognize now that NPs, ranging from 1 to 100 nm, can cross the biological membrane and they can be translocated inside of cell organelles or entities such as the mitochondria, lysosome, and nucleus. Therefore, the potential health risk will depend on the magnitude and nature of the exposures with NPs, and on the physical behavior of this particle related to dispersion, translocation, and deposition. The NPs have posed a new dilemma because they can migrate to body compartments away from the application site or deposition sites. In particular, because of their low uptake by macrophages, NPs are absorbed by endothelial cells, and they have access to cells in the epithelium, the interstitium, and the vascular endothelium [3]. The ability of low and toxic poorly soluble particulates such as carbon black and titanium dioxide ($TiO_2$) to induce chronic inflammation, fibrosis, neoplastic lesions, or lung tumors in rats has been well established [4]. Considering these challenges, it is important to understand the route taken by this new xenobiotic particulate structure (e.g., NPs). We are between the curative and toxicity impact with this new technology. Many of the exposure assessments related to a nanomaterial can be approached as a logical subset of traditional exposure assessment for chemical hazards in the workplace and the environment [5].

The objectives of this chapter are to highlight some limiting steps related to nanotoxicokinetics, and to emphasize the difficulty of finding pertinent information because there is a lack of data in toxicology. To respond to these objectives, our effort focused on the ADME steps. The absorption step explored the different routes by which NPs can reach the systemic circulation, and then target tissue in the organism. The major ways of exposure were oral, inhalation, and the cutaneous routes. Following absorption, NPs are distributed in the organism, are free to bind to proteins, and are incorporated in specialized cells. Biotransformation will only be briefly mentioned because commercial NPs are not easily degraded unless they are functionalized with a long-chain peptide or an unstable group of NPs. Section 9.4 will discuss excretion, or externalization of the NPs, and the impact of this action.

## 9.2 Absorption

Absorption is the procedure by which a xenobiotic can cross the biological barrier from the environment into the organism. Absorption of NPs can occur via the oral route from the gastrointestinal tract (GIT), in the lung (inhalation), and across the skin (cutaneous). These routes have different properties and degrees of penetration depending on the characteristics of the NPs.

## 9.2.1 Oral Absorption

According to the literature, mice, rats, sheep, pigs, and cows can absorb NPs from the GIT. Florence [6] observed that the ability of intact microparticles and NPs to be absorbed through the gut walls was different. A literature consensus mentioned that the absorption increases with decreasing particle diameter. The uptake of inert NPs has been shown to occur transcellulary through normal enterocytes and Peyer's patch (PP) via M cells and to lesser extent across paracellular pathways [7]. The absorption can also occur by a mechanism of persorption, which gave rise to contemporary studies of particulate absorption NPs, such as polystyrene latex, that have been recognized as a useful model because they do not easily degrade. This study confirmed that NPs ranging from 50 to 100 nm in diameter reached the maximal absorption rate. However, NPs >1 μm are being trapped in the PP [8,9]. It seems that at this size, NPs are not translocated to the systemic circulation.

Oral absorption is influenced by different characteristics related to the NPs (e.g., diameter, surface chemistry, surface ligands, shape and elasticity, physical and chemical stability) [7]. In general, smaller particles lead to higher absorption rates. NPs <1 μm have a limited absorption capability. Particles >3 μm are phagocytes and stay sequestered in the GIT cells. This is what we should observe in theory, but not necessarily the experimental observation. For example, even for NPs, the surface charge might limit absorption compared with nonionic NPs. Biological surfaces such as an epithelia-containing receptor at the surface can express higher absorption rates. Shape and elasticity facilitate the passage across the barrier [8].

In the GIT, it seems well established that the PP would be mostly implicated in the process of particle uptake via specialized epithelial cells. However, these specialized cells represent only approximately 10% of the cells covering the dome of these patches. Florence [8] mentioned that these immunologic cells have their analogues in the bronchus-, larynx-, and nose-associated lymphoid tissue regions (referred to as BALT, LALT, and NALT, respectively). It is not surprising that the PP part of the gut-associated lymphoid tissue (GALT) structure of the GIT wall is, as part of the lymphoid tissue, adapted for large range of phagocytes. The uptake of particles, microorganisms, and macromolecules by M cells occurs through adsorptive endocytosis by an approach of clathrin-coated pits and vesicle formation through endocytosis and phagocytosis processes [10]. This absorption route has a limitation because M cells (lymphoid tissues) occupy a relatively small region of the total GIT surface area, which is not compensated for by enhanced affinities. It has been shown that particulate systems can gain entry through normal gut epithelial cells (enterocytes); however, this absorption rate is not significant compared with the M cells. In addition, gastric mucus covers the entire wall of the GIT. Some authors have reported that mucus might inhibit the uptake of NPs through a dense structure in the viscous glycoprotein gel. However, there is a thought that entrapment of NPs in mucus actually delays the transit of these NPs down the gut and brings them closer to the absorption sites [8].

Many researchers have attempted to improve the GIT absorption rate by increasing the complexities of the NPs using different approaches called functionalization, consisting of a group change regarding the surface properties, and subsequently increasing the propensity for absorption. The functionalization approach may help raise the absorption rate, but it may also increase the size of the NPs, which reduces absorption based on our observations. Equilibrium needs to be reached because when the chemical surface of the NP is altered, the possible interaction of the NPs with the target organ and the toxicity of the NPs also change. In this scenario, even if the absorption rates increase, the new NPs must be characterized. Other techniques have been proposed, for example, coating NPs with molecules or peptides such as lectins, invasin, or internalin fragments. Even the results from such manipulation of the surface properties are often clear *in vitro*: the adhesion to the cell increases, and there is some evidence that absorption is enhanced [8]. The goal is to reach the target organ, cells (e.g., M cells, normal epithelial cells), or tissues. Thus, a lack of clarity of the outcome might result from the chemical and physical instabilities of the coated particles. The increased adhesion from the interaction of different receptors may lead to enhanced uptake into cells, but this does not necessarily translate into increased transport through and out of the cell.

In the situation in which the epithelium itself is not the target, movement of particles through the M cells or epithelial cells is only the first part of this voyage, which involves passage through the mesenteric lymph, filtration in the lymph nodes, and transfer to the blood and perhaps extravasation [8]. In a study by Carr and colleagues [11], the researchers said that estimation between the uptake and the volume of NP is not straightforward. Other factors such as maceration may overestimate the uptake into the tissue. This observation was clearly demonstrated by microscopy showing that in the small intestine, most NPs are luminal or on the surface [12]. In this study, the researchers did not find an important difference between particles; however, the sizes of the particles were >1 μm.

In a histological study by Desai and colleagues [13], the researchers demonstrated that NPs of 100 nm were diffused throughout the submucosal layers as opposed to the larger sizes, which were predominantly found in the tissue surface. Jani and colleagues [14] exposed rat GIT mucosa to different sizes of NP (i.e., 50 nm, 100 nm, 300 nm, 500 nm, 1 μm, and 3 μm) every day for 10 days. At 48 h postexposure, the researchers measured the amount of NPs in different regions. Several authors discovered that NPs <100 nm accumulated in GIT tissue; however, if the sizes were greater than this cutoff, then the accumulation rate was significantly lower [13,14]. In another study, colloidal gold was administered in water for 7 days to mice; the results showed a large distribution across several organs, including the kidney, spleen, liver, blood, and brain [15]. Even after 12 h of postexposure, NPs were still measured in the GIT, which suggests sequestration in cells or at the surfaces.

After the absorption, the amount of NPs can reach the blood circulation, and if enough of an amount is present, then this can induce a therapeutic or a toxic effect [9]. The amount of NPs absorbed is variable and depends on the size and the surface chemistry of NPs. Several studies show that between 2% and 3% of NPs orally exposed are absorbed by the GIT tissue [6]. For researchers who want to increase the intestinal absorption, they need to understand and optimize the linkage between surface chemistry of the NPs and the M cells [9]. In general, the efficiency of the uptake for NPs is ≤100 nm in size and is approximately 15- to 250-fold higher compared with a larger size [11]. In addition, from the same region, the PP tissue has 200-fold higher uptakes than non-PP tissue from the same region.

### 9.2.2 Inhalation

As described by the International Commission on Radiological Protection (ICRP) in its document, the commission measured the distribution probability of particles related to their size [16]. The ICRP study showed that NPs with a diameter of <10 μm have a greater probability of penetrating beyond the head airways. Particles <100 nm in aerodynamic diameter have a significant probability of reaching the alveolar region of the lungs. In fact, there is at least a 50% probability that particles <4 μm in aerodynamic diameter will reach this region [17]. Regarding the smaller diameter sizes of particles, another factor called inertia is secondary to Brownian diffusion in determining deposition, leading to particles penetrating deep into the lungs and diffusing to a large lung surface area presented in the alveolar region [17]. According to the ICRP, at 1 nm diameter, almost everything will be deposited onto the head and tracheobronchial region of the lung, which means that almost nothing will reach the alveolar region because the negligible mass significantly reduces the velocity of the NPs.

For NPs to deposit into the inner wall of the lungs, the particles may induce two types of toxicities (i.e., a local toxicity or a systemic toxicity), depending on their intrinsic properties. In addition to the deposition site, different factors will influence clinical observations. For instance, the deposition site will depend on the size and concentration of NPs, the durability of NPs (i.e., insoluble aqueous), and the stability of NPs (stable NPs will have higher durability and defense immune system in the lung area). The last important factor focuses on mucociliary clearance (acting in the upper airways) and the macrophages' immune system (acting in the lower airways and alveolar region), which tries to actively remove the deposition of NPs [16].

The local toxicities may cause inflammation, oxidative stress, tissue damage, and disease. Many of the biological mechanisms observed in the literature involved particle-related lung diseases (e.g., oxidative stress, inflammation, production of cytokines, chemokines, and cell growth factors) [18]. Much of our understanding about the key factors that influence the biological reactivity and toxicity of airborne particulate matter has come from animal toxicological studies. These factors, including size, surface area, surface chemistry, solubility, and shape, will influence both the deposition of NPs in the lungs and the biological responses observed. Maynard and Kuempel [17] reported that NPs, including carbon black (12 nm), elemental carbon (90 nm), and diesel exhaust particulate (120 nm), caused various cytoskeletal dysfunctions. These dysfunctions included impaired phagocytosis, inhibition of cell proliferation, and decreased cell viability in primary alveolar macrophages from dogs and mice from alveolar macrophage cell lines in 24 h, depending on the dosages [17]. Monteiro-Riviere and colleagues [19] reported an important observation, saying that if the carbon nanotubes reach the lung tissue, then they were more toxic than similarly chemically composed NPs, such as carbon black or quartz dust (actually these two NPs are known for their lung toxicities). Monteiro-Riviere and colleagues [19] argued that the observation was due to the tendency of carbon nanotubes to self-aggregate and then remove themselves from the controlled condition. These agglomerated NPs have a much higher residence time than dispersed NPs.

NPs that leave the lungs might enter the blood circulation, and then may cause endothelial cell injury (of the blood vessels) and prothrombotic effects [20]. Recent studies have indicated that NPs depositing in the nasal region may be transported to the olfactory bulb via the olfactory nerves [21]. The same group exposed rat to manganese ultrafine particles <100 nm during 12 days and observed an accumulation in the olfactive bulb. The authors concluded that the olfactory neuronal pathway is efficient for translocation. They also mentioned a nonprimate study in which the authors noted a similar observation, suggesting the plausibility of the olfactive pathway for humans [22]. The size of NPs may also penetrate cells and cellular organelles. In a study of concentrated NPs from air pollution in human bronchial epithelial cells and mouse alveolar macrophages, the ultrafine fraction (<100 nm) was found to penetrate into cells and localize in mitochondria, causing oxidative damage to mitochondrial membranes [23]. Unlike low molecular weight drugs, which penetrate cells easily, the cellular uptake of polymeric prodrugs is restricted to the endocytic route, which basically means that prodrugs are delivered to the cellular lysosomes [3]. However, other studies of drug delivery across the blood–brain barrier further confirmed the importance of surface properties, showing that particle surface components may bind to the apolipoprotein E receptor, which mediates crossing of this highly complicated tight barrier [3]. The olfactory neuronal pathway represents a significant exposure route of central nervous system (CNS) tissue to inhaled solid manganese oxide NPs. In rats, which are obligatory nose breathers, translocation of inhaled NPs along neurons seems to be a more efficient pathway to the CNS, than via the blood circulation across the blood–brain barrier for humans. Given that this neuronal translocation pathway was also demonstrated in nonhuman primates, it is likely to be operative in humans as well [24].

### 9.2.3 Cutaneous Route

The cutaneous route of exposure represents an important potential route of exposure for NPs because of the skin surfaces with workplace environment [19,25]. The risk caused by NPs or every other chemical especially after an *in vivo* exposure would depend on the skin absorption if no irritant NPs are present. The process of passage across the skin layer will depend on passive diffusion, and structural organization will influence this diffusion. The stratum corneum provides a slow diffusion capability. It is considered to be a rate-limiting step of the percutaneous absorption [26,27]. However, the dermis and epidermis have easier diffusion capabilities. The pig is a species of choice in percutaneous *in vitro* absorption studies because its skin structure is highly similar to that of humans, and numerous investigators have validated this approach [27].

The literature reports that normal skin diffusion is limited to NPs that are 100 nm in diameter. Intrinsic factors such as the chemistry surface shape of NPs can also influence the diffusion. However, more research should be conducted on this issue because there is no real consensus in the existing literature. Kohli and Alpar [28] conducted a study on percutaneous NPs and found that particles were able to permeate skin if they had a negative charge and were 50 and 500 nm in diameter. This result suggests that negative particles with sufficient charges may be ideal carriers for drugs. This is different to what we observed; usually the best particles for percutaneous permeation would be when they are lipophilic neutral and <100 nm in diameter [28]. The vehicle containing NPs is also a parameter that can influence the toxicity. However, at least one group of researchers (i.e., Schulz and colleagues [29]) found that cutaneous absorption interaction was limited to the stratum corneum.

Multiwalled carbon nanotubes are capable of entering the keratinocytes and driving interleukin-releasing effects. Tan and colleagues [30] conducted a human study on the percutaneous absorption of $TiO_2$ from sunscreens. This study was the first one to present a direct linkage between the utilization of sunscreen and the absorption of $TiO_2$ in humans. However, Gamer and colleagues [26] applied $TiO_2$ and zinc peroxide ($ZnO_2$; coated) diluted in cream (size <200 nm) on *ex vivo* pig skin for 24 h, but no significant percutaneous absorption resulted [26]. The authors concluded the absence of risk was based on the lack of systemic absorption. A similar experiment was recently repeated using sunscreen containing zinc oxide (ZnO) and $TiO_2$ NPs. The results suggest a minimal penetration and no evidence of systemic absorption [31]. The authors mentioned that ultraviolet B sunburned and damaged skin slightly enhanced the *in vitro* or *in vivo* subcutaneous penetration of $TiO_2$ or ZnO present in the sunscreen formulation [31].

Diffusion across the stratum corneum is normally the rate-limiting step for percutaneous absorption. Pig is a good model because its structure is similar to that of a human, and the technique of porcine preparation has been validated by numerous investigators. The permeation of NPs throughout the models seems to be an accurate predictive tool for human extrapolation.

## 9.3 Distribution

After absorption from oral, inhalation, or cutaneous routes, these NPs are then translocated in the systemic circulation and delivered to different organs, including the liver, spleen, kidneys, heart, and brain, where they may be deposited [24]. Many target organs are being studied to measure the impact of these exposures; however, only a few groups are working on the kinetic distribution of NPs in these organs.

A study conducted by Kreyling and colleagues [32] indicated that 1 week after inhalation, only a very small fraction of ultrafine iridium particles (18 and 80 nm in diameter) had access to systemic circulation and extrapulmonary organs. The chemical composition and physical structure of the NP surface may be an important determinant in influencing systemic translocation of ultrafine particles [32]. De Jong and Borm exposed rats aged between 6 to 8 weeks to a single oral exposure of polystyrene NPs from 10 to 250 nm in diameter at concentrations varying from 77 to 108 µg mL$^{-1}$ (25). NPs <100 nm were found mainly in the blood and liver 24 h postexposure. In addition, De Jong's group found a lower amount of NPs expressed in percentage of doses in the spleen and kidney and only trace levels in the lungs, testis, heart, brain, and thymus [25].

These studies demonstrated that NPs, after deposition, are rapidly distributed across tissue compartments of the lung, and that these NPs may move between the tissue compartments. The NPs eventually reach the capillary lumen and may penetrate into circulating cells and constituents (e.g., erythrocytes, blood macrophages). Thereby, they may be distributed into other organs of the body, such as the liver, heart, kidneys, and even the brain [14,25]. Nemmar and colleagues [33] conducted an interesting human study in which they used the inhalation of radiolabeled technetium 99 carbon NPs <100 nm in diameter. The findings showed that radiolabeled technetium 99 carbon was detected in the blood 1 min after inhalation, reached a maximum after 10–20 min, and remained for >60 min. A gamma camera showed substantial radioactivity in the liver and other organs.

## 9.4 Excretion

In a study of rats by Peters and colleagues [24], a single intravenous dose of a fullerene labeled with technetium 99 m showed a rapid distribution in different organs. The researchers measured the biodistribution in different organs in mice and rabbits. They observed a decrease of the NPs in the organ tissues only between 1 and 3 h postexposures, except for the liver at 3 h, where it was higher than at 1 h postexposure. The elimination of the fullerene was mainly via the urinary route [34]. In another comparison, Ogawara and colleagues [35] administered a single intravenous dose of polystyrene microsphere (50 and 500 nm in diameter) to rats. The distributions were independent of the size. The researchers measured the half-life ($t_{1/2}$) for the alpha phase and terminal phase at approximately 1 and 53 h, respectively [35]. The researchers believed that urinary elimination seemed to be the major elimination route. Singh and colleagues [36] exposed mice to a single intravenous dose of single-walled carbon nanotubes (1 nm in diameter and 300–1000 nm in length). The distribution was very quick across the organs, and excretion occurred via the urine pathway. In the same experiment, the researchers also studied the impact of the exposure route on the elimination half-life. Depending on the absorption route, the other local mechanism previously mentioned may also contribute to the elimination. In a study by Furumoto and colleagues [37], the researchers demonstrated that NPs can also be excreted via the biliary tract.

## 9.5 Discussion and Conclusion

The interaction between NPs and the biological system is a huge challenge in the field of toxicokinetics. The toxicokinetics discipline describes the absorption, the distribution during the metabolism process, and the excretion of the xenobiotics (the NPs). At this point, our focus is to apply the approach that we have in place in case we need to use the same kinetic approaches or need to develop new tools. However, it is important to point out that complementary approaches will be required to be able to adequately describe the experimental observation.

At the beginning of the nanotoxicokinetics observations, we believed that inhalation was the major exposure route, with negligible contribution from the skin. However, observations such as those by Ryman-Rasmussen and colleagues [38] or results from Monteiro-Riviere and colleagues [19] clearly suggest that skin is surprisingly permeable to nanomaterials with diverse physicochemical properties and may serve as a portal of entry for localized, and possibly systemic, exposure of humans to quantum dots and other engineered nanoscale materials [38]. There is a particle size dependency; thus, in the GIT, NPs with size <100 nm show significantly greater uptake in tissues [13]. For skin absorption, these findings suggest that the toxicology of these structures must be assessed before widespread public exposure so that appropriate protective measures can be developed [19]. The status of this absorption will change with the arrival of new transformer NP (NP with exotic functionalization) on the market.

This review also points out those NPs that can rapidly translocate from the lung into the cells, and then reach the systemic circulation. There is increasing evidence that the accumulation of NPs in different organs (e.g., heart, brain) shows signs of oxidative stress or other stress toxic effects. Even oxidative stress can occur for many other reasons, and this significant addition may cause a long-term health effect. A long-term study is required to quantify the long-term risk. Given that this neuronal translocation pathway was also demonstrated in nonhuman primates, it is also likely to be operative in humans [39].

New technology approaches, such as a proteomic analysis profiling approach, in which we detected much below the clinical sign effect of protein modification, will be useful to observe before the health effect is irreversible. However, these sophisticated approaches will only work if they are supported by a rigorous characterization of the NPs in medium. This overview showed that improved science in this field will span different disciplines. As a result of the improved science, we will gain insight on how NPs interact in relation to their physical and chemical properties, and will subsequently attain optimal understanding of the mode of action in the biological systems.

## References

1. Hagens, W.I. et al. What do we (need to) know about the kinetic properties of nanoparticles in the body? *Regul. Toxicol. Pharmacol.*, 49, 217–229, 2007.
2. Handy, R.D. et al. The ecotoxicology and chemistry of manufactured nanoparticles. *Ecotoxicology*, 17(4), 287–314, 2008.
3. Borm, P.J. and Kreyling, W. Toxicological hazards of inhaled nanoparticles— Potential implications for drug delivery. *J. Nanosci. Nanotechnol.*, 4(5), 521–531, 2004.
4. Nikula, K.J. Rat lung tumors induced by exposure to selected poorly soluble nonfibrous particles. *Inhal. Toxicol.*, 12(1–2), 97–119, 2000.
5. Hoover, M.D. et al. Exposure assessment considerations for nanoparticles in the workplace. In *Nanotoxicology: Characterization, Dosing, and Health Effects, First Edition* (N.A. Monteiro-Riviere and C.L. Tran, eds., CRC Press, Boca Raton, FL), pp. 71–83, 2007.
6. Florence, A.T. The oral absorption of micro- and nanoparticulates: Neither exceptional nor unusual. *Pharm. Res.*, 14(3), 259–266, 1997.
7. Hussain, N., Jaitley, V., and Florence, A.T. Recent advances in the understanding of uptake of microparticulates across the gastrointestinal lymphatics. *Adv. Drug Deliv. Rev.*, 50(1–2), 107–142, 2001.
8. Florence, A.T. Nanoparticle uptake by the oral route: fulfilling its potential? *Drug Discov. Today Technol.*, 2(1), 75–81, 2005.
9. des Rieux, A. et al. Nanoparticles as potential oral delivery systems of proteins and vaccines: A mechanistic approach. *J. Control Rel.*, 116(1), 1–27, 2006.

10. Qaddoumi, M.G. et al. Clathrin and caveolin-1 expression in primary pigmented rabbit conjunctival epithelial cells: Role in PLGA nanoparticle endocytosis. *Mol. Vis.*, 9, 559–568, 2003.

11. Carr, K.E. et al. The effect of size on uptake of orally administered latex microparticles in the small intestine and transport to mesenteric lymph nodes. *Pharm. Res.*, 13(8), 1205–1209, 1996.

12. Barrett, E.G. et al. Silica binds serum proteins resulting in a shift of the dose-response for silica-induced chemokine expression in an alveolar type II cell line. *Toxicol. Appl. Pharmacol.*, 161(2), 111–122, 1999.

13. Desai, M.P. et al. Gastrointestinal uptake of biodegradable microparticles: Effect of particle size. *Pharm. Res.*, 13(12), 1838–1845, 1996.

14. Jani, P. et al. Nanoparticle uptake by the rat gastrointestinal mucosa: Quantitation and particle size dependency. *J. Pharm. Pharmacol.*, 42(12), 821–826, 1990.

15. Hillery, A.M., Jani, P.U., and Florence, A.T. Comparative, quantitative study of lymphoid and non-lymphoid uptake of 60 nm polystyrene particles. *J. Drug Target*, 2(2), 151–156, 1994.

16. ICRP. *Human Respiratory Tract Model for Radiological Protection.* Annals of ICRP. Publication 66, pp. 1–459, 1994, Pergamon, Oxford.

17. Maynard, A.D. and Kuempel, E.D. Airborne nanostructured particles and occupational health. *J. Nanopart. Res.*, 7, 587–614, 2005.

18. Castranova, V. and Vallyathan, V. Silicosis and coal workers' pneumoconiosis. *Environ. Health Perspect.*, 108 Suppl 4, 675–684, 2000.

19. Monteiro-Riviere, N.A. et al. Multi-walled carbon nanotube interactions with human epidermal keratinocytes. *Toxicol. Lett.*, 155(3), 377–384, 2005.

20. Nemmar, A. et al. Possible mechanisms of the cardiovascular effects of inhaled particles: Systemic translocation and prothrombotic effects. *Toxicol. Lett.*, 149(1–3), 243–253, 2004.

21. Oberdorster, G. et al. Translocation of inhaled ultrafine particles to the brain. *Inhal. Toxicol.*, 16(6–7), 437–445, 2004.

22. Elder, A. et al. Translocation of inhaled ultrafine manganese oxide particles to the central nervous system. *Environ. Health Perspect.*, 114(8), 1172–1178, 2006a.

23. Li, N. et al. Ultrafine particulate pollutants induce oxidative stress and mitochondrial damage. *Environ. Health Perspect.*, 111(4), 455–460, 2003.

24. Peters, A. et al. Translocation and potential neurological effects of fine and ultrafine particles: A critical update. *Part. Fibre Toxicol.*, 3, 13, 2006.

25. De Jong, W.H. and Borm, P.J. Drug delivery and nanoparticles: Applications and hazards. *Int. J. Nanomed.*, 3(2), 133–149, 2008.

26. Gamer, A.O., Leibold, E., and van Ravenzwaay, B. The *in vitro* absorption of microfine zinc oxide and titanium dioxide through porcine skin. *Toxicol. In Vitro*, 20(3), 301–307, 2006.

27. Diembeck, W. et al. Test guidelines for *in vitro* assessment of dermal absorption and percutaneous penetration of cosmetic ingredients. European Cosmetic, Toiletry and Perfumery Association. *Food Chem. Toxicol.*, 37(2–3), 191–205, 1999.

28. Kohli, A.K. and Alpar, H.O. Potential use of nanoparticles for transcutaneous vaccine delivery: Effect of particle size and charge. *Int. J. Pharm.*, 275(1–2), 13–17, 2004.

29. Schulz, J. et al. Distribution of sunscreens on skin. *Adv. Drug Deliv. Rev.*, 54 Suppl 1, S157–S163, 2002.

30. Tan, M.H. et al. A pilot study on the percutaneous absorption of microfine titanium dioxide from sunscreens. *Australas. J. Dermatol.*, 37(4), 185–187, 1996.

31. Monteiro-Riviere, N.A. et al. Safety evaluation of sunscreen formulations containing titanium dioxide and zinc oxide nanoparticles in UVB sunburned skin: An *in vitro* and *in vivo* study. *Toxicol. Sci.*, 123, 264–280, 2011.
32. Kreyling, W.G. et al. Translocation of ultrafine insoluble iridium particles from lung epithelium to extrapulmonary organs is size dependent but very low. *J. Toxicol. Environ. Health A*, 65(20), 1513–1530, 2002.
33. Nemmar, A. et al. Passage of inhaled particles into the blood circulation in humans. *Circulation*, 105(4), 411–414, 2002.
34. Qingnuan, L. et al. Preparation of (99m)Tc-C(60)(OH)(x) and its biodistribution studies. *Nucl. Med Biol.*, 29(6), 707–710, 2002.
35. Ogawara, K. et al. Uptake by hepatocytes and biliary excretion of intravenously administered polystyrene microspheres in rats. *J. Drug Target.*, 7(3), 213–221, 1999.
36. Singh, R. et al. Tissue biodistribution and blood clearance rates of intravenously administered carbon nanotube radiotracers. *Proc. Natl Acad. Sci. U. S. A.*, 103(9), 3357–3362, 2006.
37. Furumoto, K. et al. Biliary excretion of polystyrene microspheres depends on the type of receptor-mediated uptake in rat liver. *Biochim. Biophys. Acta*, 1526(2), 221–226, 2001.
38. Ryman-Rasmussen, J.P., Riviere, J.E., and Monteiro-Riviere, N.A. Penetration of intact skin by quantum dots with diverse physicochemical properties. *Toxicol. Sci.*, 91(1), 159–165, 2006.
39. Elder, A. et al. Translocation of inhaled ultrafine manganese oxide particles to the central nervous system. *Environ. Health Perspect.*, 114(8), 1172–1178, 2006.

# 10

## Environmental Fate and Ecotoxicology of Nanomaterials

Bernard Lachance, Mahsa Hamzeh, and Geoffrey I. Sunahara

### CONTENTS

### 10.1 Introduction

Nanoecotoxicology is an emerging field of nanotechnology that is still in its infancy [1]. The peculiar nature of nanomaterials (NMs), which may underlie either greater chemical reactivity or even entirely new physico–chemical properties, relative to their bulk equivalent, is a cause of concern for potential adverse biological effects [2–4]. Nanoparticles (NPs) have been named the Jekyll and Hyde of materials science, owing to their unique chemical, electrical, optical, and physical properties [5].

NMs are already present in many industrial, household, or cosmetic products, and it seems some of these chemicals will be released and influence our environment. Agricultural practices are expected to benefit from nanotechnology through improving the efficiency and reduction in pesticide usage for crop protection [6]. However, only few studies on nanoformulation of pesticides have yet been published [7–9]. Importantly, environmental exposure may also be an issue at the end of the life cycle of some products. Therefore, to better understand the possible environmental impacts of NMs, their life cycle and fate in the environment need to be identified.

Industries of the environmental sector are presently testing NP-based remediation technologies, for example, the decontamination of groundwater (nanosized zero-valent iron, among others) [4], and the photocatalytic degradation of air pollutants or the germicidal treatment of wastewater using nanosized titanium dioxide. Still, crucial information on the environmental fate of NMs, and on their potential adverse effects individually or in combination with other common pollutants, is lacking [10].

Several reviews on the environmental behavior and toxicity of NM have been published recently [4,10–14]. In this chapter, the highlight information of those reviews, as well as the novel information obtained from various sources included on the International Council on Nanotechnology Web site (http://icon.rice.edu/research.cfm) are summarized in the present general overview of the potential ecotoxicity of NMs. This information is useful for ecological risk assessment. The assessment of the environmental impact of NMs has recently emerged as a serious issue since many of these NMs will likely enter the environment and subsequently affect environmental and human health.

## 10.2 Sources and Exposure to Nanomaterials

To understand the environmental health risks posed by NMs, one should know how the NMs can reach target organisms in the environment. Several aspects such as product life cycle, fate, and transport of NMs were described for human exposure in previous chapters. This information may also apply to ecological receptors with the exposure difference, which may occur through water column, groundwater, sediments and soil, depending on the target organism [16].

Water in the aqueous environment may be considered as a transport medium or a temporary reservoir because of the tendency of NM to agglomerate and precipitate out of solution (or of dispersion). Aquatic receptors, such as fish and invertebrates, and filter-feeding animals (benthos) are the most likely targets of NM in the aquatic and benthic media, respectively [1,14–16]. Unfortunately, few toxicity assays have been conducted using sediments.

While most of the ecotoxicity data were obtained from aquatic studies, few aquatic studies have been done under conditions resembling those found in the field, including the presence of significant amount of organic matter, high ionic strength, etc. [13,17].

The release pathways of NMs into the environment are possibly similar to those known for other environmental contaminants such as metals and organic compounds. The sources of manufactured NMs can be direct (intentional) or indirect (accidental), as discussed in the following sections.

## 10.2.1 Intentional Release into Environment

Manufactured NMs may be deliberately introduced into the environment as pesticides, or other agricultural applications, and as part of remediation technologies for decontamination of soil, water, or groundwater. Environmental remediation of nano-enabled technologies has been presented in Chapter 5 of this book. Several applications of NMs, including the removal of pesticides, organo-chlorinated solvents, or explosives from groundwater, and reclamation of land lost to forest fires have been investigated; however, the potential ecotoxicological risks associated with the use of NMs in groundwater or their dispersion on the soil surface remains a concern [10,18–20]. For instance, following their dispersion into soil, NMs could become part of aerosols formed by wind erosion. Once in the environment, NMs could possibly impair key ecological functions, such as nutrient recycling, water depuration, and biomass production [10]. Ecological receptors at risk would encompass all sensitive species that are exposed to NMs through air, water, or soil. Geochemical cycles such as carbon ($CO_2$ fixation by plants and algae) and nitrogen cycle may also be affected.

The carbon cycle could be affected as it has been speculated that some NMs (e.g., $TiO_2$) with photo-oxidizing activity could enhance the turnover rate of the stable organic matter in soil [16]. In addition, NMs introduced in soils could modify soil hydrophilicity and decrease wettability, and lead to increased problems with erosion, loss of soil fertility, and water pollution [10]. Finally, NMs in soil, sediments, and water may also affect the bioavailability of certain essential nutrients (e.g., phosphate) and change growth rates (biomass production) in algae, phytoplankton, soil bacteria, and plants. Soil respiration rates would then be modified, as well as soil texture-related processes such as transport of gases (soil $CO_2$ transport, evapotranspiration) or water (infiltration, soil moisture transport, surface runoff) [10].

## 10.2.2 Accidental Release into Environment

A significant part of the environmental contamination will occur via indirect routes. The industrial NMs producers and manufacturers of products containing NM are among the largest sources of NM contamination. Atmospheric emissions and effluents of conventional industrial pollutants have entered the environment for centuries; products of the nanotechnology may follow in a similar manner. For instance, million tons of production of nanosized $TiO_2$ (and other NMs in less amounts) will inevitably be accompanied by release into effluents, and one may also expect that accidental spills during production or transport will become more likely with increased production [10]. In addition, manufactured NMs will also enter the environment by using cosmetics, household products (e.g., cleansing aids, fabrics, washing machines, toys, etc.), paints (especially on buildings), and as various surface treatments, such as self-cleansing windows or other surfaces (self-cleaning condensers in air conditioners). The wear and tear of NM-containing objects by natural erosion processes will result in transfer into the atmosphere (NMs becoming airborne), in which they are either subsequently settled down or removed by rain and transported by storm water. Other sources might be the effluents of wastes sites (discharge water) where degradation and leaching of NP-containing objects may occur. In this respect, it is noteworthy to mention that the Wilson Woodrow International Center for Scholars has identified >1000 consumer products containing NMs or nanotechnology [21]. Of these products, nanosilver was the most commonly used NM (in 200 items), mainly as an antimicrobial agent. Finally, various dispersive compounds such as fuel additives (case of $CeO_2$) may contribute to the environmental burden [22].

The potential contamination resulting from leaching of NMs present in surface coating of buildings has been recently studied [23]. The presence of $TiO_2$ in water has been reported earlier (albeit without determination of the source and concentration of the NP) [35], while a recent study presents the first evidence that NP incorporated in paints can be transported by facade runoff and discharged into aquatic systems [23]. Approximately half of the $TiO_2$ amount could originate from facades and the larger aggregates could presumably come from other sources, such as road paints or other types of coatings. These studies do not cover all forms of transport of man-made NPs into the environment, but they identify some impacts of nanotechnology on our environment. In fact, using a life cycle model to calculate the predicted environmental concentrations for nanosilver, nano-Ti, and carbon nanotubes (CNTs), it is concluded that presence of $TiO_2$ may be a risk to aquatic life, based on its low predicted no-effect concentration (PNEC) value and relatively high predicted environmental concentrations (PEC) in the environment [24].

Other studies have used environmental exposure models to estimate environmental concentrations ranges of various NMs used in consumer products [27]. While the estimated results show relatively low concentrations, it should be noted that in some countries, industrial uses may multiply these estimates by many orders of magnitude. For example, a million metric tons of production is forecasted for nano-$TiO_2$ that will eventually completely replace the micro-$TiO_2$ production [26]. In a different approach, the PECs were used for sludge-treated soil in Europe and the United States [27]. It is reported that the

PECs of nano-Ag, nano-TiO$_2$, and nano-ZnO in sewage treatment effluents could pose a risk for aquatic receptors. At the same time, it was admitted that prediction of toxicological risk is complicated because of the lack of reliable ecotoxicity data, especially for the nano-Ag and nano-ZnO.

Recently, many researches have dealt with silver contamination [27–36]. As mentioned above, the antimicrobial effect of nanosilver is already exploited in washing machines, and in a vast assortment of household products, including wound dressing and even footwear. The increased use of nanosilver has been the subject of many debates, especially for the environmental defense community [28], concerning its effects on soil (or sediment) microbes as well as on the biomass in wastewater treatment plants [29]. However, a study conducted on nanosilver fate suggests that this NM may be detoxified when present in wastewater, by transformation into an innocuous form (Ag$_2$S) [36]. Still, fate issues remain to be identified for other NMs. Moreover, it is not known if the biosolids coming from wastewater treatment plants will exert toxic effects when dispersed on surface soil. The geochemical cycles of carbon and nitrogen are largely dependent on microbial activity and it has been reported that bacteria such as nitrifiers and denitrifiers are highly sensitive to xenobiotics [31,37]. The possible effect of nanosilver acting as a mutagen on the genetic diversity of exposed microbial populations has been investigated, suggesting that nanosilver would influence neither the genetic diversity nor antibiotic resistance, at least in a marine sediment environment [32,33]. Because these results were obtained from short-term exposure assays, the chronic exposure effects remain to be verified.

Likewise, the presence of carbonaceous or organic NP in industrial effluents and in leachates coming from landfill sites has been suspected to have an impact on the aquatic environment. On the basis of mathematical modeling, a recent study predicted that manufactured carbon nanoparticles (MCNPs) would not contribute significantly to toxicity or to transport of cocontaminants because the MCNPs should remain in a small fraction compared with black carbon NP that resulted from other human activities (coal combustion) or even from natural sources such as forest fires [38].

Nanotechnology has also been used in the defense sector for several applications, for example, using CNTs for various purposes, including smokes, fogs, and obscurants [40–41]. Following the unintentional release of NMs into the environment during their production, testing, and training activities, a series of environmental (transport, toxicity, and fate) studies have been initiated [41].

Finally, very few studies have addressed the issue of particle emission from coated materials. Significant transfer to the atmosphere takes place when the surfaces coated by nano-TiO$_2$ are eroded by wind, UV light, or direct contact by the users; therefore, particle emission should be evaluated for materials coated with nano-TiO$_2$ [43]. Studies on surface preparation and potential release of NMs from functional clothes and nanocomposite filters are also recommended [43].

### 10.2.3 Parameters Affecting Environmental Fate and Translocation

An important question is how NM interactions with the environmental matrices can exert a toxic effect on the environmental receptors. The behavior of NPs in the environment may follow the same laws as for natural colloids; their stability should depend on (a) physical properties (including particle size, solubility, state of aggregation, concentration, shape, crystal structure, surface area, zeta-potential or surface charge, and pHpzc—the pH at which the net particle surface charge is zero); (b) the nature of the surface chemistry of the NMs (including elemental composition, presence of impurities, presence of coating); and (c) environmental conditions such as solution chemistry (pH, composition, and ionic strength of solution), redox potential, and possibly biochemical reactions over time (aging properties) [23,25,39,42].

Nano-TiO$_2$ is one of the best-studied NMs from the standpoint of environmental fate, and is considered to be a possible sentinel NM [44]. It is found that the pH of the milieu can affect surface charge properties, and subsequently the aggregation, agglomeration, potential "bioavailability," and reactivity of nano-TiO$_2$ [45], and high concentrations of Na$^+$ and K$^+$ (high ionic strength) could promote its aggregation [46]. The presence of surfactants (bronchoalveolar lavage fluid or combinations of albumin and complex lipids) can also stabilize the TiO$_2$ NPs [47]. The interaction between TiO$_2$ and organic matter (as humic acid or equivalents) was found to increase the stability of the NP [48]. In studies conducted with soil columns, both surface potential and aggregate size influenced the mobility of TiO$_2$ NPs [49–51]. As expected for colloids, the smaller particles could be transported for longer distances. Similarly, results from several studies indicate that nano-TiO$_2$ particles and their aggregates/agglomerates might be very mobile in subsurface and in groundwater [39,49]. In fact, results from a recent study suggest that transport of TiO$_2$ NP would be favored by low ionic strength and by the presence of large soil particles; conversely, high clay content, natural organic matter, and salinity would favor soil retention of the same particles [52]. Studies with other NMs, such as nanoaluminum, yield similar conclusions [53]. Transport of aluminum particles also depends on the size, surface charge, and agglomeration rate, which is inversely related to the size of agglomerates and can be affected over time by the ionic strength of the medium. Additionally, the surface charge of the particles and that of the receiving matrices (e.g., soil) are important for small agglomerates, in which they tend to bind to large soil particles of opposite charge [53].

In another study, the mobility of zero-valent iron was found to be enhanced by natural organic matter [54]. This effect was completely evident at high particle loads, but was still measurable at low concentrations. Likewise, the stability of CNTs can be greatly improved by the presence of natural organic matter or humic acids [41,42]. It seems that untreated CNTs as received from producers are undispersable in water [42]. Owing to their hydrophobicity, it was thought earlier that CNTs could not be sufficiently bioavailable to cause harm to aquatic organisms. In contrast, CNTs were found to be suspended at fairly high concentrations in turbulent stream waters containing natural organic matter [42]. Whether NMs can induce toxicity in environmental health is described below.

## 10.3 Ecotoxicity of Nanomaterials

Most of the toxicological studies of NMs have been carried out using laboratory animals or mammalian cells *in vitro*. Animal studies have shown that inhaled NPs (e.g., polystyrene beads, airborne ultrafine particles) are removed less efficiently than larger particles by the macrophage clearance mechanisms in their lungs, thereby causing lung damage; NPs can translocate through the circulatory, lymphatic, and nervous systems to many tissues and organs, including the brain [2,55]. It can be anticipated that these effects shown in laboratory animals (rat and mouse) would also be observed in animals in the wild life upon exposure, with respect to the dose and similar routes of exposure. On the other hand, *in vitro* results cannot be directly extrapolated to environmental conditions because additional factors, such as bioavailability and uptake by biota, are not considered.

In regard to the role of NPs on the ecotoxicity, little or no data can be found for protists, fungi, birds, reptiles, and amphibians. Most of the studies therefore refer to aquatic receptors (microbes, alga, invertebrates, and freshwater or marine water fish) or to terrestrial receptors (invertebrates and plants). The information presented here are according to six general classes of NMs: metals/metal oxides/semiconductors, carbonaceous compounds, and pharmaceutical and industrial organic polymers. The US Environmental Protection Agency uses a fourth class of NMs called composites. Two examples of composites (Ag-doped $TiO_2$ and Pt-loaded $TiO_2$) were presented under the metal/metal oxide section because only limited ecotoxicity data are available [56]. Ecotoxicity information for other types of composites such as nanocarbon or nanocellulose fiber-based materials is not available.

### 10.3.1 Metal, Metal Oxide, and Semiconductor-Based Nanoparticles

Several metal and especially metal oxide NMs have been in production for a relatively long time and they are therefore a priority to be studied. Tables 10.1 and 10.2 summarize the available toxicological information. Nominal (or in some cases estimated) diameters of test particles are reported, when available. These NMs could be toxic when bioavailability is favored (e.g., in a low salt medium, absence of organic matter, or solid matrices). According to the data, bacteria and plants seem to be comparatively resistant (using mass-based concentrations for exposure) relative to algae and aquatic invertebrates.

**TABLE 10.1**

Summary of Ecotoxicity for Metallic and Semiconductor Nanoparticles

| Nanomaterial (Size) | Test Organism | Effect | References |
|---|---|---|---|
| Silver | | | |
| 9–62 nm | Bacteria[a] | 24–96 h, Growth inhibition | [14] |
| <5 nm | Nitrifying bacteria | Toxic $EC_{50} = 0.14$ mg $L^{-1}$ | [31] |
| 2 nm | Mar. bacteria[b] | 30 min, no effect at 45 mg $L^{-1}$ | [64] |
| | Bact. consortium[c] | 21 days, no effect at 16 mg $L^{-1}$ | [64] |
| ~10 nm | Mar. Phy.[d] | Growth inhibition, reduced PSII quantum yield, reduction in chlorophyll content | [10] |
| | FW alga[e] | Growth inhibition | [10] |
| 20–30 nm | FW alga[f] | 96-h $EC_{50} = 0.19$ mg $L^{-1}$ | [30] |
| | *Daphnia pulex* | 48-h $LC_{50} = 0.04$ mg $L^{-1}$ | [30] |
| | *Ceriodaphnia dubia* | 48-h $LC_{50} = 0.07$ mg $L^{-1}$ | [30] |
| | Zebrafish (adult) | 48-h $LC_{50} = 7.1$ mg $L^{-1}$ | [30] |
| | Nematode[g] | Reproduction inhibition at 0.5 mg $L^{-1}$ | [65] |
| 100 nm | Zucchini | 15 days, 75% mass reduction at 1000 mg $L^{-1}$ | [56] |
| 13 nm | Mouse | Liver inflammatory response by ingestion | [66] |
| 18–19 nm | Sprague–Dawley rats | Alveolar inflammation after inhalation | [67] |
| Ag-doped $TiO_2$ or $Al_2O_3$ | Bacteria[a] | Growth inhibition | [14] |
| Copper | | | |
| 15–80 nm | Bacteria[h] | Growth inhibition | [14] |
| 15–45 nm | FW alga[f] | 96-h $EC_{50} = 0.54$ mg $L^{-1}$ | [30] |
| | *D. pulex* | 48-h $LC_{50} = 0.06$ mg $L^{-1}$ | [30] |
| | *C. dubia* | 48-h $LC_{50} = 0.42$ mg $L^{-1}$ | [30] |
| | Zebrafish (adult) | 48-h $LC_{50} = 0.94$ mg $L^{-1}$ | [30] |
| 80 nm | Zebrafish | 48-h $LC_{50} = 1.5$ mg $L^{-1}$ | [68] |
| 50 nm | Zucchini | 15 days, 90% biomass loss at 1000 mg $L^{-1}$ | [56] |
| 25–70 nm | Higher plants[i] | Root growth inh., $EC_{50} = 335$ mg $L^{-1}$ | [69] |
| Pt-loaded $TiO_2$ | Bacteria[j] | Growth inhibition | [14] |
| Gold 10 nm | Mar. bacteria[b] | 30 min, no effect at 28 mg $L^{-1}$ | [64] |
| | Bact. consortium[c] | 21 days, no effect at 10 mg $L^{-1}$ | [64] |
| Aluminum | Microtox[k] | 30 min, $EC_{50} = 5000$ mg $L^{-1}$ | [71] |

*(continued)*

**TABLE 10.1 (Continued)**

Summary of Ecotoxicity for Metallic and Semiconductor Nanoparticles

| Nanomaterial (Size) | Test Organism | Effect | References |
|---|---|---|---|
| 100 nm | Higher plants[l] | No effect on growth at 10–10,000 mg kg$^{-1}$ | [71] |
| 18 nm | Higher plants[m] | 25%–50% root growth inh. at 2000 mg L$^{-1}$ | [70] |
| Ligand-coated Al | Microtox[k] | 30 min, EC$_{50}$ = 17,500 mg L$^{-1}$ | [71] |
| Nickel 5–20 nm | FW alga[f] | 96-h EC$_{50}$ = 0.35 mg L$^{-1}$ | [30] |
| | D. pulex | 48-h LC$_{50}$ = 3.89 mg L$^{-1}$ | [30] |
| | C. dubia | 48-h LC$_{50}$ = 0.67 mg L$^{-1}$ | [30] |
| | Zebrafish | 48-h LC$_{50}$ > 10 mg L$^{-1}$ | [30] |
| Cobalt 10–20 nm | D. pulex | 48-h LC$_{50}$ > 10 mg L$^{-1}$ | [30] |
| | C. dubia | 48-h LC$_{50}$ = 1.67 mg L$^{-1}$ | [30] |
| CoCr alloy 30 nm | Human cells | Genotoxic, comet assay | [72] |
| Zinc 35 nm | Higher plants[m] | Germination inh. 40% at 2000 mg L$^{-1}$ | [70] |
| | Higher plants[m] | 90% Root growth inh. at 2000 mg L$^{-1}$ | [70] |
| *Semiconductors (Core Size)* | | | |
| CdSe 4–5 nm | Bacteria[n] | Bacteriostatic effects | [73] |
| CdSe ligand capped | *Pseudomonas aeruginosa* | Membrane damage at 50 mg L$^{-1}$ | [61] |
| CdSe/ZnS | Bacteria[n] | Bacteriostatic effects | [59,74] |
| | *Pseudokirchneriella subcapitata* | 96-h LC$_{50}$ = 37 μg L$^{-1}$ | [75] |
| | C. dubia | No effect at 110 μg L$^{-1}$ | [75] |
| CdSe/ZnS | *Xenopus blastomer*[o] | Viability and motility loss (~0.23 pmol/cell) | [73] |
| CdSe/ZnS MPA/TOPO | D. magna[p] | Toxicity changed by coating and light | [76] |
| CdSe/ZnS PEG coated | Mouse | Not toxic at 20 pmol g$^{-1}$, 133-day study | [73,77] |
| Weathered CdSe/ZnS | Bacteria[q] | Bactericidal (95% inh. at 20 nM) | [59] |
| CdTe MPA capped | Bacteria[r] | 10-h IC$_{50}$ ~0.3–0.6 μM | [78] |
| CdTe TGA capped | *Elliptio complanata* | Immunocompetence loss at 1.6 mg L$^{-1}$ | [79] |
| 2–6 nm | *E. complanata* | 1.4-fold gill LPO increase at 8 mg L$^{-1}$ | [79] |

(*continued*)

**TABLE 10.1 (Continued)**

Summary of Ecotoxicity for Metallic and Semiconductor Nanoparticles

| Nanomaterial (Size) | Test Organism | Effect | References |
|---|---|---|---|
| | Mouse | Neurotoxic, locomotor effects, 24-h postadministration | [77] |
| | Mouse | Not toxic, 40-day clearance study | [80] |
| CdHgTe TGA capped | Mouse | Not toxic, 40-day clearance study | [80] |

*Note:* Inh., inhibition; LPO, lipid peroxidation; MPA, mercaptopropionic acid; TGA, thioglycolic acid (or mercaptoacetic); TOPO, tri-*n*-octylphosphine.

a Including *Escherichia coli, Pseudomonas aeruginosa, Vibrio cholera, Bacillus subtilis, Staphylococcus aureus, Listeria monocytogenes,* and *Micrococcus lylae.* Ag-loaded polystyrene is also toxic. Note that smaller silver particles (9 nm) are more active than large ones (62 nm).
b Marine bacteria *Photobacterium phosphoreum.*
c Bacterial consortium taken from an industrial anaerobic digester, matrix may bind nano Ag/Cu.
d Marine phytoplankton *Thalassiosira weissflogii.*
e Freshwater alga *Chlamydomonas reinhardtii.*
f Freshwater alga *Pseudokirchneriela subcapitata.*
g Nematode *Caenorhabditis elegans.*
h Including *E. coli, B. subtilis, S. aureus,* and *L. monocytogenes.*
i Exposure in agar gel, *Phaseolus radiatus* (bean) and *Triticum aestivum* (wheat).
j Including *E. coli, S. aureus,* and *Enterococcus faecalis.*
k Microtox bacteria, tested as soil–nanoparticle suspension.
l California red kidney bean (*Phaseolus vulgaris*) and ryegrass (*Lolium perenne*).
m Radish *Raphanus sativus,* rape *Brassica napus,* ryegrass *Lolium perenne,* lettuce *Lactuca sativa,* corn *Zea mays,* and cucumber *Cucumis sativus.*
n Bacteria *E. coli* and *B. subtilis.*
o Direct injection of CdSe/ZnS quantum dots encapsulated in phospholipid block–copolymer micelles.
p MPA coating much less toxic than TOPO coating. Toxicity increased by UV light.
q Following 48-h exp. *E. coli* and *B. subtilis,* only 20% inhibition in metal-tolerant *P. aeruginosa.*
r Increased order of sensitivity: *B. subtilis, P. aeruginosa, E. coli,* and *S. aureus.*

Bacteriostatic effects are common for microbes, whereas bactericidal effects were reported only upon coexposure of the NM with UV radiation (for $TiO_2$) or halides (for MgO) [57]. Most of the antimicrobial NPs belong to the group of metals (i.e., silver) and metal oxides [55]. Metal NPs (e.g., copper, silver) are often found more toxic to environmental receptors such as bacteria, alga, *Daphnia,* and zebrafish in comparison with metal oxides (e.g., $TiO_2$, $SiO_2$, $Al_2O_3$, $Fe_2O_3$). There are exceptions for some metal oxides that dissociate easily (e.g., MgO, CuO, ZnO) [22].

Semiconductors containing known toxic metals, such as the cadmium selenide quantum dots, are also toxic for a range of receptors, whereas semiconductors made from nontoxic metals exhibit much lower toxicity, at least

**TABLE 10.2**

Summary of Ecotoxicity for Metallic Oxide Nanoparticles

| Nanomaterial (Size) | Test Organism | Effect | References |
|---|---|---|---|
| $Al_2O_3$ | Bacteria[a] | 57%, 36%, 70% killing at 20 mg $L^{-1}$ | [81] |
| <50 nm | Microtox | Nontoxic at 100 mg $L^{-1}$ | [82] |
| | *C. elegans* | 24-h $LC_{50}$ = 82 mg $L^{-1}$ | [83] |
| | Zebrafish | Nontoxic | [84] |
| 13 nm | Plants[b] | $EC_{20}$ = 2 g $L^{-1}$ (root growth) | [85] |
| MgO, CaO ± Hal | *E. coli* | Bactericidal (with halides) | [57] |
| MgO 4–11 nm | Bacteria[c] | Most active oxide, even w/o light | [86] |
| $CeO_2$ | Bacteria | Bactericidal | [14] |
| 7 nm | *E. coli* | $EC_{50}$ = 5 mg $L^{-1}$ | [87] |
| | Microtox, Chydotox | Nontoxic at 100 mg $L^{-1}$ | [82] |
| 14, 20, 29 nm | *P. subcapitata* | $EC_{10}$ = 2.6–5.4 mg $L^{-1}$ (14–29 nm) | [88] |
| | Crustaceans[d] | DNA damage, strand breaks | [89] |
| CuO 30 nm | *Vibrio fischeri* | 30 min $EC_{50}$ = 79 mg $L^{-1}$ | [5] |
| CuO | Yeast[e] | 24-h $EC_{50}$ = 13.4 mg $L^{-1}$ | [90] |
| | Protozoa[f] | 4-h $EC_{50}$ = 128 mg $L^{-1}$ | [91] |
| | *P. subcapitata* | 72-h $EC_{50}$ = 0.7 mg Cu $L^{-1}$ | [92] |
| 30 nm | *D. magna*[g] | 48-h $LC_{50}$ = 3.2 mg Cu $L^{-1}$ | [5] |
| | *Thamnocephalus platyurus*[g] | 24-h $EC_{50}$ = 2.1 mg $L^{-1}$ | [5] |
| $Er_2O_3$ <100 nm | Microtox | 15 min $EC_{25}$ ~1–10 mg $L^{-1}$ | [93] |
| | *P. subcapitata* | 72-h-$IC_{25}$ ~1–10 mg $L^{-1}$ | [93] |
| $Fe_3O_4$ 7 nm | Marine bacteria[h] | 30 min, no effect | [64] |
| | Bact. consortium[i] | 21 days, no effect | [64] |
| $NiZnFe_4O_4$ <50 nm | *P. subcapitata* | 72-h $IC_{25}$ ~0.1–1 mg $L^{-1}$ | [93] |
| $CuZnFe_4O_4$ <100 nm | *P. subcapitata* | 72-h $IC_{25}$ ~1–10 mg $L^{-1}$ | [93] |
| $Cu/NiZnFe_4O_4$ | *T. platyurus* | 24-h $LC_{50}$ ~10–100 mg $L^{-1}$ | [93] |
| $CuZnFe_4O_4$ <100 nm | Cnidarian test[j] | 96-h $EC_{50}$ ~0.1–1 mg $L^{-1}$ | [93] |
| $HO_2O_3$ <100 nm | *P. subcapitata* | 72-h $IC_{25}$ ~1–10 mg $L^{-1}$ | [93] |
| | Cnidarian test[j] | 96-h $EC_{50}$ ~0.1–1 mg $L^{-1}$ | [93] |
| Indium tin oxide <50 nm | *P. subcapitata* | 72-h $IC_{25}$ ~1–10 mg $L^{-1}$ | [93] |
| | *T. platyurus* | 24-h $EC_{50}$ ~10–100 mg $L^{-1}$ | [93] |
| | Cnidarian test[j] | 96-h $EC_{50}$ = 0.3 mg $L^{-1}$ | [93] |
| $Sm_2O_3$ <100 nm | MARA[k] | 18-h MTC ~1–10 mg $L^{-1}$ | [93] |
| $SiO_2$ 14 nm | *B. subtilis, E. coli*[l] | + Bactericidal | [94] |

*(continued)*

**TABLE 10.2 (Continued)**

Summary of Ecotoxicity for Metallic Oxide Nanoparticles

| Nanomaterial (Size) | Test Organism | Effect | References |
|---|---|---|---|
| | Bacteria[a] | 40%, 58%, 70% killing at 20 mg L$^{-1}$ | [81] |
| 12.5, 27 nm | P. subcapitata | 72-h EC$_{20}$ = 20 mg L$^{-1}$ (12.5 nm) | [95] |
| TiO$_2$ <100 nm | Bacteria | Bactericidal | [14] |
| 66 nm | B. subtilis, E. coli[l] | ++ Bactericidal | [94] |
| | V. fischeri | Nontoxic at 20 g L$^{-1}$ | [5] |
| | Yeast[c] | Nontoxic | [90] |
| | E. coli | LD$_{50}$ = 1105 mg L$^{-1}$ | [96] |
| 79 nm | E. coli | + Light; 75% killing at 100 mg L$^{-1}$ | [97] |
| 50–150 nm | Microtox | Nontoxic at 100 mg L$^{-1}$ | [82] |
| 25–100 nm | Alga[m] | EC$_{50}$ = 44 mg L$^{-1}$ (25 nm diam) | [98–100] |
| 140 nm | P. subcapitata | 72-h EC$_{50}$ = 21 mg L$^{-1}$ | [101] |
| | P. subcapitata | 72-h EC$_{50}$ = 5.8 mg Ti L$^{-1}$ | [92] |
| 25–100 nm | D. magna[n] | 48-h LC$_{50}$ = 5.5 mg L$^{-1}$ | [102,103] |
| 25–70 nm | D. magna | Nontoxic (48-h; no light) | [5] |
| | D. magna[o] | Mortality, reproductive defects | [104] |
| | C. elegans | 24-h LC$_{50}$ = 80 mg L$^{-1}$ | [83] |
| 21 nm | Rainbow trout | Oxidative stress at 1 mg L$^{-1}$ | [105] |
| 21 nm | Zebrafish embryo | Not toxic up to 10 mg L$^{-1}$ | [30,84] |
| 25, 100 nm | Willow tree | Nontoxic at 100 mg L$^{-1}$ | [106] |
| 25, 100 nm | Eisenia fetida | Nontoxic at 1000 mg kg$^{-1}$ | [107] |
| | Collembola | Reproduction, IC$_{50}$ ~1000 mg kg$^{-1}$ | [107] |
| 15 nm | Isopods[p] | Sublethal effects, antioxidant enzymes at 2 mg g$^{-1}$ food | [108] |
| 21 nm | Mouse[q] | Genotoxic at 500 mg kg$^{-1}$ | [109] |
| [109] Pt$^{IV}$-modified TiO$_2$, | Bacteria | Bactericidal | [14] |
| C-doped TiO$_2$, | | Bactericidal | |
| N-doped TiO$_2$, | | C and N doped particles | |
| N-doped ZrO$_2$ | | active under sunlight | |
| ZnO | Bacteria | Bactericidal | [14] |
| 67 nm | B. subtilis, E. coli[l] | +++ Bactericidal | [94] |
| 30 nm | V. fischeri | 30 min EC$_{50}$ = 1.9 mg L$^{-1}$ | [5] |
| | Yeast[c] | 24-h EC$_{50}$ = 158 mg L$^{-1}$ | [90] |
| | Protozoa[d] | 4-h EC$_{50}$ = 5 mg L$^{-1}$ | [91] |

*(continued)*

**TABLE 10.2 (Continued)**

Summary of Ecotoxicity for Metallic Oxide Nanoparticles

| Nanomaterial (Size) | Test Organism | Effect | References |
|---|---|---|---|
| | Bacteria[a] | 100% killing at 20 mg $L^{-1}$ | [81] |
| | E. coli | $LD_{50} = 21$ mg $L^{-1}$ | [96] |
| | P. subcapitata | 72-h $EC_{50}$ ~5–10 mg $L^{-1}$ | [110] |
| | P. subcapitata | 72-h $EC_{50}$ ~0.04 mg $L^{-1}$ | [92] |
| 50–70 nm | D. magna | 48-h $LC_{50} = 3.2$ mg $L^{-1}$ | [5] |
| | T. platyurus | 24-h $EC_{50} = 0.18$ mg $L^{-1}$ | [5] |
| | C. elegans | 24-h $LC_{50} = 2.3$ mg $L^{-1}$ | [83] |
| | Zebrafish embryo | 48-h $LC_{50} = 1.8$ mg $L^{-1}$ | [84] |
| 20 nm | Plants[r] | Root elongation $IC_{50}$ < 50 mg $L^{-1}$ | [70] |
| $ZrO_2$ < 100 nm | Microtox | Nontoxic at 100 mg $L^{-1}$ | [82] |

*Note:* Hal, adsorbed halides (iodine, bromine, chlorine); MTC, microbial toxic action (50% effect) [93].

[a] Killing efficiency given for three strains: *B. subtilis, E. coli*, and *Pseudomonas fluorescens* [81].

[b] Seedlings (corn, cucumber, *Brassica oleracea*, and carrot *Daucus carota*). No effect for bulk alumina. Size for NP aggregates, 200 nm.

[c] Activity increase with decrease in nanoparticle diameter, *B. subtilis var. niger, S. aureus* [86].

[d] Freshwater crustaceans *D. magna* and *Chironomus riparius*.

[e] *Saccharomyces cerevisiae*. Bulk and nano Zn similar toxicity, Nano-Cu more toxic than bulk.

[f] Protozoa *Tetrahymena thermophila*.

[g] Use of natural waters containing dissolved organic matter decreased toxicity up to 140-fold compared with artificial freshwater [111].

[h] Marine bacteria *P. phosphoreum*.

[i] Bacterial consortium taken from an industrial anaerobic digester, matrix may bind nano-Ag/Cu.

[j] Morphological changes in *Hydra attenuata*.

[k] MARA = microbial array for risk assessment, growth inhibition of 11 microbial strains.

[l] Antimicrobial potency increases from $SiO_2$ to $TiO_2$ to ZnO. $TiO_2$ activity increased by light.

[m] Alga *Chroococcus* sp. [98,99] or freshwater alga *Desmodesmus subspicatus* [100].

[n] Value for 0.22 μm filtered material [102] Sonicated $TiO_2$ without effects at 100 mg $L^{-1}$.

[o] Chronic (21-day) exposure resulted in severe growth retardation, mortality, and reproductive defects.

[p] Terrestrial isopod *Porcellio scaber*, decrease in antioxidant enzymes GST and catalase.

[q] Inhalation study, DNA damage by comet assay, genetic instability as double-strand breaks.

[r] For plants such as radish, rape, and ryegrass.

in the absence of sunlight or UV light [58]. Weathering of NM such as quantum dots generally increases the toxicity; however, little is known about the weathering of most of the NMs [59–61]. Gold NPs are relatively innocuous in bacterial assays (although gold compounds can retard growth of tubercle bacillus) [62]; however, a recent study suggests that higher organisms may respond differently [62]. Gold in colloidal state is not bio-inert as it shows potent antiarthritic activity in rats, approximately 1000 times more potent than sodium aurothiomalate, a classic drug used against rheumatoid arthritis and nondisseminated lupus erythematosus [62].

Finally, a word of caution should be said about the use of nanoscale zero-valent iron for the remediation of contaminated groundwater, a most widely studied environmental application of nanotechnology [19,42,54,63]. The ecological evaluation of nanoiron is not available; however, the possible neurotoxicity of nanoscale zero-valent iron has been studied in rodent cells [63]. Complete or partial oxidation of nanoscale zero-valent iron was found to be effective in decreasing the toxicity, as well as agglomeration, sedimentation rate, and "redox" activity [63]. These results suggest that weathering or aging of the nanoiron will decrease the environmental burden at treated sites, although ecotoxicological data are still essential.

### 10.3.2  Carbon-Based Nanomaterials

Localization of redox-active carbon-based NMs into cell membranes prompted additional research on their toxicity for aquatic receptors [112]. Because underivatized fullerenes ($C_{60}$) and single-walled or multiwalled CNTs are almost insoluble in water, it is difficult to measure their toxicity in aqueous medium [4,112]. The earlier study on tetrahydrofuran (THF) as a cosolvent and carrier of $C_{60}$ (and nanotubes) has shown high toxicity, whereas recent toxicological data suggest that water-stirred fullerene has a low toxicity for a number of ecological receptors. The toxicity observed for THF-$C_{60}$ was later shown to be due to the presence of $C_{60}$-bound degradation products of THF, notably gamma-butyrolactone [13]. Further investigations on the bioavailability of environmental contaminants bound to $C_{60}$ or CNT may be warranted as these NMs can transport toxicants across cell membranes [113]. From the data summarized in Table 10.3, fish appear particularly sensitive to the effect of carbon-based NPs, and bacteria are quite resistant. As discussed for other NPs, exposure to $C_{60}$ in complex medium (soil, humic matter) strongly reduced the toxicity [14,114,115].

### 10.3.3  Organic Nanomaterials, Nanopesticides, Polymers, and Dendrimers

In addition to pesticides, organic NMs in the general class of nanopharmaceuticals may also become environmental contaminants, similar to hormonally active drugs (known as an endocrine disruptors), when released into the environment through wastewaters. It is not apparent whether the nano-based drugs emerging from biomedical nanotechnology will have to be tested for ecotoxicity. While preliminary toxicological information is available for polymers and dendrimers (polycationic organic NP), little information is known for the nanopesticides, including their fate. Despite the constant NM development, the prior knowledge existing on these general classes of compounds suggests that they may have an impact on the environment.

**TABLE 10.3**

Summary of Ecotoxicity for Carbon-Based Nanomaterials

| Nanomaterial (Size) | Test Organism | Effect | References |
|---|---|---|---|
| $C_{60}$ fullerene (THF-s) | Bacteria | 100% kill at 140 μM | [97] |
| (Nominal 0.72 nm) | Soil bacteria | No effect in silt clay loam at 1 mg kg$^{-1}$ | [14] |
| (10–20 nm) | B. subtilis, E. coli[a] | Reduced growth in MD at 0.4 mg L$^{-1}$ | [114] |
|  | D. magna | $LC_{50}$ = 0.46 mg L$^{-1}$ | [102] |
| (50–300 nm) | Zebrafish | $LC_{50}$ = 0.8 mg L$^{-1}$ | [116] |
|  | Mouse | Cancer promoter, immune suppressor | [117] |
| $C_{60}$ fulllerene (WS) | B. subtilis | Growth inhibition | [118] |
| (average 84 nm) | Bacteria | No effect at 140 μM | [97] |
|  | Soil bacteria[b] | Short-duration inhibition at 50 mg kg$^{-1}$ | [119] |
|  | Soil bacteria[b] | Slight (20%–30%) diversity loss at 14 days | [119] |
|  | Microtox | No effect at 1 mg L$^{-1}$ | [82] |
|  | D. magna | No effect at 35 mg L$^{-1}$ | [120] |
|  | D. magna[c] | $LC_{50}$ = 7.9 mg L$^{-1}$ | [102] |
|  | D. magna[d] | 21-day $LC_{40}$ = 2.5 mg L$^{-1}$ | [121] |
|  | Hyalella azteca, copepod | No effect at 22.5 mg L$^{-1}$ | [121] |
|  | Fathead minnow[e] | Metabolic change (fatty acids) | [121] |
|  | Medaka | No effect at 0.5 mg L$^{-1}$ | [121] |
|  | Zebrafish | No effect at 25 mg L$^{-1}$ (nominal) | [116] |
|  | Freshwater fish[f] | LPO in liver, body weight loss at 1 mg L$^{-1}$ | [122] |
|  | Marine fish[g] | Minute effects, GSH, LPO, at 10 mg L$^{-1}$ | [123] |
|  | Earthworm | 33% mortality at 1000 mg L$^{-1}$ | [124] |
| $C_{60}$ waste solids leachate | C. dubia | 48-h $LC_{50}$ = 5% dilution | [125] |
|  | P. promelas | 48-h $LC_{50}$ = 54% dilution | [125] |
| Fullerol $C_{60}(OH)_{24}$ | Bacteria | No effect at 140 μM | [97] |
| 122 nm | Zebrafish | No effect at 50 mg L$^{-1}$ | [126] |
| Carbon nanohorns | E. coli | Inhibition in liquid low-salt medium | [14] |
| Soot | K. pneumoniae | Inhibition in liquid low-salt medium | [14] |
| SWCNT | Bacteria | Inhibition in liquid low-salt medium | [14] |
|  | Copepods[h] | 64% reduced fertilization rate at 10 mg L$^{-1}$ | [127] |
|  | D. magna[i] | No effect on feeding on lipids | [128] |
|  | P. subcapitata | 72-h $IC_{25}$ values between 1 and 10 mg L$^{-1}$ | [93] |
|  | H. attenuata | 96-h $EC_{50}$ values between 1 and 10 mg L$^{-1}$ | [93] |
|  | Zebrafish[j] | Hatching delay at 120 mg L$^{-1}$ | [129] |

(*continued*)

**TABLE 10.3 (Continued)**

Summary of Ecotoxicity for Carbon-Based Nanomaterials

| Nanomaterial (Size) | Test Organism | Effect | References |
|---|---|---|---|
| | Rainbow trout[k] | Respiratory toxicant at 0.5 mg $L^{-1}$ | [130] |
| MWCNT | C. dubia[l] | 48-h $LC_{50}$ = 50.9 mg $L^{-1}$ | [41] |
| | Invertebrates[m] | $LC_{50}$ = 68 mg $kg^{-1}$ | [41] |
| | Protozoan[n] | Growth inhibition by d-MWCNT | [113] |
| | Zucchini[o] | 15-day 60% biomass red. at 1000 mg $L^{-1}$ | [56] |
| | Mouse (IV inj.)[p] | Accumulation in spleen, not toxic | [131] |
| | Mouse (inh.)[q] | Immune suppression, lung to spleen signal | [132] |
| Hydroxylated MWCNT | C. dubia | No effect at 120 mg $L^{-1}$ | [41] |
| Carbon black (20–25 nm) | Invertebrates[r] | $LC_{50}$ = 27/22 mg $kg^{-1}$ | [41] |

*Note:* See Tables 10.1 and 10.2 for previous abbreviations. MD, liquid low-salt minimal Davis medium; GSH, glutathione *S*-transferase; IV inj., intravenous injection; inh., inhalation; LPO, lipid peroxidation; d-MWCNT, decylamine-conjugated multiple-walled carbon nanotubes; Red., reduction; THF-s, tetrahydrofuran solubilization; WS, water stirred.

[a] Size of filtered aggregates. Effect noted only in minimal Davis medium, no effect noted in Luria broth [114]. No toxic effect noted upon addition of soil suspension or 0.05 mg $L^{-1}$ humic acids [115].

[b] Inhibition was no longer detected after 1 week of exposure [119].

[c] Sonicated fullerene.

[d] Water-stirred fullerene aggregates with average diameter 349–1394 nm, also produced delayed molting (at 2.5 mg $L^{-1}$) and 75% decreased offspring production at 5 mg $L^{-1}$.

[e] Downregulation of the PMP70 gene, suggesting fatty acid metabolism inhibition, oxidative stress.

[f] Freshwater fish *Carassius auratus*, 32-day study.

[g] Marine fish model *Fundulus heteroclitus* embryos. Animals can withstand small oxidative stress.

[h] Estuarine copepods *Amphiascus tenuiremis*, unpurified material caused 34% reduction molting success, 36% mortality at 10 mg $L^{-1}$ but purified material was nontoxic.

[i] Lipid-coated nanotubes.

[j] Nonsignificant effect as 99% of exposed embryo hatched by 75-h postfertilization.

[k] SDS-solubilized SWCNT, surfactant may have caused observed toxicity after 10 days [130].

[l] Nanotubes were stabilized with 100 mg $L^{-1}$ natural organic matter.

[m] Sediment tests with *Leptocheirus plumulosus* and *Hyalella azteca*. Value shown for *L. plumulosus*, no $LC_{50}$ value could be obtained for *H. azteca* (more tolerant species).

[n] Protozoan *Tetrahymena pyriformis*, glucosamine, and decylamine-coated tubes. The d-MWCNT liberated toxic decylamine upon ingestion by organisms.

[o] *Cucurbita pepo*, root growth inhibition was observed only for copper nanoparticles [56].

[p] Study duration, 2 months.

[q] Immune suppression observed at 1 mg $m^3$, no effect at 0.3 mg $m^3$.

[r] Exposure in sediments, 27 for *L. plumulosus*, 22 for *H. azteca*.

### 10.3.3.1 Nanoformulated Pesticides

The advent of nanopesticides (or nanoformulated pesticides) created debate recently, including the regulatory issues that are applied to these chemicals [9]. Industries in the agricultural sector will probably exploit the alleged advantages of the NP-based pesticides; that is, the novel nanopesticide delivery systems, including nanocapsules, nanocontainers, and nanocages, could replace conventional emulsifiable concentrates, thus reducing organic solvent content in agricultural formulations, and enhancing dispersibility, wettability, and the penetration strength of the droplets [9]. It is also expected that enhanced use of smart systems could diminish runoff and avert unwanted movement of pesticides [133]. Smart field systems detect, locate, and report/apply, as needed, pesticide and fertilizers before the onset of symptoms [133]. Available chemical or toxicity information on commercial nanopesticides is limited, probably due to proprietary reasons. A study by Cao et al. [7] indicated that a chlorfenapyr nanoformulation has a slightly higher degradation rate compared with the standard suspension (half-lives of 4.3 and 3.9 days, respectively); their effects on nontarget organisms were not studied. Liu et al. [8] reported that nanosized pesticide particles could produce better spatial distribution of the agent on the surface of leaves, as well as increase the absorption of the pesticide by leaf-chewing organisms. Another proposed advantage is a reduced risk of exposure for workers by elimination of handling of pesticide solutions in oil, which have a high potential to be absorbed transdermally. Ecotoxicological effects have not been reported.

**TABLE 10.4**

Summary of (Eco)toxicity Studies of Polymers and Dendrimers

| Nanomaterial (Size) | Test Organism | Effect | References |
|---|---|---|---|
| NIPAM/BAM (50–70 nm) | Microtox, alga | Toxicity proportional to zeta-potential | [134] |
| | Salmonid cells | Nontoxic up to 1000 mg $L^{-1}$ | [134] |
| NIPAM/BAM | *D. magna* | Proportional to reduction in zeta-potential | [134] |
| PAMAM (5 nm) | Mouse | Kidney accumulation (possible renal failure) | [15] |
| Chitosan | Human cells | Cell necrosis, LPO, ROS production | [135] |
| G5NH₂ PAMAM | Animal cells | Membrane damage $EC_{20}$ ~500 nM | [136] |
| G7NH₂ PAMAM | Animal cells | Membrane damage $EC_{20}$ ~50–150 nM | [136] |
| G5 Ac PAMAM | Animal cells | Nontoxic at 500 nM | [136] |

*Note:* LPO, lipid peroxidation; NIPAM, poly-*N*-isopropylacrylamide; NIPAM/BAM, *N*-isopropylacrylamide/*N-tert*-butylacrylamide copolymer nanoparticles; PAMAM, poly-(amidoamine) dendrimers; G5 NH₂/G7 NH₂ PAMAM, generation 5 (or 7) cationic PAMAM (10–20 nm); G5 Ac PAMAM, generation 5 neutral PAMAM (5 nm diameter).

### 10.3.3.2 Polymers and Dendrimers

A range of polymers, either artificial or made from natural building blocks, is being developed for drug delivery (e.g., copolymers, dendrimers) or as active drugs (e.g., chitosan). A few of these NMs have been tested for ecotoxicity; information available is summarized in Table 10.4.

## 10.3.4 Factors Affecting Toxicity

These factors can be divided into two types, those pertaining to the NPs themselves, such as the presence of coatings or any other type of surface modification, and those pertaining to the medium (water, soil, or sediment) or to the ecological receptor itself. Surface coating or surface derivatization has been used to modify inherently toxic materials (e.g., uncoated CdTe quantum dots) and makes them usable in medical applications (as tested in animals). Dunphy Guzmaän et al. [39] questioned whether the surface coating reduces the bioavailability (thus toxicity) and limits the solubility of some toxic NMs. In fact, such coatings may not be persistent after release into the environment. For instance, in the case of toxic cadmium selenide NP, the coating (e.g., ZnS) can be oxidized over time, leading to the subsequent release of the toxic core materials.

Surface modifications are another method to alter the physico–chemical and ultimately the toxicity of some NMs. Fullerene has been subjected to several types of surface modifications, for example, partial oxidation (producing fullerol) that improves water dispersibility and diminishes its toxicity to living organisms, possibly via a lower affinity for hydrophobic lipid membrane sites [41]. Whether the lower toxicity could be due to a reduced capacity to generate reactive oxygen species (ROS) has been questioned because the production of ROS (as superoxide and singlet oxygen production under UV light) is, in fact, greater for fullerol than for fullerene [97]. It is suggested that NMs have to be in the vicinity of the cells to induce toxicity through ROS generation.

Soil and the aquatic media, including sediments, contain several constituents such as clays and organic matter that may bind NM and change their bioavailability compared with their suspension in pure water. These constituents have high specific surface areas (300–500 $m^2$ $g^{-1}$ typically), and the surface charge allows them to interact with charged particles [16]. In addition, uncharged hydrophobic NP can interact with hydrophobic domains of natural organic matter such as humic and fulvic acids present in water, soil, and sediments [16]. For example, the presence of natural organic matter improved the stability of multiwalled NT suspensions in water [41,131]. As mentioned earlier, most laboratory-based aquatic toxicity studies are using simple or well-defined aquatic media that are not representative of diverse natural waters. Similarly, conditions are optimized in some plant toxicity studies, for instance using filter paper in aquatic test and response endpoints, such as germination and root elongation, or effects on plant transpiration flux in hydroponics setting. These model systems were used because of their "simplicity" and ease of certain measurements (e.g., elongation of plant roots); however, toxicity tests conducted for soil or sediments as substrate would be more reliable and environmentally relevant under field conditions. In fact, few available data regarding the exposure of organisms (plants, invertebrates) in soil or sediments suggest that the toxicity of various NPs is strongly reduced compared with those in aquatic media. Apart from direct binding to medium constituents, aggregation (or agglomeration) may occur, that leads to a reduction of bioavailability and therefore ecotoxicity, even if NP aggregates (or agglomerates) can be toxic by itself [24,39]. As described earlier for nano-$TiO_2$, factors that reduce the transport of particles (such as aggregation caused by variations in ionic strength or pH, binding to larger particles) may reduce the toxicity as well, at least for live organisms in the water column [16].

Lastly, it is noteworthy to highlight the bacteria–NP interactions, that bacteria might modify the environmental fate of NMs, that is, through the production of proteins that could change their aggregation state and consequently their transport in the environment [138]. It is also reported that bacteria may influence the chemical degradation of NPs, or the stability of NMs coated with biodegradable coatings [138]. This ability of bacteria may be shared by other ecological receptors such as *Daphnia magna* [128].

## 10.3.5 Adequacy of Current Ecotoxicity Testing Methods

While novel physico–chemical properties of engineered NMs may induce different toxicity mechanisms (as described below), one wonders whether the short-term ecotoxicity assays are adequate for the detection of all modes of toxicity. According to a review by Stern and McNeil [139], the available toxicity data demonstrate a lack of size-specific mechanisms [i.e., toxicological profile shared by all NMs], with an overall picture of "material-specific rather than nanogeneralized risk." Until now, the toxicological properties of NMs are known to be similar to that of ultrafine particles [25]. Some aspects of testing methods are still unknown. For instance, using the deionized water and harsh NM suspension methods may not be realistic in comparison with NM dispersion and suspension in natural waters because they vary significantly with respect to the water chemistry and the reactivity of NMs [35]. The use of sonication as a suspension method is questionable, as it leads to unpredictable results (enhanced or reduced activity) according to the test material [35,124]. The physico–chemical characterization of the test materials is thus an important issue (for more details, refer to the website: http://characterizationmatters.org/), as toxicity results of identical materials have been shown to be contradictory. Insufficient chemical characterization may explain, at least in part, some of those discrepancies [140].

Assay sensitivity should also be considered for the adequacy of the ecotoxicity test. Stampoulis et al. [56] indicated that standard root germination and elongation assays might not be sufficiently sensitive to detect the toxicity of the test NMs (e.g., Ag, ZnO, multiwall CNTs), suggesting the use of longer-term assays such as biomass changes. In addition, testing issues regarding the genotoxicity of NMs have been raised as well [141,142]. Unexpected interactions with test reagents (e.g., colorimetric and fluorimetric dyes) generate misleading data sets. Similarly, a nanogenotoxicity test of NMs such as metals and their oxides on bacteria indicates that the current microbial assays (e.g., Ames) may not be suitable, possibly owing to the presence of the bacterial cell wall that prevents the entry of NM into the cells [141]. The most sensitive assays were the comet and the micronucleus assays, using eukaryotic cells. The use of a battery of standard genotoxicity tests is recommended, including *in vivo* assays to correlate *in vitro* results [141].

## 10.4 Mechanisms of Ecotoxicity

On the basis of available studies, NPs may act on biological systems by known pathways (as described below) depending on their chemical surface characteristics and chemical reactivity related to their increased surface area. Physical effects, such as shading, have been postulated as a mechanism of growth inhibition, exemplified by adsorption of nano-$TiO_2$ to algal cells [10]. Several authors demonstrated the relation between NM size (surface area) and magnitude of the toxic outcome, generally using binary physico–chemical comparisons (e.g., nanosized vs. bulk, or ultrafine vs. fine). For example, Van Hoecke et al. [88,95] recently demonstrated a relation between surface area and toxic effect, using $SiO_2$ and $CeO_2$ NP (all <30 nm diameter). Algal toxicities differed when expressed on a mass basis, but these effects were identical among materials of different sizes when corrected for surface area.

Differences in toxicity between bulk and nanosized materials have shed some light on modes of toxic action. In metals (Ag, Cu, Zn) and metal oxides (CuO, ZnO), toxicity could be related to particle solubility (or solubilization rate). Owing to the high solubility, all forms of ZnO have the same toxicity for a given ecoreceptor [5,90,110]. For less soluble materials, nanosized particles are generally more toxic than the bulk counterpart, because of their increased specific surface area, leading to increased chemical surface reactivity and possibly ROS generation. Auffan et al. [143] reviewed in depth the size effect and suggested that the size limit for the change from bulk to nano properties could lie around 30 nm, causing the difference between small particles and NPs. The atypical surface structure (e.g., crystallinity for inorganic compounds) and reactivity of NPs may enhance chemical processes including dissolution and redox reactions (such as ROS generation) compared with bulk materials. Also, environmental parameters such as dissolved organic carbon and ionic strength can affect the toxicity of metals for aquatic receptors [35].

Interestingly, prokaryotes (e.g., microbial fauna), in contrast to eukaryotes, may be protected against the uptake of many types of NPs because they do not have mechanisms for colloidal transport across their cell wall; they are nevertheless susceptible to toxic effects mediated by ROS production ($C_{60}$ + UV light, $TiO_2$), metal ion leakage ($Ag^+$, $Cu^{2+}$, $Zn^{2+}$, $Cd^{2+}$, $Ni^{2+}$), or even to the generation of by-products [14,39,144,145]. Because the release of $Cd^{2+}$ did not explain the observed toxicity of quantum dots, it was suggested that other possible major contributors to bacterial toxicity could include $TeO_2$ and $CdO$ (or in some cases $SeO_3^{2-}$ ions) [144]. Further studies indicated that in intact quantum dots, the main mechanism of bactericidal action is ROS production, and not $Cd^{2+}$ release [78]. Algal nanotoxicity is also related in part to metal dissociation or leakage (e.g., ZnO) and/or to ROS production (e.g., $TiO_2$ in the presence of light), or to specific particle–membrane interactions (Ag), depending on the type of NM [10].

It is possible that some invertebrates and other animals may share common modes of toxicity, except that exposure may be increased through the biomagnification phenomena, as discussed later. Filter-feeding invertebrates (e.g., *Daphnia*) were found to be more sensitive to nanometals than zebrafish. This may be explained by the separate feeding strategies employed, daphnids being particulate filter feeders that would be expected to be more intimately exposed to large numbers of particles during exposure [30]. This difference in sensitivity could not be verified for other NMs because of a lack of data. Soluble forms of the metals (salts) were more toxic to *Daphnia* species (e.g., *D. pulex*) than the particulate metals using mass-based concentrations of exposure. In contrast, the same metal salts were less toxic to *Ceriodaphnia* sp. (e.g., *C. dubia*). In the latter case, nano-Ag or nano-Cu may exert their toxicity through ROS production or other unidentified mechanisms.

In some cases in plants, the cell wall limits the passage of NMs; however, the NMs may be translocated from roots to shoots depending on the type of material [56]. Similar to bacteria, plant cells are sensitive to the released metal ions ($Ag^+$, $Cu^{2+}$), as well as to ROS generation [56]; however, the uptake of toxic NPs appears to be limited. For instance, zucchini exposed to 1000 mg $L^{-1}$ nanosilver in hydroponic conditions contained approximately 9.5 mg Ag $kg^{-1}$ tissue [56]. In another study, a 2.5-fold increase in aluminum levels in ryegrass leaves (but not in red kidney beans) was measured at the highest concentration of 10,000 mg $kg^{-1}$ in soil [71].

The mode of toxicity of organic NMs and polymers may differ compared with those for inorganic NMs. For interpretation of toxicity studies on carbon-based NMs, one should consider the effects of the concentration of functional groups, the hydrophilicity of functionalized NPs (nanotubes or fullerenes), and the sequential nonspecific interactions between the NMs and the organisms or constituents in the culture medium (113). The importance of the cotransporting activity of $C_{60}$ and multiwalled NTs that could lead to detrimental effects on ecological receptors has been studied [13,113]. In higher animals, $C_{60}$ (and perhaps other carbon-based materials) has been shown to have hazardous consequences, due to inflammatory response accompanied by release of nitric oxide, ultimately resulting in immune suppression and cancer [117].

## 10.4.1 Photoreactivity

Light-triggered ROS production or redox reactions are viewed as important modes of toxicity for some NMs, such as quantum dots, several metals and metal oxides, fullerenes, and possibly dendrimers. While redox reactions might occur in the dark for NMs such as zero-valent iron, the toxicity of most other NMs is strongly enhanced in the presence of light (e.g., the bactericidal effects of photoactivated $TiO_2$) [86]. Differences in testing methods (i.e., carrying out the experiment in the presence or absence of light, or light intensity) may explain some of the different outcomes reported in the literature for the same NP (e.g., $TiO_2$) tested in the same species (e.g., *D. magna*).

The photoactivity of some NMs is a relevant mode of toxicity for photosynthetic organisms [99], and also for bacteria. Dumas et al. [78] reported that a 30-min exposure of blue light to bacteria simultaneously exposed to CdTe quantum dots totally inhibited bacterial growth, whereas only weak bacteriostatic effects were observed following exposure in the dark. Interestingly, nanosized $TiO_2$ can exhibit a specific toxicity on algal cells, without affecting the photosynthetic bacteria [99]. This differential sensitivity was explained by the fact that alga can release oxygen, which is then activated by the nano-$TiO_2$ (in the presence of UV light) to produce toxic superoxide ions [99].

Light-induced genotoxicity has also been observed in studies using $TiO_2$ [146]. In the absence of visible or UV light, $TiO_2$ is not (or only weakly) genotoxic to mammalian cells or to *Salmonella typhimurium*; however, coexposure to UV light causes DNA damage as detected by the comet assay (12.5–200 mg$^{-1}$ for nano-$TiO_2$; 50–3200 mg$^{-1}$ for microscale $TiO_2$), as well as chromosomal aberrations in Chinese hamster cells (3–50 mg$^{-1}$ nano-$TiO_2$). Negative results were found for nano-$TiO_2$ (microscale $TiO_2$ not tested) using the mouse lymphoma L5178Y mutation assay (250–2000 mg$^{-1}$). At concentrations from 5000 to 40,000 mg$^{-1}$, *S. typhimurium* bacteria showed decreased mutant yield upon exposure to nano-$TiO_2$ (21 nm average diameter, mixture of anatase and rutile nano-$TiO_2$) relative to UV light illumination only ($TiO_2$ added), suggesting that photo-activated nano-$TiO_2$ can cause toxicity to bacteria without genotoxicity [146].

## 10.4.2 Interactions with Xenobiotics: A Carrier Effect

Even if a given NM is not toxic to living organisms, its presence in the environment can modify the toxicity of other toxicants. Either increased or decreased toxicities have been reported depending on particular combinations. Highly hydrophobic compounds that are poorly available to organisms might be delivered more efficiently when transported by NMs. For instance, a 60% increase in phenanthrene toxicity was found in *D. magna* that are coexposed to $C_{60}$ [147]. In addition, $Cd^{2+}$ toxicity to algae can be increased in the presence of 2 mg L$^{-1}$

nano-$TiO_2$ but not with bulk $TiO_2$. These results suggest a "carrier" effect of the NMs, in that the combination of the NM–xenobiotic can facilitate adsorption or absorption into the cells [148]. Similarly, in the carp, a 132% increase in arsenic accumulation was found following coexposure to 0.2 mg $L^{-1}$ As and 10 mg $L^{-1}$ $TiO_2$ for 25 days [149]. On the other hand, it is possible that water-soluble toxicants become greatly adsorbed onto an NM, causing a decrease in the bioavailable fraction of the toxicant to organisms and subsequently less toxicity; this was evidenced by the formation of newly formed complexes, for example, pentachlorophenol and $C_{60}$, or diuron and carbon black [147]. The detailed mechanism(s) by which the bioavailability of xenobiotics can be modified when adsorbed onto NMs are not well known and further studies are warranted.

### 10.4.3 Bioaccumulation and Trophic Transfer

Many authors have discussed the mechanisms underlying the trophic transfer and biomagnification of NMs. For instance, Baun and colleagues [1] suggested that a possible route for nano-$TiO_2$ biomagnification is the ingestion of NP-coated alga by planktonic species, such as *D. magna*. The inefficient elimination of $TiO_2$ by *D. magna* resulted in significant bioaccumulation (72 h or longer exposure) that may lead to a direct effect on the organism following food intake [104]. Transfer of quantum dots 545 ITK carbonyl to *Daphnia* fed by exposed alga was detected by fluorescence microscopy, and quantified by means of an increase in light (pixel) intensity [75]. A food web based on bacteria, ciliates, and rotifers was used by Holbrook et al. [150]. This food web was not optimal, as bacteria could not absorb the test NPs (e.g., carboxylated quantum dots). It was noted, however, that the quantum dots adhered to ciliates and resulted in significant bioconcentration with bioconcentration factor (BCF) values in the range of 1000 to 1400 ($kg^{-1}$ wet weight), depending on the coating of the quantum dots. Surprisingly, further ingestion of ciliates by rotifers did not lead to biomagnification.

In a bioaccumulation study of $TiO_2$ in carp, Zhang et al. [151] reported a BCF value around 600 $kg^{-1}$ wet weight (whole body, accumulation mainly in viscera and gill; 25-day exposure to 3 or 10 $mg^{-1}$). The transfer of gold nanorods was demonstrated by Ferry et al. [152] using a mesocosm that contained seawater, sediment, sea grass, microbes, biofilms, snails, clams, shrimp, and fish. After a 12-day exposure period, clams and bacterial biofilms accumulated the highest amounts of gold NP, suggesting that NPs can readily pass from the water column to the food web.

## 10.5 Concluding Remarks

There is no doubt that some NMs have the ability to adversely affect different environmental receptors (at least in conditions of high bioavailability);

however, it remains to be identified how this toxic potential can be influenced by biotic and abiotic environmental factors. Knowledge gaps for aquatic toxicology have been described [12]. There is no general consensus on the "dose-metric" or the measure of exposure, or of bioaccumulation in wild fish. Most of the available toxicity data were obtained under controlled laboratory settings using standard test species such as freshwater fish or invertebrates. Whether these results can be extrapolated to ecological receptors under field conditions is not known. It is essential to validate these effects using marine and estuarine fish, and also on sediment-dwelling fish species and invertebrates [147]. A similar type of interpretation can be applied for terrestrial toxicology, where only a limited number of laboratory species are in use. Further, some studies have involved terrestrial receptors (microbes, plant seeds) without using soil as the exposure medium.

Standard and research-based techniques need to be developed to measure NMs in environmental samples, including animal and vegetal tissues. While a few approaches have been proposed, it is still difficult to distinguish between the manufactured NMs and natural NMs. Other knowledge gaps include the effects of abiotic factors (salinity, hardness, dissolved organic matter, pH) on the bioavailability of NMs to ecological receptors. It is anticipated that advances in the chemistry of the individual NM will make it possible for a better prediction of NM bioavailability. Some data are available concerning the uptake of NMs by fish; however, information on the distribution, metabolism, and excretion of these particles is still lacking [12].

Fate and transport, as well as bioavailability of NMs in the environment and in biota are not presently well known, and a better knowledge concerning these aspects will increase the scientific value of future ecological risk assessments for NMs [12,147]. Likewise, there are numerous information gaps related to algae, plants, and fungi as environmental receptors, including the development of mechanistic models to explain NM passage through their cell membranes and walls, and trophic transfer of NM in their food chain [10], as well as a better understanding of specific properties of NM related to their toxicity.

Clearly, the field of nanoecotoxicology is a young and evolving discipline. Presently, toxicological observations are NM specific based on the available data, and it is very difficult to make broad conclusions with great certainty. Nevertheless, it seems that the putative effects of NPs on soil bacterial communities may not be really an issue, as it seems that soil bacteria might be protected from the toxic effect of NMs through the strong binding capacity of the soil (or sediments), plus the fact that the bacterial cell wall limits passage on NMs inside the cells [14,153]. Higher organisms might be more susceptible than bacteria to the toxic effects of NMs, as observed in aquatic assays using invertebrates or algal cells. Terrestrial receptors, plants, and soil invertebrates appear relatively insensitive in most assays done for NM, although only a very limited number of compounds have been examined.

In addition, the type of assay and duration of exposure are also important for conclusive evidence. For example, nano-$TiO_2$ showed negative results using a battery of short-term screening tests, such as the 15-min Microtox and the PAM (photosystem-II inhibition assay) [82]. The same NM was, however, repeatedly found to be a strong inhibitor of algal growth, using a 4-day exposure [92,100,101]. Similar limitations have been observed for many short-term exposure assays, suggesting that components of a valuable test battery should be selected with care.

Chronic toxicity assays should be implemented for NM studies. Such effects are not well studied, except for immune toxicity (inflammatory response) reported in animal inhalation studies. Genotoxic effects might also be examined because changes in genetic diversity are considered important endpoints for the ecological perspective, as they could alter the ability of populations to adapt to new conditions or stressors [154]. In case of bacteria, such mutations may alter their resistance to metals or even antibiotics, and the mutants could subsequently act as new pathogens for higher animals and humans.

To avoid possible risks, a complete evaluation should be made of human and/or environmental exposure resulting from emission throughout the NM life cycle, including the manufacturing process, the various expected use situations, and the final disposal or recycling processes. This information may be beneficial for the potential risks assessment and hazard identification of NMs. In addition, the early recognition of potential risks, at all stages of product life cycles, will provide better opportunities for risk mitigation and management.

## References

1. Baun, A. et al. Ecotoxicity of engineered nanoparticles to aquatic invertebrates: A brief review and recommendations for future toxicity testing. *Ecotoxicology*, 17, 387, 2008.
2. Oberdörster, G., Oberdörster, E., and Oberdorster, J. Nanotoxicology: An emerging discipline evolving from studies of ultrafine particles. *Environ. Health Perspect.*, 113, 823, 2005.
3. Nel, A. et al. Toxic potential of materials at the nanolevel. *Science*, 311, 622, 2006.
4. Farré, M. et al. Ecotoxicity and analysis of nanomaterials in the aquatic environment. *Anal. Bioanal. Chem.*, 393, 81, 2009.
5. Heinlaan, M. et al. Toxicity of nanosized and bulk ZnO, CuO and TiO$_2$ to bacteria *Vibrio fischeri* and crustaceans *Daphnia magna* and *Thamnocephalus platyurus*. *Chemosphere*, 71, 1308, 2008.
6. Kuzma, J. and VerHage, P. *Nanotechnology in Agriculture and Food Production: Anticipated Applications*, Woodrow Wilson International Center for Scholars, Washington DC, 2006, Available at: http://www.nanotechproject.org/process/assets/files/2706/94_pen4_agfood.pdf, accessed October 2009.
7. Cao, Y. et al. HPLC/UV analysis of chlorfenapyr residues in cabbage and soil to study the dynamics of different formulations. *Sci. Total Environ.*, 350, 38, 2005.

8. Liu, Y., Tong, Z., and Prud'homme, R.K., Stabilized polymeric nanoparticles for controlled and efficient release of bifenthrin. *Pest. Manag. Sci.*, 64, 808, 2008.
9. ABA, *The Adequacy of FIFRA to Regulate Nanotechnology-Based Pesticides.* American Bar Association; Section of Environment, Energy, and Resources. May 2006. Publication 505.33 (FIFRA Nano Paper_.doc) Chicago, IL.
10. Navarro, E. et al. Environmental behavior and ecotoxicity of engineered nanoparticles to algae, plants, and fungi. *Ecotoxicology*, 17, 372, 2008.
11. Handy, R.D. et al. The ecotoxicology and chemistry of manufactured nanoparticles. *Ecotoxicology*, 17, 287, 2008.
12. Handy, R.D., Owen, R., and Valsami-Jones, E. The ecotoxicology of nanoparticles and nanomaterials: Current status, knowledge gaps, challenges, and future needs. *Ecotoxicology*, 17, 315, 2008.
13. Klaine, S.J. et al. Nanomaterials in the environment: Behavior, fate, bioavailability, and effects. *Environ. Toxicol. Chem.*, 27, 1825, 2008.
14. Neal, A.L. What can be inferred from bacterium–nanoparticle interactions about the potential consequences of environmental exposure to nanoparticles. *Ecotoxicology*, 17, 362, 2008.
15. Borm, P.J.A. et al. The potential risks of nanomaterials: A review carried out for ECETOC. *Part. Fibre Toxicol.*, 3, 1, 2006.
16. Norwegian Pollution Control Authority, *Environmental Fate and Ecotoxicity of Engineered Nanoparticles*, Report TA 2304/2007, Joner, E.J., Hartnik, T., and Amundsen, C.E., eds., Bioforsk, Ås., 2008, 64 pp.
17. Handy, R.D. et al. Manufactured nanoparticles: Their uptake and effects on fish—A mechanistic analysis, *Ecotoxicology*, 17, 396, 2008.
18. Higarashi, M.M. and Jardim, W.F. Remediation of pesticide contaminated soil using $TiO_2$ mediated by solar light. *Catal. Today*, 76, 201, 2002.
19. Quinn, J. et al. Field demonstration of DNAPL dehalogenation using emulsified zero-valent iron. *Environ. Sci. Technol.*, 39, 1309, 2005.
20. Monteil-Rivera, F. et al. Reduction of octahydro-1,3,5,7-tetranitro-1,3,5,7-tetrazocine by zerovalent iron: Product distribution. *Environ. Sci. Technol.*, 39, 9725, 2005.
21. Rejeski, D. *CPSC FY2010 Agenda and Priorities*, Woodrow Wilson International Center for Scholars, Available at: http://www.nanotechproject.org., accessed October 2009.
22. Tran, C.L. et al. *A Scoping Study to Identify Hazard Data Needs for Addressing the Risks Presented by Nanoparticles and Nanotubes*, IOM Research Report, Edinburgh, UK, 2005.
23. Kaegi, R. et al. Synthetic $TiO_2$ nanoparticle emission from exterior facades into the aquatic environment. *Environ. Pol.*, 156, 233, 2008.
24. Mueller, N.C. and Nowack, B. Exposure modeling of engineered nanoparticles in the environment. *Environ. Sci. Technol.*, 42, 4447, 2008.
25. Tiede, K. et al. Considerations for environmental fate and ecotoxicity testing to support environmental risk assessments for engineered nanoparticles. *J. Chromatogr. A*, 1216, 503, 2009.
26. Ogilvie Robichaud, C. et al. Estimates of upper bounds and trends in nano-$TiO_2$ production as a basis for exposure assessment. *Environ. Sci. Technol.*, 43, 4227, 2009.
27. Gottschalk, F. et al. Modeled environmental concentrations of engineered nanomaterials ($TiO_2$, ZnO, Ag, CNT, Fullerenes) for different regions. *Environ. Sci. Technol.*, 43, 9216, 2009.

28. Senjen, R. *Nanosilver, A Threat to Soil, Water and Human Health?* Friends of the Earth, FOE, Australia, 2007.
29. Benn, T.M. and Westerhoff, P. Nanoparticle silver released into water from commercially available sock fabrics. *Environ. Sci. Technol.*, 42, 4133, 2008.
30. Griffitt, R.J. et al. Effects of particle composition and species on toxicity of metallic nanomaterials in aquatic organisms. *Environ. Toxicol. Chem.*, 27, 1972, 2008.
31. Choi, O. and Hu, Z.Q. Size dependent and reactive oxygen species related nanosilver toxicity to nitrifying bacteria. *Environ. Sci. Technol.*, 42, 4583, 2008.
32. Mühling, M. et al. An investigation into the effects of silver nanoparticles on antibiotic resistance of naturally occurring bacteria in an estuarine sediment. *Mar. Environ. Res.*, 68, 278, 2009.
33. Bradford, A. et al. Impact of silver nanoparticle contamination on the genetic diversity of natural bacterial assemblages in estuarine sediments. *Environ. Sci. Technol.*, 43, 4530, 2009.
34. Roh, J.Y. et al. Ecotoxicity of silver nanoparticles on the soil nematode *Caenorhabditis elegans* using functional ecotoxicogenomics. *Environ. Sci. Technol.*, 43, 3933, 2009.
35. Gao, J. et al. Dispersion and toxicity of selected manufactured nanomaterials in natural river water samples: Effects of water chemical composition. *Environ. Sci. Technol.*, 43, 3322, 2009.
36. Nowack, B. Nanosilver revisited downstream. *Science*, 330, 1054, 2010.
37. Siciliano, S.D., Roy, R., and Greer, C.W. Reduction in denitrification activity in field soils exposed to long term contamination by 2,4,6-trinitrotoluene. *FEMS Microbiol. Ecol.*, 32, 61, 2000.
38. Koelmans, A.A., Nowack, B., and Wiesner, M.R. Comparison of manufactured and black carbon nanoparticle concentrations in aquatic sediments. *Environ. Pollut.*, 157, 1110, 2009.
39. Dunphy Guzmaän, K.A., Taylor, M.R., and Banfield, J.F. Environmental risks of nanotechnology: National Nanotechnology Initiative funding, 2000–2004. *Environ. Sci. Technol.*, 40, 1401, 2006.
40. Gartner, J. *Military Reloads with Nanotech*, Technology Review, MIT, 2005, accessed May 2007.
41. Kennedy, A.J. et al. Factors influencing the partitioning and toxicity of nanotubes in the aquatic environment. *Environ. Toxicol. Chem.*, 27, 1932, 2008.
42. Nowack, B. and Bucheli, T.D. Occurrence, behavior and effects of nanoparticles in the environment. *Environ. Pollution*, 150, 5, 2007.
43. Hsu, L.-Y. and Chein, H.-M. Evaluation of nanoparticle emission for $TiO_2$ nanopowder coating materials. *J. Nanopart. Res.*, 9, 157, 2007.
44. Kiser, M.A. et al. Titanium nanomaterial removal and release from wastewater treatment plants. *Environ. Sci. Technol.*, 43, 6757, 2009.
45. Ridley, M.K., Hackley, V.A., and Machesky, M.L. Characterization and surface-reactivity of nanocrystalline anatase in aqueous solutions. *Langmuir*, 22, 10972, 2006.
46. Long, T.C. et al. Titanium dioxide (P25) produces reactive oxygen species in immortalized brain microglia (BV2): Implications for nanoparticle neurotoxicity. *Environ. Sci. Technol.*, 40, 4346, 2006.
47. Sager, T.M. et al. Improved method to disperse nanoparticles for *in vitro* and *in vivo* investigation of toxicity. *Nanotoxicology*, 1, 118, 2007.
48. Yang, K., Lin, D., and Xing, B. Interactions of humic acid with nanosized inorganic oxides. *Langmuir*, 25, 3571, 2009.

49. Lecoanet, H.F., Bottero, J.Y., and Wiesner, M.R. Laboratory assessment of the mobility of nanomaterials in porous media. *Environ. Sci. Technol.*, 38, 5164, 2004.
50. Domingos, R.F. et al. Characterizing manufactured nanoparticles in the environment—Multimethod determination of particle sizes. *Environ. Sci. Technol.*, 43, 7277–7284, 2009.
51. Domingos, R.F., Tufenkji, N., and Wilkinson, K.J. Aggregation of titanium dioxide nanoparticles: Role of a fulvic acid. *Environ. Sci. Technol.*, 43, 1282–1286, 2009.
52. Fang, J. et al. Stability of titania nanoparticles in soil suspensions and transport in saturated homogeneous soil columns. *Environ. Pollut.*, 157, 1101, 2009.
53. Darlington, T.K. et al. Nanoparticle characteristics affecting environmental fate and transport through soil. *Environ. Toxicol. Chem.*, 28, 1191, 2009.
54. Johnson, R.L. et al. Natural organic matter enhanced mobility of nano zerovalent iron. *Environ. Sci. Technol.*, Article ASAP DOI: 10.1021/es900474f, 43, 5455, 2009.
55. Buzea, C., Pacheco, I.I., and Robbie, K. Nanomaterials and nanoparticles: sources and toxicity. *Biointerphases*, 2, MR17, 2007.
56. Stampoulis, D., Sinha, S.K., and White, J.C. Assay-dependent phytotoxicity of nanoparticles to plants. *Environ. Sci. Technol.*, 43, 9473, 2009.
57. Koper, O.B. et al. Nanoscale powders and formulations with biocidal activity toward spores and vegetative cells of *Bacillus* species, viruses, and toxins. *Curr. Microbiol.*, 44, 49, 2002.
58. Male, K.B. et al. Assessment of cytotoxicity of quantum dots and gold nanoparticles using cell-based impedance spectroscopy. *Anal. Chem.*, 80, 5487, 2008.
59. Mahendra, S. et al. Quantum dot weathering results in microbial toxicity. *Environ. Sci. Technol.*, 42, 9424, 2008.
60. Metz, K.M. et al. Engineered nanomaterial transformation under oxidative environmental conditions: Development of an *in vitro* biomimetic assay. *Environ. Sci. Technol.*, 43, 1598, 2009.
61. Priester, J.H. et al. Effects of soluble cadmium salts versus CdSe quantum dots on the growth of planktonic *Pseudomonas aeruginosa*. *Environ. Sci. Technol.*, 43, 2589, 2009.
62. Brown, C.L. et al. Colloidal metallic gold is not bio-inert. *Inflammopharmacology*, 16, 133, 2008.
63. Phenrat, T. et al. Partial oxidation ("aging") and surface modification decrease the toxicity of nanosized zerovalent iron. *Environ. Sci. Technol.*, 43, 195, 2009.
64. Barrena, R. et al. Evaluation of the ecotoxicity of model nanoparticles. *Chemosphere*, 75, 850, 2009.
65. Roh, J.Y. et al. Ecotoxicity of silver nanoparticles on the soil nematode *Caenorhabditis elegans* using functional ecotoxicogenomics. *Environ. Sci. Technol.*, 43, 3933, 2009.
66. Cha, K. et al. Comparison of acute responses of mice livers to short-term exposure to nano-sized or micro-sized silver particles. *Biotechnol. Lett.*, 30, 1893, 2008.
67. Sung, J.H. et al. Subchronic inhalation toxicity of silver nanoparticles. *Toxicol. Sci.*, 108, 452, 2009.
68. Griffitt, R.J. et al. Exposure to copper nanoparticles causes gill injury and acute lethality in zebrafish (*Danio rerio*). *Environ. Sci. Technol.*, 41, 8178, 2007.
69. Lee, W.-M. et al. Toxicity and bioavailability of copper nanoparticles to the terrestrial plants mung bean (*Phaseolus radiatus*) and wheat (*Triticum aestivum*): Plant agar test for water-insoluble nanoparticles. *Environ. Toxicol. Chem.*, 27, 1915, 2008.

70. Lin, D. and Xing, B. Phytotoxicity of nanoparticles: Inhibition of seed germination and root growth. *Environ. Pollut.*, 150, 243, 2007.

71. Doshi, R. et al. Nano-aluminum: Transport through sand columns and environmental effects on plants and soil communities. *Environ. Res.*, 106, 296, 2008.

72. Papageorgiou, I. et al. The effect of nano- and micron-sized particles of cobalt-chromium alloy on human fibroblasts *in vitro*. *Biomaterials*, 28, 2946, 2007.

73. Hardman, R. A toxicologic review of quantum dots: Toxicity depends on physicochemical and environmental factors. *Environ. Health Perspect.*, 114, 165, 2006.

74. Kloepfer, J.A., Mielke, R.E., and Nadeau, J.L. Uptake of CdSe and CdSe/ZnS quantum dots into bacteria via purine-dependent mechanisms. *Appl. Environ. Microbiol.*, 71, 2548, 2005.

75. Bouldin, J.L. et al. Aqueous toxicity and food chain transfer of quantum dots in freshwater algae and *Ceriodaphnia dubia*. *Environ. Toxicol. Chem.*, 27, 1958, 2008.

76. Lee, J. et al. Acute toxicity of two CdSe/ZnSe quantum dots with different surface coating in *Daphnia magna* under various light conditions. *Environ. Toxicol.*, DOI: 10.1002/tox.20520, 25, 593, 2010.

77. Zhang, Y. et al. *In vitro* and *in vivo* toxicity of CdTe nanoparticles. *J. Nanosci. Nanotechnol.*, 7, 497, 2007.

78. Dumas, E.M. et al. Toxicity of CdTe quantum dots in bacterial strains. *IEEE Trans. Nanobiosci.*, 8, 58, 2009.

79. Gagné, F. et al. Ecotoxicity of CdTe quantum dots to freshwater mussels: impacts on immune system, oxidative stress and genotoxicity. *Aquat. Toxicol.*, 86, 333, 2008.

80. Liu, L. et al. *In vitro* and *in vivo* assessment of CdTe and CdHgTe toxicity and clearance. *J. Biomed. Nanotechnol.*, 4, 524, 2008.

81. Jiang, W., Mashayekhi, H., and Xing, B. Bacterial toxicity comparison between nano- and micro-scaled oxide particles. *Environ. Pollut.*, 157, 1619, 2009.

82. Velzeboer, I. et al. Aquatic ecotoxicity tests of some nanomaterials. *Environ. Toxicol. Chem.*, 27, 1942, 2008.

83. Wang, H., Wick, R.L., and Xing, B. Toxicity of nanoparticulate and bulk ZnO, $Al_2O_3$ and $TiO_2$ to the nematode *Caenorhabditis elegans*. *Environ. Pollut.*, 157, 1171, 2009.

84. Zhu, X.S. et al. Comparative toxicity of several metal oxide nanoparticle aqueous suspensions to zebrafish (*Danio rerio*) early developmental stage, *J. Environ. Sci. Health Pt-A-Toxic Hazard. Subst. Environ. Eng.*, 43, 278, 2008.

85. Yang, L. and Watts, D.J. Particle surface characteristics may play an important role in phytotoxicity of alumina nanoparticles. *Toxicol. Lett.*, 158, 122, 2005.

86. Huang, L. et al. Controllable preparation of nano-MgO and investigation of its bactericidal properties. *J. Inorg. Biochem.*, 99, 986, 2005.

87. Thill, A. et al. Cytotoxicity of $CeO_2$ nanoparticles for *Escherichia coli*. Physico-chemical insight of the cytotoxicity mechanism. *Environ. Sci. Technol.*, 40, 6151, 2006.

88. Van Hoecke, K. et al. Fate and effects of $CeO_2$ nanoparticles in aquatic ecotoxicity tests. *Environ. Sci. Technol.*, 43, 4537, 2009.

89. Lee, S.W., Kim, S.M., and Choi, J. Genotoxicity and ecotoxicity assays using the freshwater crustacean *Daphnia magna* and the larva of the aquatic midge *Chironomus riparius* to screen the ecological risks of nanoparticle exposure. *Environ. Toxicol. Pharmacol.*, 28, 86, 2009.

90. Kasemets, K. et al. Toxicity of nanoparticles of ZnO, CuO and TiO$_2$ to yeast *Saccharomyces cerevisiae. Toxicol. In Vitro*, 23, 1116, 2009.

91. Mortimer, M., Kasemets, K., and Kahru, A. Toxicity of ZnO and CuO nanoparticles to ciliated protozoa *Tetrahymena thermophila. Toxicology*, DOI: 10.1016/j.tox.2009.07.007, 269, 182, 2010.

92. Aruoja, V. et al. Toxicity of nanoparticles of CuO, ZnO and TiO$_2$ to microalgae *Pseudokirchneriella subcapitata. Sci. Total Environ.*, 407, 1461, 2009.

93. Blaise, C. et al. Ecotoxicity of selected nano-materials to aquatic organisms. *Environ. Toxicol.*, 23, 591, 2008.

94. Adams, L.K., Lyon, D.Y., and Alvarez, P.J.J. Comparative eco-toxicity of nanoscale TiO$_2$, SiO$_2$, and ZnO water suspensions. *Water Res.*, 40, 3527–3532, 2006.

95. Van Hoecke, K. et al. Ecotoxicity of silica nanoparticles to the green alga *Pseudokirchneriella subcapitata*: Importance of surface area. *Environ. Toxicol. Chem.*, 27, 1948, 2008.

96. Hu, X. et al. *In vitro* evaluation of cytotoxicity of engineered metal oxide nanoparticles. *Sci. Total Environ.*, 407, 3070, 2009.

97. Brunet, L. et al. Comparative photoactivity and antibacterial properties of C60 fullerenes and titanium dioxide nanoparticles. *Environ. Sci. Technol.*, 43, 4355, 2009.

98. Wong, S.L., Nakamoto, L., and Wainwright, J.P. Detection and toxicity of titanium from pulp and paper effluents. *Bull. Environ. Contam. Toxicol.*, 55, 878, 1995.

99. Hong, J. and Otaki, M. Association of photosynthesis and photocatalytic inhibition of algal growth by TiO$_2$. *J. Biosci. Bioeng.*, 101, 185, 2006.

100. Hund-Rinke, K. and Simon, M. Ecotoxic effect of photocatalytic active nanoparticles (TiO$_2$) on algae and daphnids. *Environ. Sci. Pollut. Res.*, 13, 225, 2006.

101. Warheit, D.B. et al. Development of a base set of toxicity tests using ultrafine TiO$_2$ particles as a component of nanoparticle risk management. *Toxicol. Lett.*, 171, 99, 2007.

102. Lovern, S.B. and Klaper, R. *Daphnia magna* mortality when exposed to titanium dioxide and fullerene (C$_{60}$) nanoparticles. *Environ. Toxicol. Chem.*, 25, 1132, 2006.

103. Lovern, S.B., Strickler, J.R., and Klaper, R. Behavioral and physiological changes in *Daphnia magna* when exposed to nanoparticle suspensions (titanium dioxide, nano-C$_{60}$, and C60HxC70Hx). *Environ. Sci. Technol.*, 41, 4465, 2007.

104. Zhu, X., Chang, Y., and Chen, Y. Toxicity and bioaccumulation of TiO$_2$ nanoparticle aggregates in *Daphnia magna. Chemosphere*, 78, 209, 2010.

105. Federici, G., Shaw, B.J., and Handy, R.D. Toxicity of titanium dioxide nanoparticles to rainbow trout (*Oncorhynchus mykiss*): Gill injury, oxidative stress, and other physiological effects. *Aquat. Toxicol.*, 84, 415, 2007.

106. Seeger, E.M. et al. Insignificant acute toxicity of TiO$_2$ nanoparticles to willow trees. *J. Soils Sediments*, 9, 46, 2008.

107. Hund-Rinke, K. and Simon, M. *Ecotoxicity of Photoactive Nanoparticles (TiO$_2$)*, Presented at the SETAC Europe, 16th Annual Meeting, The Hague, May 7–11, 2006.

108. Jemec, A. et al. Effects of ingested nano-sized titanium dioxide on terrestrial isopods (*Porcellio scaber*). *Environ. Toxicol. Chem.*, 27, 1904, 2008.

109. Trouiller, B. et al. Titanium dioxide nanoparticles induce DNA damage and genetic instability *in vivo* in mice. *Cancer Res.*, 69, 8784, 2009.

110. Rogers, N.J. et al. The importance of physical and chemical characterization in nanoparticle toxicity studies. *Integr. Environ. Assess. Manag.*, 3, 303, 2007.
111. Blinova, I. et al. Ecotoxicity of nanoparticles of CuO and ZnO in natural water. *Environ Pollut.*, DOI: 10.1016/j.envpol.2009.08.017, 158, 41, 2010.
112. Oberdörster, E. Manufactured nanomaterials (fullerenes, $C_{60}$) induce oxidative stress in the brain of juvenile largemouth bass. *Environ. Health Perspect.*, 112, 1058, 2004.
113. Guo, J. et al. The different bio-effects of functionalized multi-walled carbon nanotubes on *Tetrahymena pyriformis*. *Curr. Nanosci.*, 4, 240, 2008.
114. Fortner, J.D. et al. $C_{60}$ in water: Nanocrystal formation and microbial response. *Environ. Sci. Technol.*, 39, 4307, 2005.
115. Li, D. et al. Effects of soil sorption and aquatic natural organic matter on the antibacterial activity of a fullerene water suspension. *Environ. Toxicol. Chem.*, 27, 1888, 2008.
116. Henry, T.B. et al. Attributing effects of aqueous $C_{60}$ nano-aggregates to tetrahydrofuran decomposition products in larval zebrafish by assessment of gene expression. *Environ. Health Perspect.*, 115, 1059, 2007.
117. Zogovic, N.S. et al. Opposite effects of nanocrystalline fullerene ($C_{60}$) on tumour cell growth *in vitro* and *in vivo* and a possible role of immunosuppression in the cancer-promoting activity of C60. *Biomaterials*, 30, 6940, 2009.
118. Lyon, D.Y. et al. Antibacterial activity of fullerene water suspensions: Effects of preparation methods and particle size. *Environ. Sci. Technol.*, 40, 4360, 2006.
119. Johansen, A. et al. Effects of $C_{60}$ fullerene nanoparticles on soil bacteria and protozoans. *Environ. Toxicol. Chem.*, 27, 1895, 2008.
120. Zhu, S., Oberdörster, E., and Haasch, M.L. Toxicity of an engineered nanoparticle (fullerene, $C_{60}$) in two aquatic species, *Daphnia* and fathead minnow. *Mar. Environ. Res.*, 62 Suppl S, S5, 2006.
121. Oberdörster, E. et al. Ecotoxicology of carbon-based engineered nanoparticles: effects of fullerene ($C_{60}$) on aquatic organisms. *Carbon*, 44, 1112, 2006.
122. Zhu, X. et al. Oxidative stress and growth inhibition in the freshwater fish *Carassius auratus* induced by chronic exposure to sublethal fullerene aggregates. *Environ. Toxicol. Chem.*, 27, 1979, 2008.
123. Blickley, M. and Mc-Clellan-Green, P., Toxicity of aqueous fullerene in adult and larval *Fundulus heteroclitus*. *Environ. Toxicol. Chem.*, 27, 1964, 2008.
124. Chan-Remillard, S., Kapustka, L., and Goudey, S. Nano in nanotechnology does size matter? In: *34th Annual Aquatic Toxicity Workshop*, 30th Sept.–3rd October, Halifax, Nova Scotia, 2007.
125. Hull, M.S. et al. Release of metal impurities from carbon nanomaterials influences aquatic toxicity. *Environ. Sci. Technol.*, 43, 4169, 2009.
126. Zhu, X. et al. Developmental toxicity in zebrafish (*Danio rerio*) embryos after exposure to manufactured nanomaterials: Buckminsterfullerene aggregates ($nC_{60}$) and fullerol. *Environ. Toxicol. Chem.*, 26, 976, 2007.
127. Templeton, R.C. et al. Life-cycle effects of single-walled carbon nanotubes (SWNTs) on an estuarine meiobenthic copepod. *Environ. Sci. Technol.*, 40, 7387, 2006.
128. Roberts, A.P. et al. *In vivo* biomodification of lipid-coated carbon nanotubes by *Daphnia magna*. *Environ. Sci. Technol.*, WEB, A, 2007.
129. Cheng, J., Flahaut, E., and Cheng, S.H. Effects of carbon nanotubes on developing zebrafish (*Danio rerio*) embryos. *Environ. Toxicol. Chem.*, 26, 708, 2007.

130. Smith, C.J., Shaw, B.J., and Handy, R.D. Toxicity of single walled carbon nanotubes to rainbow trout (*Oncorhynchus mykiss*): Respiratory toxicity, organ pathologies, and other physiological effects. *Aquat. Toxicol.*, 82, 94, 2007.

131. Deng, X. et al. The splenic toxicity of water soluble multi-walled carbon nanotubes in mice. *Carbon*, 47, 1421, 2009.

132. Mitchell, L.A. et al. Mechanisms for how inhaled multiwalled carbon nanotubes suppress systemic immune function in mice. *Nat. Nanotechnol.*, DOI: 10.1038/nnano.2009.151, 4, 451, 2009.

133. Bergeson, L.L. Nanotechnologies and FIFRA, *Gradient Corp. EH&S Nano News*, 1, 3, 2006.

134. Naha, P.C. et al. Preparation, characterization of NIPAM and NIPAM/BAM copolymer nanoparticles and their acute toxicity testing using an aquatic test battery. *Aquat. Toxicol.*, 92, 146, 2009.

135. Qi, L., Xu, Z., and Chen, M. *In vitro* and *in vivo* suppression of hepatocellular carcinoma growth by chitosan nanoparticles. *Eur. J. Cancer*, 43, 184, 2007.

136. Leroueil, P.R. et al. Nanoparticle interaction with biological membranes: Does nanotechnology present a Janus face? *Acc. Chem. Res.*, 40, 335, 2007.

137. Chappell, M.A. et al. Surfactive stabilization of multi-walled carbon nanotube dispersions with dissolved humic substances. *Environ. Pollut.*, 157, 1081, 2009.

138. Aruguete, D.M. and Hochella, M.F. Bacteria-nanoparticle interactions and their environmental implications. *Environ. Chem.*, 7, 3, 2010.

139. Stern, S.T. and McNeil, S.E. Nanotechnology safety concerns revisited. *Toxicol. Sci.*, 101, 4, 2008.

140. Boverhof, D.R. and David, R.M. Nanomaterial characterization: Considerations and needs for hazard assessment and safety evaluation. *Anal. Bioanal. Chem.*, DOI 10.1007/s00216-009-3103-3, 396, 953, 2010.

141. Landsiedel, R. et al. Genotoxicity investigations on nanomaterials: Methods, preparation and characterization of test material, potential artifacts and limitations—Many questions, some answers. *Mutat. Res.*, 681, 241, 2009.

142. Doak, S.H. et al. Confounding experimental considerations in nanogenotoxicology. *Mutagenesis*, 24, 285, 2009.

143. Auffan, M. et al. Towards a definition of inorganic nanoparticles from an environmental, health and safety perspective. *Nat. Nanotechnol.*, 4, 634, 2009.

144. Schneider, R. et al. The exposure of bacteria to CdTe-core quantum dots: The importance of surface chemistry on cytotoxicity. *Nanotechnology*, 20, 225101, 2009.

145. Fenoglio, I. et al. Structural defects play a major role in the acute lung toxicity of multiwall carbon nanotubes: Physicochemical aspects. *Chem. Res. Toxicol.*, 21, 1690, 2008.

146. Nakagawa, Y. et al. The photogenotoxicity of titanium dioxide particles. *Mutat. Res.*, 394, 125, 1997.

147. Baun, A. et al. Ecotoxicity of engineered nanoparticles to aquatic invertebrates: A brief review and recommendations for future toxicity testing. *Ecotoxicology*, 17, 387, 2008.

148. Hartmann, N.B. et al. Algal testing of titanium dioxide nanoparticles—Testing considerations, inhibitory effects and modification of cadmium bioavailability. *Toxicology*, Aug 15. [Epub ahead of print], 269, 190, 2010.

149. Sun, H.W. et al. Enhanced accumulation of arsenate in carp in the presence of titanium dioxide nanoparticles. *Water Air Soil Pollut.*, 178, 245, 2007.

150. Holbrook, R.D. et al. Trophic transfer of nanoparticles in a simplified invertebrate food web. *Nat. Nanotechnol.*, 3, 352, 2008.
151. Zhang, X.Z., Sun, H.W., and Zhang, Z.Y. Bioaccumulation of titanium dioxide nanoparticles in carp. *Huan Jing Ke Xue*, 27, 1631, 2006.
152. Ferry, J.L. et al. Transfer of gold nanoparticles from the water column to the estuarine food web. *Nat. Nanotechnol.*, 4, 441, 2009.
153. Li, D. et al. Effects of soil sorption and aquatic natural organic matter on the antibacterial activity of a fullerene water suspension. *Environ. Toxicol. Chem.*, 27, 1888, 2008.
154. Kleinjans, J.C.S. and van Schooten, F.-J. Ecogenotoxicology: The evolving field. *Environ. Toxicol. Pharmacol.*, 11, 173, 2002.

# Section VI

# Life Cycle

# 11

# *Life Cycle Risks and Impacts of Nanotechnologies*

**Olivier Jolliet, Ralph K. Rosenbaum, and Alexis Laurent**

## CONTENTS

## 11.1  Introduction to Life Cycle Assessment

On the basis of a life cycle perspective, we analyze how Life Cycle Assessment (LCA) has been addressing the trade-offs between the risks and benefits of nanotechnologies, as a replacement for conventional technologies. This chapter starts by shortly describing the LCA approach and its use to compare the impacts of products for readers that are not familiar with LCA. It then discusses how the LCA approach applies to nano-based products. It comprehensively reviews the existing LCA literature of case studies applied to nano-based products. Finally, it identifies the main questions that need to be addressed.

LCA evaluates the environmental impact of a product, a service, or a system in relation to a particular function, and considers all of its life cycle stages. It helps identify where improvements can be made in a product's life cycle and helps in designing new products. Primarily, this tool is used to compare the environmental load of various products, processes, or systems, and a particular product's different life cycle stages.

### 11.1.1  LCA and Other Environmental Tools

Different environmental tools are incorporated into policy and decision making. Preliminary choices and evaluations of technological systems can be based on concepts such as life cycle thinking (qualitative consideration of the whole life cycle of a good), environmental design (consideration of environmental parameters when designing a good), or industrial ecology (consideration of the economic life cycle, accounting for the possibility that the waste of one industry can become a resource for another). These tools generally do not provide quantified assessments but help properly set up the problem. More quantitative procedures and tools are used to support decision making by different end users. Environmental impact assessments are used as legal authorization to assess the local impacts of a proposed project.

Environmental audits and environmental management systems provide and structure information to guide industrial decision makers. Environmental labeling (e.g., organic labels or carbon footprints) and environmental certification (an official statement of environmental performance, such as building certification by the Leadership in Energy and Environmental Design Green Building Rating System) is used to communicate information to the consumer.

These end-user tools rely on quantified analytical methods such as substance flow analysis, risk assessment, and LCA, which differ mainly in the focus of the analysis. Substance flow analysis quantifies flows and reservoirs of a given substance (e.g., lead) or of a group of substances (e.g., inorganic nitrogen compounds) for a given region and time duration. Risk assessment concentrates on the probabilistic risk for large production facilities (e.g., nuclear power plants) or for the local impacts of toxic chemicals in a region. The focus of LCA is to relate environmental impacts to the function of a product over its whole life cycle, from cradle to grave, considering a wide range of pollutants and impacts. Because of this broad application, the results are more comprehensive but with higher uncertainties. As these analytical tools are all based on common elements, such as mass balance and multimedia modeling, LCA developments are performed in collaboration with specialists from the other domains described above. As discussed by Jolliet and Small,[1] the human health component of Life Cycle Impact Assessment (LCIA) aims to assess in a comparative way the multiple impacts and large number of toxic substances that are involved in the life cycle of products. This often differs from the scope of regulatory toxicological assessments, which generally focus on ensuring that safe doses are not surpassed by exposures at any location or point in time.

## 11.1.2 Different Steps of LCA

According to the definition provided in the ISO standards and SETAC, an LCA consists of four steps. *Goal definition* defines the product or system function and the functional unit to which emissions will be related, as well as the boundary of the system that meets this function. The next stage in LCA is *inventory*, which lists the resources extracted and pollutant emissions to air, water, and soil for all the processes needed to achieve this functional unit. The third stage, *impact assessment*, estimates the environmental impacts of these emissions. Finally, *interpretation* identifies key processes and pollutants; performs sensitivity, uncertainty, and cost–benefit analyses; and can assess the improvement potential (Figure 11.1). LCA is meant to be an iterative procedure (Figure 11.1), performed in at least two iterations. First, a screening should be performed, covering all LCA phases, to assess the orders of magnitude of emissions and related impacts. Then, focusing on the most damaging processes, emissions, and life cycle phases, a more detailed analysis should be carried out to improve the assessment quality. In the context of nano-based applications,

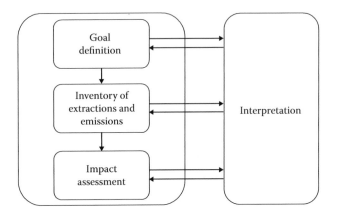

**FIGURE 11.1**
General scheme of four stages of LCA (ISO 14040). (From International Organization for Standardization ISO 14040 International Standard. In *Environmental Management—Life Cycle Assessment—Principles and Framework*. Geneva, Switzerland, 2006.)

this is particularly important to initially identify the hot spots by location and process and then find more location-specific data where necessary.

The four steps of LCA are further defined as follows (adapted from Shaked and Jolliet[2]).

### 11.1.2.1 Goal and Scope Definition

In this initial step, the problem is described, and the objectives and the scope of the study are defined. A number of crucial elements are determined at this point. Because the goal of LCA is to assess the environmental impacts of the function of the product, it begins by defining the main function and the main service offered by the system. Products or systems can only be compared on the basis of a similar specific function.

On the basis of the determined function, it is possible to define the *functional unit* of all scenarios, which is the common unit representing the function of the system (the offered service), serving as the basis for scenario comparison (e.g., a single use of 1 m$^3$ of packaging material for a filling material or 100 days of use of a T-shirt). The functional unit is the same for all scenarios, and it is a quantified and additive value (i.e., not a ratio). This is an important choice because inventory emissions are calculated and compared per functional unit. A low-quality T-shirt (scenario 1) can then be compared with a high-quality T-shirt (scenario 2) by determining the type and number of products needed to be purchased to achieve the functional unit. Assuming a low-quality T-shirt lasts for 50 days of use and a high-quality one lasts for 200 days of use, the reference flow for scenario 1 is 2 low-quality T-shirts, whereas the reference flow for scenario 2 is only 0.5 high-quality T-shirt. In addition, assuming that T-shirts are washed every 2 days of use, 50 washing/drying are accounted for as reference flow. This small example shows that it is essential to include the duration or number of uses in the definition of the functional unit.

The second crucial step of the LCA goal definition is the determination of the system and *system boundaries*, which are also based on the product function. A system consists of a set of processes that combine to perform one or several functions. Each process in the system can have inputs from the environment (consumption of resources, energy, or land area) and outputs to the environment (emissions to air, water, or soil). Theoretically, the system boundary should include all economic processes required to achieve the system function, from cradle to grave (creation to disposal), which generally involves the following phases: extraction of energy and raw materials, manufacturing (infrastructure production, input products, product manufacturing), transportation (e.g., to the consumer), use phase (including maintenance), and the short- and long-term emissions and extractions associated with waste treatment. In practice, the system boundaries cannot include all necessary processes. For example, to model the function of 100 days of use of a T-shirt, the T-shirt manufacturing process should be included, but should the manufacturing of the T-shirt-manufacturing machine also be included? And the machine that manufactured this machine? System boundaries should cover the same functional reality in all scenarios, with a cutoff percentage that only includes processes that contribute more than this percentage of the total mass of extractions or emissions for each scenario. System boundaries are particularly important in the context of nanoproducts to ensure that alternative and innovative materials are evaluated within the same framework even if their production chains are extremely different.

### 11.1.2.2 Inventory of Extractions and Emissions

Once the system boundary has been determined, all processes are detailed in a Process LCA. For each process, the inventory of resource extractions and environmental emissions (e.g., the carbon dioxide emissions at the T-shirt production plant in India) must be recorded, as well as the intermediary flows that link the different unit processes together (e.g., the quantity of cotton used in T-shirt manufacturing). To also estimate the inventories associated with indirect processes in the supply chain (e.g., electricity production in India), LCA experts have created large inventory databases, such as the EcoInvent database,[4] that grandly facilitate the realization of the inventory and enable the practitioner to mostly focus on the core manufacturing processes, using existing data for the supply chain in a first screening.

For applications such as services, it is difficult to assess what is actually important. One way to ensure that all relevant processes are included is to use a method known as Input–Output LCA (IO LCA). Rather than using physical fluxes, IO LCA inventories the monetary fluxes between different economic sectors involved in the production chain for a given product, process, or activity. Each sector is studied to determine the resource extraction and pollutant emissions associated with each dollar spent in this sector. Since the expenditure of each sector on all other sectors is included, it is possible to exhaustively describe the chain of suppliers and impacts for a given service. The disadvantage compared with Process LCA is that IO LCA is not able to differentiate products from the same sector (e.g., it is not able to distinguish T-shirt A from T-shirt B if they have the same price), which is a main issue for the manufacturing phase of nano-based materials.

### 11.1.2.3 Life Cycle Impact Assessment

Inventories are useful for comparing the environmental emissions of different products, but are not sufficient to compare, for example, one product that uses more detergent to another that generates some nanosilver emissions. Impact assessment estimates the environmental and human health impacts associated with these emissions so that the impacts can then be compared between different chemicals.

Impact assessment evaluates the impact on the environment from the emissions inventoried previously. It can be broken down into three steps[5]:

- Classification determines which emissions contribute to which environmental impacts (greenhouse effect, human toxicity, ecotoxicity, resource use, etc.).
- Midpoint characterization weighs the emissions for each impact category.
- Damage characterization aggregates impact categories into damage categories (damage to human health, ecosystems, climate equilibrium, resources, and ecosystem services) corresponding to areas that deserve protection.

An additional normalization step can be carried out to show the contribution of the studied product to the global impact, for a given impact category. Environmental impact assessment can be completed in the interpretation phase with a social-based weighting of impacts or damages to evaluate the relative importance of intermediate classes of impact or damage categories.

Many different methods exist (see review by Hauschild et al.[6]). For human toxicity and ecotoxicological impacts, impact assessment methods estimate chemical impacts using environmental and exposure models that simulate the fate (transport, dilution, and degradation), exposure (e.g., human intake), and effects (e.g., dose–response and severity) of many chemicals in a consistent manner such as with the United Nations Environment Programme (UNEP)—Society of Environmental Toxicology and Chemistry (SETAC) consensus toxicity model (USEtox™ model[7,8]; Figure 11.2).

The various cause–effect models yield a list of characterization factors expressing the impact in kilogram of a reference substance per kilogram of

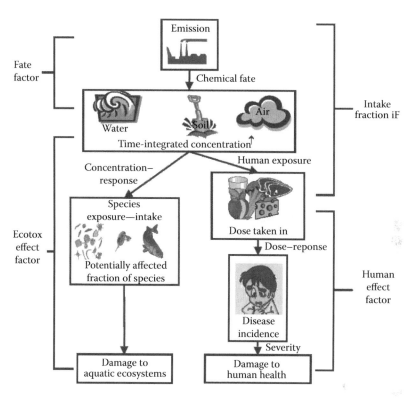

**FIGURE 11.2**
USEtox source-to-impact diagram from emission to human and ecosystem health damage.

the substance emitted. Human toxicity (a midpoint category) is expressed as the equivalent kilogram of chloroethylene emitted to air, and the human health endpoint damage is in units of disability-adjusted life years (DALYs), which are the sum of the years of life lost and years of life disabled (as defined by the World Health Organization). The advantage of endpoint factors is that they aggregate midpoint impacts and are therefore easier to interpret. However, more assumptions and models are necessary to link the midpoint units to the endpoint units (e.g., the assumption that each equivalent kilogram of chloroethylene corresponds to a given number of DALYs), making them more uncertain than midpoint factors. Because none of the impact assessment methods is recognized as a standard, a robust LCA will use several in parallel to determine the dominant impacts in all methods.

### 11.1.2.4 Interpretation and Uncertainty

Interpretation is a key step in the iterative process of LCA, determining what can be neglected and what must be examined in more depth. A factor should be explored further if it leads to a relatively high impact or if the system is sensitive to this value (i.e., small changes in the factor lead to large variations in calculated impacts). To determine these factors, the interpretation stage involves a systematic look at each stage of the assessment (inventory and impact assessment), each life cycle phase (manufacturing, use, and disposal), and each product component (e.g., boots and shoelaces), identifying the dominant processes, substances, and impact categories. Interpretation can be taken further by looking at cost-effectiveness or ease of acting see Cost-effectiveness and Rebound Effects. Processes that have small impact contributions but can be easily improved should also be identified, as reducing many of these small contributions can lead to large benefits.

Many of the assumptions made during an LCA are consistently applied to all scenarios, yielding valuable comparison results; however, these assumptions can yield large uncertainties, so the field has developed methods for estimating uncertainty for individual scenarios and for scenario comparisons. Parameter uncertainty propagation has mainly been studied using Monte Carlo[9] or Taylor series expansion[10] techniques to evaluate the distribution of outcomes (impacts, in this case) given uncertainty distributions for the input parameters (e.g., amount of formaldehyde emissions per kilowatt-hour of electricity used).

LCA only deals with the environmental impacts of a product, but sustainability also refers to economic and social aspects, which can be compared with and balanced against the environmental aspects. To address the economic aspects, LCA could be complemented by performing a life cycle costing to calculate the costs to the consumer associated with each step in the life cycle of a product and to guide a decision maker to make more cost-effective decisions. For example, the construction costs of a well-insulated and energy-efficient building may be higher than those of a conventional building, whereas its energy consumption costs will be reduced during operation. To address the social aspects, social LCA is being developed, which quantifies various social indicators associated with goods and services, such as wages, gender equality, child labor, and health insurance.

### 11.1.3 A Short LCA Example

As an example, polystyrene packing peanuts are made with nonrenewable raw materials (oil) and are not biodegradable; therefore, popcorn has been proposed as a substitute packaging material.[11] To compare the two, the differences in environmental impacts must be quantified and the responsible key variables must be determined.

Using LCA techniques, the emissions over the life cycle of each option can be inventoried to quantify the subsequent environmental impacts in a manner consistent with the product function. Many materials are compared according to the environmental impacts per mass. The use of popcorn packaging results in fewer emissions per mass over its life cycle, making it three to four time less damaging than polystyrene, according to the chosen impact weighting method (Figure 11.3a). However, the comparison should be based on the function of this material rather than on its weight. The function of packaging is to occupy volume. Since popcorn is 4.6 times denser than polystyrene peanuts, more mass is needed to fill the same volume, making popcorn comparable to or less environmentally friendly than polystyrene on a per volume basis (Figure 11.3b).

On the basis of this analysis, key parameters can be identified to guide future decisions on reducing impacts of packaging materials. Initially, the key parameters for popcorn production appear to be the quantities of nitrates and fertilizers used for growth, of diesel used for tractors, or of gas used to make the popcorn, as these are all major sources of key emissions and subsequent impacts. This analysis shows that due to the function of this product, the key parameter is actually the density of the materials. The industrial process of extracting starch and blowing it into polystyrene results in more chemical emissions per mass than popcorn, but it is able to sufficiently decrease the key parameter of density to make the impacts of the more industrial product comparable or even less than those of the "natural" one. This example shows the importance of considering the product function as the basis for comparing products. It also shows the potentially existing synergy between technological optimization (here the reduction of weight and of used material quantity) and energetic and environmental optimization.

How does the classic and standardized LCA approach apply to the specific of a nano-based product?—that is the question addressed in our next section!

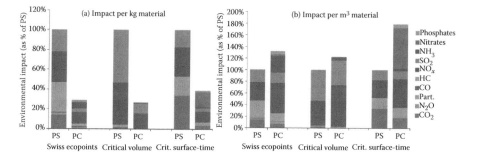

**FIGURE 11.3**
Comparison of impacts of popcorn (PC) packaging versus polystyrene (PS) packaging on per kilogram basis (a) and per volume basis (b). Impacts are weighted according to three impact assessment methods (critical volume, critical surface-time, and Swiss ecopoints methods). (From Jolliet, O. et al., *Agric. Ecosyst. Environ.*, 49, 253, 1994.)

## 11.2 Application of LCA to Nanomaterials and Nanotechnologies

### 11.2.1 Adaptation of LCA Approaches to Nano-Based Products

An expert workshop on the LCA of nanotechnologies was co-organized by the US Environmental Protection Agency and the European Union in 2006 at the Washington DC Wilson Center. The main outcome of this workshop[12] showed that (i) LCA is well suited to study and compare the benefits and impacts of nanoparticles and the ISO-framework for LCA (ISO 14040:2006) is fully suitable to the case of nanotechnologies and nanomaterials; (ii) there is no generic LCA of nanomaterials, just as there is no generic LCA of chemicals; (iii) processes are under development and may be rapidly evolving, leading to a similar situation as, for example, the electronic industry; and (iv) the main challenges and gaps in the LCIA of nanoparticles is linked to the direct toxicity of nanoparticles, which should be the focus of further research.

As discussed in the earlier chapter, LCA relates environmental impacts and performances to the function of the product in which nanomaterials are embedded. This concurs with point (ii) above and also with the comparative nature of LCA, meaning that it is not possible nor relevant to characterize the intrinsic impact of a nanomaterial, nor to answer questions such as "are nanotubes acceptable from an environmental point of view?" What can be characterized is the environmental performance of a nanomaterial within a given product with a specific function or range of potential function, enabling to address questions such as "does the use of carbon nanotubes as fiber reinforcement reduces impacts compared with classic fibers, and what are the key processes on which to focus further improvements?"

### 11.2.2 Evolution of LCA Nano-Studies and Development of Nanotechnologies: A Parallel?

By 2011, the Woodrow Wilson International Centre for Scholars—Project on Emerging Nanotechnologies had listed more than 1300 commercialized nanomaterial-embedded products or "nanoproducts" (Figure 11.4a). By early 2012, about 43 LCA-claimed studies were identified in the scientific litera-ture, most of them being post-2008 studies (Figure 11.4b). Several of them did not focus on a specific application, but merely looked at the production of nanomaterials. Figure 11.4b shows the repartition of the LCA studies per categories of investigated products or services. The electronics sectors (e.g., semiconductor or photovoltaic modules) and the automotive industry (poly-mer composites) are the two major fields of application. Surprisingly, other types of products such as personal care products, home and garden prod-ucts, or sporting goods have not drawn interest among LCA practitioners in spite of a current domination of these products on the market. This tends

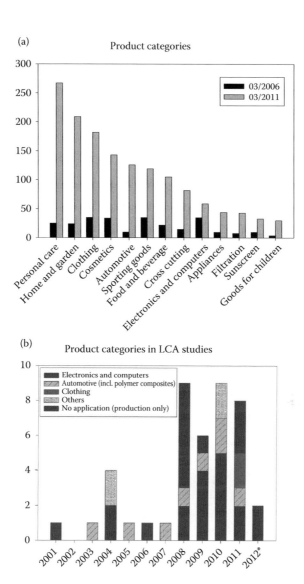

**FIGURE 11.4**
Evolution of LCA studies in parallel with commercialization of nanomaterials. (a and c: Retrieved from the Woodrow Wilson International Centre for Scholar—Project on Emerging Nanotechnologies, 04/2012.)

to indicate that the application of LCA to nanoproducts has lagged behind the booming expansion of the field of nanotechnologies (note the many-fold increases in number of commercialized products per category in Figure 11.4a).

Among the major nanomaterials that were investigated (as such or as part of a product), half of the studies related to carbon-based nanomaterials, with

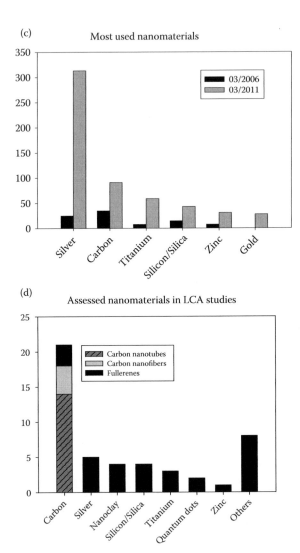

**FIGURE 11.4 (Continued)**
Evolution of LCA studies in parallel with commercialization of nanomaterials. (a and c:
Retrieved from the Woodrow Wilson International Centre for Scholar—Project on Emerging
Nanotechnologies, 04/2012.)

strong focus on carbon nanotubes, while silver, nanoclay, silicon and silica,
and titanium were the focus of less than five studies each (Figure 11.4d).
Comparing with the use of nanomaterials on the market, as in Figure 11.4c,
this observed distribution appears to better correlate to the situation in 2006
than to that of 2011.

This confirms the existence of a lag time between LCA practice and
the commercialization of the nanoproducts. It also tends to indicate the

unfortunate absence of LCA application at the early stages of the nanoproduct development, which is one of the major intended uses of LCA.

### 11.2.3 Review of LCA Applied to Nanomaterials and Nanotechnologies

In spite of being a standardized tool (ISO 14040[3] and ISO 14044[13]), the use of LCA undergoes many distorted interpretations and uses, which can be encountered in the scientific literature. The overview of the 43 LCA studies presented in Table 11.1 embraces studies where the authors have claimed conducting a "life cycle analysis" or "life cycle assessment."

Taking these LCA studies as a whole, a number of general findings can be drawn. A substantial amount of studies shares the conclusion that, on a same produced mass basis, the manufacture of nanomaterials is found to be more energy intensive than the production of conventional materials such as aluminum or steel. Although large discrepancies exist between figures reported for a same type of nanomaterial, higher energy requirements of one up to several orders of magnitude have been reported for carbon nanofibers,[14–16] carbon nanotubes,[17,18] fullerenes,[19–21] titanium dioxide,[22] and nanosilver.[23,24] In contrast, the production of other nanomaterials such as nanoclays appear to be low energy demanding,[25,26] which still calls for a case-by-case treatment of nanomaterials.

However, nanomaterials are not final products as such and are often used in small quantities in order to improve the functionalities of a given product, such as an increased stiffness or a lighter weight. The low percentage of mass of nanomaterials over the total mass of the product, mainly ranging below 5 wt.%, thus tends to reduce the contribution of nanoparticles to the whole product environmental burden. However, it does not make it negligible. In a study assessing fullerene used in organic solar cells, Anctil et al.[21] showed that, while only the mass of fullerene accounted for 0.3% in the total weight, its embodied energy accounted for 19% of the total embodied energy of the solar cells. As concluded by the authors, this demonstrates the need for overruling the typical 5 wt.% cutoff rules when setting up inventories for assessing nanoproducts.

These high energy requirements, mainly stemming from the large use of solvents or other chemicals for the purification and functionalization of the nanomaterials, drive many nontoxic impact categories. In studies assessing a broad range of impact categories, nonrenewable resource depletion, global warming, acidification, and impacts caused by airborne inorganics were found to be dominating after performing normalization and weighting of the results.[17,22,28,33]

A very limited number of studies attempted to investigate the toxicity-related impacts caused by the releases of nanoparticles into the environment. Walser et al.[24] and Meyer et al.[37] performed the assessments of nanosilver-embedded T-shirts and socks, respectively. To estimate the releases of nanosilver to the freshwater environment during the washing process (use stage), Walser et al.[24] used literature sources and measurements and evaluated the

**TABLE 11.1**

Overview of LCA Studies Dedicated to Nano-Based Products[a]

| Nanomaterials | Application/Product Category[b] | LC Stages Included[c] | | | | 'Impact' Assessment Coverage[d] | | | | References |
|---|---|---|---|---|---|---|---|---|---|---|
| | | RM | P | U | D | Energy | Nontoxic Impacts[e] | Toxic Impacts[e] | NP-Specific Toxicity[f] | |
| Carbon nanofibers | NA (production) | x | x | – | – | – | +++ | +++ | – | Khanna et al.[14] |
| Carbon nanofibers | Polymer composites used in automotive body panel | x | x | – | – | +++ | – | – | – | Khanna et al.[15] |
| Carbon nanofibers | Glass fibre/epoxy composite used in wind turbine blades | x | x | (x) | – | +++ | – | – | – | Merugula et al.[16] |
| Carbon nanofibers[g] | Polymer composites used in automotive body panel | x | x | x | (x) | +++ | – | – | – | Dhingra et al.[27] |
| Carbon nanotubes | Field Emissions Display screen | x | x | x | x | +++ | +++ | – | – | Bauer et al.[28] |
| Carbon nanotubes | NA (production via CVD, HiPCO, Arc Ablation) | x | x | – | – | – | – | + (FE) | +++ | Eckelman et al.[29] |
| Carbon nanotubes | Styrene production | x | x | – | – | +++ | – | – | – | Steinfeldt et al.,[30] von Gleich et al.[31] |
| Carbon nanotubes | Field Emissions Display screen | x | x | x | – | +++ | – | – | – | Steinfeldt et al.,[30] von Gleich et al.[31] |
| Carbon nanotubes | NA (production) | x | x | – | – | +++ | – | – | – | Kushnir et al.[19] |
| Carbon nanotubes | NA (production) | x | x | – | – | – | +++ | +++ | – | Singh et al.[32] |

| Material | Application | | | | | | | Reference |
|---|---|---|---|---|---|---|---|---|
| Carbon nanotubes | CNT switch | x | - | - | +++ | +++ | - | Dahlben et al.[33] |
| Carbon nanotubes | CNT-polymer mesh used as electromagnetic interference shielding | x | - | - | +++ | +++ | - | Dahlben et al.[33] |
| Multiwalled carbon nanotubes | Conductive polycarbonate foil | x | - | +++ | +++ | - | - | Steinfeldt[34] |
| Single-walled carbon nanotubes | NA (production) | x | - | - | +++ | +++ | - | Healy et al.[17] |
| Single-walled carbon nanotubes | Anodes in lithium-ion batteries | x | x | +++ | - | - | - | Wender et al.[18] |
| Single-walled carbon nanotubes | NA (production via laser vaporisation) | x | - | +++ | - | - | - | Ganter et al.[35] |
| Fullerenes[g] | Bulk heterojunction organic solar cells | x | (x) | +++ | + (GW) | - | - | Garcia-Valverde et al.[36] |
| Fullerenes | NA (production) | x | - | +++ | - | - | - | Kushnir et al.[19] |
| Fullerenes | NA (production via plasma or pyrolisis) | x | - | +++ | - | - | - | Anctil et al.[20,21] |
| Nanosilver | T-shirts | x | x | +++ | +++ | +++ | + (Conv-Ag) | Walser et al.[24] |
| Nanosilver | Socks | x | (x) | - | +++ | +++ | + (Conv-Ag) | Meyer et al.[37] |
| Nanosilver | NA (production) | x | - | +++ | + (GW) | - | - | Kuck et al.[23] |

*(continued)*

**TABLE 11.1 (Continued)**

Overview of LCA Studies Dedicated to Nano-Based Products[a]

| Nanomaterials | Application/Product Category[b] | LC Stages Included[c] | | | | Energy | 'Impact'[f] Assessment Coverage[d] | | | References |
|---|---|---|---|---|---|---|---|---|---|---|
| | | RM | P | U | D | | Nontoxic Impacts[e] | Toxic Impacts[e] | NP-Specific Toxicity[f] | |
| Nanosilver (nanowires); SWCNT | Transparent conductors used in organic photovoltaic modules | x | x | (x) | – | +++ | – | – | – | Emmott et al.[38] |
| Nanoclay | Polypropylene composite used in automotive panels | x | x | x | – | – | + (GW, Inv.) | + (Inv.) | – | Lloyd et al.[39] |
| Nanoclay | Polypropylene composite used in packaging film, agricultural film, and automotive panels | x | x | x | x | – | +++ | – | – | Roes et al.[25] |
| Nanoclay | Biopolymers | x | x | – | – | +++ | + (GW, Inv.) | + (Inv.) | – | Joshi et al.[26] |
| Nanoclay, $SiO_2$, CNT | Polymers | x | x | x | x | +++ | + (GW) | – | – | Roes et al.[40] |
| Quantum dots | White-light emitting LEDs | x | x | x | – | +++ | + (GW) | – | – | Steinfeldt et al.,[30] von Gleich et al.[31] |
| Quantum dots | Photovoltaic systems | x | x | x | – | +++ | + (GW, AC) | + (Inv.) | – | Sengul et al.[41] |
| Nanocrystalline silicon | Multi-junction photovoltaic modules | x | x | (x) | – | +++ | – | – | – | Kim et al.[42] |

| | | | | | | | | | |
|---|---|---|---|---|---|---|---|---|---|
| Nanocrystalline silicon; Nano CdTe; nanosilver | Photovoltaic systems | x | x | – | +++ | – | – | – | Fthenakis et al.[43] |
| Silica | Epoxy silica composite used in photovoltaic modules | x | (x) | – | +++ | +++ | – | – | Roes et al.[44] |
| Nanocrystalline dye (from nano-TiO$_2$ and carbon powder) | Sensitized solar cell systems | x | x | x | – | + (GW, Inv.) | + (Inv.) | – | Greijer et al.[45] |
| Titanium dioxide | NA (production) | x | – | – | +++ | + (GW) | – | – | Osterwalder et al.[46] |
| Titanium dioxide | NA (production) | x | – | – | +++ | +++ | +++ | – | Grubb et al.[22] |
| Zinc oxide | Polymer solar cell modules | x | x | (x) | +++ | + (GW) | – | – | Espinosa et al.[47,48] |
| Titannitride, titan-aluminium-nitride | Surface coating (via Physical Vapor Deposition) | x | – | – | – | +++ | +++ | – | Bauer et al.[28] |
| Nanocoating (unspecified) | Nanovarnish | x | x | x | +++ | + (GW, AC) | – | – | Steinfeldt et al.[30,34] von Gleich et al.[31] |
| Nanoscale platinum-group metals | Platinum automotive catalyst | x | x | – | – | + (GW, Inv.) | + (Inv.) | – | Lloyd et al.[49] |
| Organic metal (nanoscale polyanilin + silver) | Surface finishing of circuit boards | x | x | x | +++ | +++ | – | – | Steinfeldt[34] |

(continued)

**TABLE 11.1 (Continued)**

Overview of LCA Studies Dedicated to Nano-Based Products[a]

| Nanomaterials | Application/Product Category[b] | LC Stages Included[c] | | | | 'Impact' Assessment Coverage[d] | | | | References |
|---|---|---|---|---|---|---|---|---|---|---|
| | | RM | P | U | D | Energy | Nontoxic Impacts[e] | Toxic Impacts[e] | NP-Specific Toxicity[f] | |
| Yttria-stabilized zirconia | Surface coating (via different plasma spray techniques) | x | x | – | – | – | +++ | +++ | – | Moign et al.[50] |
| Complementary metal–oxide–semiconductor (CMOS) | Wafer (semiconductor) | x | x | – | – | +++ | + (GW) | – | – | Krischnan et al.[51] |
| Fe- and Al-nanoparticles (energetic NPs)[g] | Nanofuel | x | x | x | x | +++ | – | – | – | Wen et al.[52] |

a   Retrieved in April 2012 from Meyer et al.,[53] Gavankar et al.,[54] Steinfeld et al.,[55] Upadhyayula et al.,[56] Olsen and Miseljic,[57] Hischier and Walser,[58] and own search.

b   "NA" indicates a study that focuses on the production of the nanomaterial without considering its application to a specific product.

c   '(x)' in use stage indicates that the use stage is comprehended in the assessment only as energy/impact payback time, i.e. time required for an energy generation plant or device to produce the same amount of energy as was invested to fabricating it; '(x)' in disposal stage indicates that the assumptions made in the studies led to ruling out the assessment of the disposal stage.

d   Marked with "+++": complete 'impact' assessment. Marked with "+": partial assessment. Marked with "−": no assessment.

e   Nontoxic impacts include global warming (GW), acidification (AC), eutrophication, photochemical ozone formation, stratospheric ozone depletion and resource depletion including water and nonrenewable resources; toxic impacts include ecotoxicity (FE: freshwater ecotoxicity) and human toxicity-related impact categories; some authors reported aggregated emission inventories of different pollutants: they are marked as 'Inv.'

f   Indications refer to quantitative impact assessment of the released nanoparticles (NP) in one or several life cycle stages; 'Conv-Ag' indicates that authors regarded the released nanosilver as elemental/ionic silver and not as a nanoparticle in the impact assessment phase.

g   These studies used already-published data about nanomaterials production to conduct their assessments; Dinghra et al.[27] used data for the CNF production from Khanna et al.,[14] Garcia-Valverde et al.[36] used data for the production of fullerenes from Kushnir et al.[19]

dissolved fraction of emitted silver, while Meyer et al.[37] assumed that 100% of the nanosilver contained in the socks was released. Using the characterization factors available for colloidal silver, both studies concluded on the minor contribution from the releases of nanosilver to ecotoxicity-related impacts over the entire life cycle. In a third study, Eckelman et al.[29] compared the freshwater ecotoxicity impacts caused by the production of carbon nanotubes and those caused by their emissions to the environment. Using the USEtox model,[7,59] the characterization factor for carbon nanotubes was determined on the basis of existing literature and assuming two scenarios—realistic and worst-case—with regard to emission, fate, transport, and effects in the freshwater environment. In the unrealistic worst-case scenario, the ecotoxicity exerted by carbon nanotubes in freshwater was approximately equivalent to the ecotoxicity caused during the production of the nanotubes, while it ranged three orders of magnitude lower under the realistic scenario. Although other exposure routes have not been investigated in these studies, like exposure of workers and users to nanosilver or carbon nanotubes during the production, use, or disposal stage, these results tend to lower the anticipated risks related to the use of nanomaterials. These studies, dating from 2011 to 2012, also constitute signals that the field of LCA has started to bridge the gaps in the life cycle toxicity assessment of nanoparticles.

## 11.2.4 Limitations in Application of LCA in Studies

Despite the fact that all the identified LCA studies claim to perform an LCA—sometimes improperly termed "life cycle analysis"—only a few meet the holistic dimensions of LCA in both the completeness of the life cycle (scope of the studies) and the breadth of impact coverage (impact assessment).

### 11.2.4.1 Goal and Scope of Studies

One major shortcoming of the LCA studies lies in the extent to which the life cycle perspective is encompassed. To fulfill its purpose and avoid environmental problem shifting, an LCA should include all life cycle stages. However, as Figure 11.5 shows, a large number of studies are mere cradle-to-gate studies, thus stopping after the production stage. Less than half of them include the use stage, while only 20% go to complete the life cycle up to its disposal stage.

This choice in the system boundaries has large implications on the results obtained throughout the study and on their interpretation by LCA practitioners. Eventually, it is the whole decision-making process that ends up being at stake—let us see how.

Cradle-to-gate studies typically use functional units defined by either (i) a mass of produced nanomaterials or (ii) a mass of manufactured nanoproduct. Let us first take case (i). This situation has led many studies to compare the impacts caused by producing a given mass of nanomaterials with those from producing a same mass of conventional materials such as aluminum or steel.

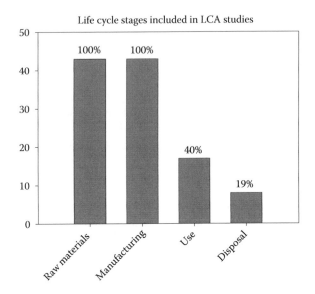

**FIGURE 11.5**
Life cycle stages included in inventoried LCA studies.

However, these are just materials to be fed into the manufacture of a finished product or good. Typically nanomaterials will amount to small percentages, that is, <5%, relative to the final mass of the nanoproduct. Therefore, comparing for instance 1 kg of steel with 1 kg of carbon nanotubes is inappropriate. Figure 11.6a illustrates the large differences of magnitude that can result from conducting such an improper assessment; note the order-of-magnitude differences in the results between the nanomaterial-embedded polymers (dark grey) and the nanomaterials alone (black).

Yet, comparing results for producing a given mass of nanomaterial-embedded polymers and those for manufacturing a same mass of steel of aluminum is still inappropriate—this exemplifies case (ii). These materials indeed possess different physico–chemical properties that are exploited in their different applications. For instance, 1 kg of steel is not equivalent to 1 kg of carbon-nanofiber-embedded polypropylene (CNF/PP nanocomposite)—and even not to 1 kg of aluminum. Aluminum has a much lower density than steel; the CNF/PP nanocomposite offers more strength and stiffness than steel in addition to exhibiting other properties such as electrical conductivity. These properties have a strong influence on the type of application they will be used in and hence are determinant in the settings of the functional unit if one wants to ensure an adequate comparability of the assessed products or materials. Figure 11.6b shows how the results can be affected by the choice of the functional unit. The assessment of the switch from the use of steel to the use of nanocomposites in automotive body paneling should be based on the main function of the materials, which is primarily driven by

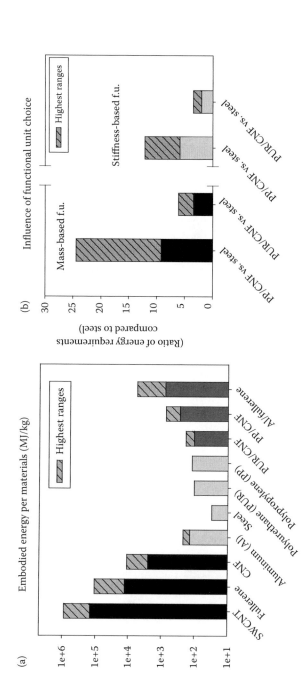

**FIGURE 11.6**

(a) Selection of energy requirements (logarithmic scale) for production of carbon-based nanomaterials (black), conventional materials (light grey), nanocomposites (dark grey). SWCNT, single-walled carbon nanotubes; CNF, carbon nanofibers. (From Khanna, V. et al., *J. Ind. Ecol.*, 12, 394, 2008; Khanna, V. and Bakshi, B.R., *Environ. Sci. Technol.*, 43, 2078, 2009; Anctil, A. et al., *Environ. Sci. Technol.*, 45, 2353, 2011; Healy, M.L. et al., *J. Ind. Ecol.*, 12, 376, 2008; and own computation.) (b) Change in energy requirements for production of PP/CNF and PUR/CNF, used for automotive body paneling, compared with that for steel production, using a product mass-based functional unit (black) or a product property-based functional unit (light grey; in the example, stiffness is used). Lowest and highest ranges dependent on percent weight of nanomaterials in product. f.u., functional unit. (From Khanna, V. and Bakshi, B.R., *Environ. Sci. Technol.*, 43, 2078, 2009.)

their mechanical properties and not by their mass. Although the ranking of the three options (PUR/CNF and PP/CNF are each compared with steel) in Figure 11.6b appears the same no matter how the functional unit is defined, conclusions could still differ if one was to investigate and include uncertainty ranges; for example, the use of an appropriate functional unit according to stiffness could lead to the performances of PUR/CNF nanocomposite ranging within those of steel (not shown in figure).

Adopting a property-based functional unit is also a first step to encompass the use stage, which is so lacking in many LCA studies performed until now. In practice, the substitution of an existing product by a nanoproduct occurs because the latter offers more advantages related to the function it is entitled to fulfill. Those advantages are primarily expressed during the use stage as well as in the disposal stage to a lesser extent (e.g., to improve material/thermal recovery).

Including those stages is thus crucial if one strives toward a comprehensive and accurate overview of the impacts and benefits of nanoproducts over conventional products. On the basis of data from Khanna et al.,[15] Figure 11.7 illustrates how conclusions of an LCA can radically change when including the use stage to a "cradle-to-gate" assessment of automotive components. Relying on the cradle-to-gate study (black on graph), an LCA practitioner would conclude on the too large impacts caused by the nanoproducts over the steel-based

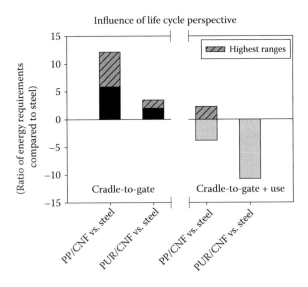

**FIGURE 11.7**
Change in energy requirements in life cycle of PP/CNF- and PUR/CNF-based automotive components compared with that of steel, using cradle-to-gate perspective (black) and including influence of use stage (light grey; influence is here characterized by fuel consumption savings due to utilization of lighter materials than steel). Lowest and highest ranges dependent on percent weight of nanomaterials in product. (Retrieved from Khanna, V. and Bakshi, B.R., *Environ. Sci. Technol.*, 43, 2078, 2009; Design inspired by Hischier, R. and Walser, T., *Sci. Total Environ.*, 425, 271, 2012.)

alternative, which would fall onto the highly energy intensive production of the carbon nanofibers, whereas just including some of the savings generated in the use stage (here the lighter weight causing less fuel consumption) would lead to the opposite conclusion. Ultimately, the outcome of the decision-making process could be deeply influenced by such misleading results.

### 11.2.4.2 Inventory of Emissions

For the background data, most LCA studies have relied on available life cycle inventory (LCI) databases. However, to build inventories for nanoproduct-specific processes, the data used are mainly computations or measurements from laboratory-scaled studies, which have been reported in the publicly available literature; very few studies have used data from actual pilot or commercialization plants (see Hischier and Walser[58]). This is paradoxical when one considers the amount of nanoproducts already available on the market. One cause may stem from the potential of the market for nanotechnologies, which, along with driving their rapid development (see Figure 11.4a), has simultaneously raised a number of barriers from industries that are not inclined to share process information. Facing a rapidly evolving sector where most data are kept confidential is a difficult challenge for the creation of inventory databases, and one that is going to be essential for the consistency of future LCA studies.

By assessing immature and nonoptimized processes, most of the existing studies on nanoproducts are thus likely to have reported overestimated results (e.g., energy requirements for in the production of nanomaterials). This shortcoming may have large consequences on the interpretation of the results when the LCA practitioner compares the thus-biased performances of a nanoproduct with those of a product already well established on the market. A way to address this issue could be by conducting prospective LCA studies that include a foresight of the impacts caused by nanoproducts in a mass production context (e.g., Walser et al.[24]).

### 11.2.4.3 Impact Assessment

An LCA aims at addressing all relevant environmental problems related to the product life cycle. However, as displayed in Figure 11.8, about two-thirds of the LCA studies identified in the scientific literature have focused on energy requirements, with some of them solely addressing this indicator. Studies assessing environmental impacts as such have concentrated on the assessment of global warming (accounting for nearly all the partial assessment in the non-toxic impact categories in Figure 11.8). As a consequence of such trend, only 15 out of the 43 listed studies have conducted a complete assessment of nontoxic impacts, and 10 out of those 15 have included toxic impacts (among which three have addressed the toxicity exerted by the released nanoparticles).

Several reasons can be advanced for such a pattern. The most obvious one is likely to be the paucity of available data. In an emerging and quickly

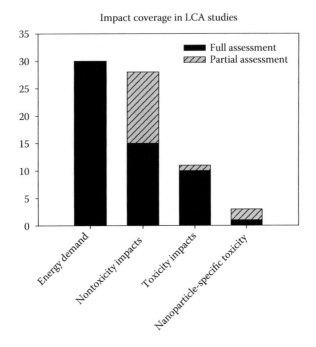

**FIGURE 11.8**
Impact categories covered by inventoried LCA studies.

evolving field, data are difficult to gather—see Section 11.2.4.2. On the other hand, the assessment of nontoxic impacts does not require much data as these impacts are typically caused by a limited number of substances, which have been identified and are relatively well monitored. For ruling out the assessment of toxicity-related impacts, many authors have argued the lack of reliability in the obtained results. This is primarily caused by the limited coverage of substances in the characterization factor databases and by the strong dependence of the results on the choice of the characterization models.[60–63]

Nevertheless, this pattern of excluding several impact categories is worrying in the sense that such truncated LCA may be too limited to avoid any burden shifting across impact categories. Several studies have investigated the representativeness of stand-alone indicators such as the cumulative energy demand (accounting for energy requirements) or the carbon footprint (accounting for climate change impacts). Huijbregts et al.[64,65] have found significant correlations between the cumulative energy demand and the total environmental burden for a majority of products taken from different sectors and recommended its use as a screening tool, particularly useful for emerging fields because of its low data requirements, but advised against its use as a stand-alone indicator because of the too high uncertainties from nonfossil-energy-related emissions and land use. Laurent et al.[66] have demonstrated the limitations of the carbon footprint to account for the entire environmental burden, particularly failing to predict toxicity-related impacts and resource depletion (e.g., metals), thus eventually leading to high risks in decision-making processes if used as a stand-alone indicator to quantify and manage environmental sustainability.

These studies thus counter the apparent trend of the LCA studies to focus on energy requirements and climate change, and call for the use of these indicators as mere facilitators or catalysts for conducting full LCAs. The increasing gain in credibility of the models assessing toxicity-related impacts, for example, with the advent of the USEtox consensus model,[7,59] as well as the recent advances that start emerging in the assessment of impacts caused by nanoparticles (e.g., Eckelman et al.[29]) are signals that some hurdles, which render a difficult broadly encompassing LCA, may soon fall and eventually allow the results of LCA studies to be more consistent and usable.

### 11.2.4.4 Interpretation

The main limitations in the LCA studies conducted thus far are in fact due to missing life cycle stages and impact categories. More generally speaking, very few of the case studies provide assessment of uncertainties, a crucial point in a rapidly evolving field.

### 11.2.5 Gaps and Further Needs

Table 11.2 summarizes the gaps identified in the literature review of LCA studies on nanoproducts. The next section will propose and further discuss for each step of the LCA potential strategies to meet these needs, addressing the following questions: (i) how to identify the required LCA scope and the life cycle risks of new nanomaterials and nanoproducts compared with conventional products; (ii) how to better assess the inventory of emissions associated with nanomaterial engineering compared with the processing of conventional products; (iii) which mechanisms affect the fate, exposure, and biological effects of nanoparticles; and (iv) how to interpret results for fast-changing technologies, with limited data availability and high uncertainties.

---

## 11.3 Recommendations and Strategies for Improving Nano-Specific LCAs

### 11.3.1 Nano-Specificities for Scope and Goal Definition

#### 11.3.1.1 Identification of LCA Scope and of Main Risk of Nanomaterials

We first need to refine the assessment framework, relating impacts to functional units—the unit that characterizes the service offered by the final product as the basis to compare nano- and classic technologies.

**TABLE 11.2**

Gaps in Present Studies and Proposed Actions and Path Toward Improving Quality of Available Data and Models

| Gaps from Literature Review on Nano-LCA | Proposed Paths and Strategies to Address These Gaps |
|---|---|
| *(a) Goal and Scope Definition* | |
| Incomplete scope, especially for the use and disposal phase | Simplified matrix to identify study scope and main impacts and trade-offs to be covered in comparing nano-based with conventional applications |
| *(b) Life Cycle Inventory* | |
| Lack of systematic life cycle inventory data on manufacturing process unit for nanomaterials | – Life cycle inventory database characterizing main nanomaterial and nanoproduct manufacturing pathways and technologies, including lithography, precipitation, SPM, and depositions |
| Lack of direct emission data about nanoparticle releases during use and disposal of nanomaterials | – Method for assessing the nanoparticle releases from the nanomaterial samples during the whole life cycle under use conditions (simulating the use of the samples by accelerated aging in different environmental conditions), until the end of life |
| *(c) Life Cycle Impact Assessment* | |
| Lack of life cycle impact characterization factors for impact of direct emissions of nanoparticles on human health covering fate, exposure, and dose–response | – Modeling of fate of transport of nanoparticles in the air and of fraction inhaled in the respiratory tract as a function of particle sizes<br>– Multimedia modeling of exposure to nanoparticles in food and through various media<br>– Dose–response slope based on $ED_{50}$ extrapolated from NOAEL or *in vivo* toxic doses 50% ($TD_{50}$)<br>– Determination of the influence of particle size and surface modification on biodistribution via pharmacokinetic modeling<br>– Creation of a set of USEtox compatible characterization factors |
| Lack of life cycle impact characterization factors for ecosystem | Creation of a set of hazard concentrations 50% ($HC_{50}$) for nanoparticles, based on the geometric mean on all available $LC_{50}$ measured on aquatic species, to determine concentration–response |
| *(d) Interpretation* | |
| Lack of systematic uncertainty study | First estimate of coefficients of variation for each multiplicative component of the assessment (emission, fate, exposure, and dose–response) |

We therefore developed a matrix approach (Table 11.3) to identify the main risks and benefits associated with nanotechnologies over the whole product life cycle (raw material extraction, manufacturing, use phase, disposal, and recycling) compared with those of conventional products. This framework considers (i) additional risks and benefits directly due to nanotechnologies, and (ii) indirect risks and impacts (e.g., through greenhouse gas and particulate emissions during electricity production for nanomaterial

**TABLE 11.3**

Identification of Life Cycle Impacts and Benefits Linked to Nanomaterial Manufacturing and Use, Compared with Traditional Products

| | Emissions and Impacts/Benefits Directly due to Nanoparticles | Indirect Emissions, Risks and Impacts: Nano vs. Conventional | Key Factors |
|---|---|---|---|
| Raw material extraction | – | Impacts linked to energy preparation/combustion, criteria pollutant emissions | Energy and material use for a given function and application |
| Manufacturing | Potentially important for workers' health Emission to ecosystems | Impacts and risks linked to chemical exposure in manufacturing/accidental rates | – Nanomaterial manufacturing process emissions<br>– Indoors exposure of workers<br>– Pharmacokinetics and bioeffects of nanoparticle |
| Use phase | Dominant for medical applications and in case of direct releases in exposed environment Direct benefits in terms of human health by improved diagnostic/treatment | Impacts and risks linked to other chemical releases/combustion/medical interventions | – Releases indoors and in the environment during use phase<br>– Pharmacokinetics and biological effects<br>– Surface desorption of nanoparticles |
| Disposal and Material recycling | Exposure of overall population and ecotoxicological risks due to nanomaterial releases in the environment | Exposure to conventional chemical and drugs in the disposal phase | Long-range transport of nanoparticles, environmental fate, and chemical properties Feasibility to collect and recycle |

manufacturing) of nanotechnologies compared with (iii) those of conventional technologies. For each case, the key factors of influence are identified.

Table 11.3 shows that both direct and indirect effects of nanoparticles need to be considered. Compared with classic application, the following issues are expected to be nanospecific, of high relevance, and need to be addressed in priority:

- The approach should enable the assessment of direct exposure of both workers and general population exposure.
- Nanoparticle emissions during the manufacturing and use phases, indoors or through direct dermal contact, should be considered in a specific way.

- Direct impacts of nanoparticles on both human health and ecosystems need to be addressed. In this respect, knowledge and modeling of fine and ultrafine particles is a good starting basis to model the exposure.
- The assessment method needs to be consistent between impacts of classic chemicals and technologies and the direct impacts of nanoparticles.

**TABLE 11.4**

Identification of Life Cycle Impacts and Benefits of a Nanosilver T-shirt

| | Emissions and Impacts/Benefits Directly due to Nanosilver Particles | Indirect Emissions, Risks and Impacts: Nano T-shirt vs. Conventional T-shirt | Key Factors |
|---|---|---|---|
| Raw material extraction | – | – Electricity production emissions <br> – Silver extraction and mining | Electricity use per washing cycle |
| Manufacturing | Direct intake of silver nanoparticles by workers during nanosilver and T-shirt manufacturing | – Washing powder manufacturing <br> – Nanosilver production energy and chemicals | – Nanomaterial manufacturing process emissions <br> – Indoors exposure of workers <br> – Pharmacokinetics and bioeffects of nanoparticle |
| Use phase | – Dermal uptake of silver nanoparticle through skin contact during use <br> – Potential reduction in bacterial risks for consumer (unlikely to be dominant) <br> – Direct emissions of nanosilver to wastewater treatment plant and surface water | Indirect impacts linked to decrease in number of washing cycle per functional unit: <br> – Reduction in powder and washing and drying electricity due to antibacterial effect <br> – Subsequent reduction in impacts of detergents | – Reduction in washing frequency due to antibacterial effect (can use the T-shirt one more day without odors before washing = reuse!) <br> – Fraction of nanosilver released to the environment <br> – Fate and ecotoxicological effects of nanosilver and of detergents in the environment |
| Disposal and recycling | Direct releases during T-shirt end-of-life (e.g., incinerator or landfill) or when recycling | Indirect change in wastewater treated per functional unit | – Fraction of nanosilver released to environmental media during wastewater treatment |

- Effects on living organisms are highly dependent on the specific nanoparticle properties and will differ significantly between different particle types (nanotubes, fullerenes, $TiO_2$, polyacrylamide nanoparticles, etc.).

Applying this matrix to the nanosilver T-shirt case study yields Table 11.4. It already preidentifies that the impact during use phase will directly depend on the consumer behavior: if the nanosilver T-shirt is used one or several more days before being washed than a conventional T-shirt (assuming that bacterial growth and therefore odors are delayed), all impacts linked to washing and drying will be reduced when considered per day of T-shirt use. This leads to a trade-off between reduced indirect impacts of washing versus additional direct impacts due to, for example, impacts of dissolved nanosilver on ecosystem quality.

### 11.3.1.2 Nano-Specificities of LCA Goal Definition

The goal definition is not intrinsically different from other LCAs; however, certain features are even more important to consider to avoid strong biases:

- *Functional unit*: It is crucial to address impacts per functional unit rather than per kilogram of material. With nanomaterials and nano-based products, despite the often high impact per kilogram of nanomaterials, the overall impact per functional unit can be limited compared with other conventional materials, since quantities of nanomaterial purchased per functional unit are often limited.
- *Nanomaterial versus nano-based product*: From an LCA perspective, it is not possible nor desirable to judge the intrinsic environmental performance of a nanomaterial or in fact of any material as such. A (nano-)material assessment can only be assessed within the context of its application to a given product with its corresponding function and functional unit (e.g., for a nanosilver T-shirt).
- *System boundaries*: Including direct nanomaterial releases during nanoproduct manufacturing, use, and disposal is crucial to ensure a fair comparison with other traditional chemicals.

### 11.3.2 Nano-Specificities for Life Cycle Inventory

When quantifying and collecting emission data to build an LCI for nanomaterial-embedded products, a number of specific aspects need to be considered, adding to the complexity this task already demands for any LCA. In general, the inventory database to be built for nanoproducts can be divided into three major groups of data, comprising (i) the indirect resources and emissions associated with the supply of inputs into the life cycle of the

**TABLE 11.5**

Generic Matrix of Most Needed Inventory Efforts[a]

|  | Raw Materials | Manufacturing | Use | Disposal |
|---|---|---|---|---|
| Indirect processes – inventory components | – Idem conventional | – Idem conventional | – Idem conventional | – Idem conventional |
| "Nano-product"-specific processes – inventory components | NA / | +++ To be developed | ++ To be developed in some cases/ Idem conventional | + Idem conventional processes until now |
| Direct nanoparticle emissions | NA / | +++ To be characterized | +++ To be characterized | +++ To be characterized |

[a] The importance of inventory efforts is reflected by the following code in decreasing order: +++ > ++ > + > –. NA: not applicable.

nanoproducts; (ii) the nanoproduct-specific inventory components that focus on direct material and energy inputs, and classic toxic emissions for the main manufacturing pathways, as well as during the use stage and disposal of the nanoproducts; and (iii) the direct nanoparticle emissions from the considered processes in each of the life cycle stages. Table 11.5 shows the general importance of these three inventory components through the nanoproduct life cycle in terms of required efforts (in the present context).

The processes associated with the supply of inputs into the nanoproduct life cycle (e.g., the matrix in which a nanomaterial is to be embedded) are the least demanding in terms of data collection, as they typically refer to processes used in conventional materials, and hence are already well covered by publicly available LCI databases or LCA software/tools. On the other hand, the two other inventory components—direct nanoparticle emissions and nanoproduct-specific process inventory—require further efforts (see color-coding in Table 11.5); these are developed in the following, after a brief status of the quantification of nanoparticle releases throughout the life cycle.

### 11.3.2.1 Quantification of LC Emissions of Nanoparticles: A Status

*11.3.2.1.1 Measurements of Nanoparticle Emissions: Many Challenges Left*

What would be the needed information for quantifying releases and allowing characterization in LCA studies? To allow a proper assessment of toxicity exerted by the nanoparticles (see Section 11.3.3), more information than bulk chemicals are needed. Ideally, apart from a proper characterization of the process under study, knowledge on the size distribution of the emitted nanoparticles, including distinction between the (i) aggregated nanoparticles, (ii) the matrix-bound nanoparticles, (iii) the single nanoparticles, and (iv) the nanoparticles already present in the background, is required. Additionally, the emitted mass and number of particle concentration are needed along with knowledge about the physico–chemical properties of the nanoparticles, which include the shape, surface area, surface chemistry, composition (including coatings), solubility, charge, crystal structure, and state of agglomeration of the nanoparticles.[67–71]

However, until now, little is known about the exact magnitude of the emissions.[72–74] Although several measurements are currently performed in the workplace and during laboratory simulations, not all studies are able to distinguish between background and nanoproduct-induced emissions,[75,76] and techniques do not allow for consistent monitoring and characterization of nanoparticle emissions.[74] In several studies, it was therefore not possible to assign consistently the part of nanoparticle emissions arising from the nanoproduct itself to the measured occupational concentrations. Among the few studies that report emissions of nanoparticles, some detected nano-$TiO_2$ in water leaching from exterior painted facades[77] or releases of nanosilver from textiles, for example, during washing.[24,53] Other studies also reported emissions during the manufacturing stage[78] and at the disposal stage, for example, recycling.[79]

Difficulties also arise in characterizing the physico–chemical properties of the nanoparticles, primarily due to (i) the variations in the importance of the different properties among nanoparticles that prevent any generic treatment, for example, the crystallinity for nano-$TiO_2$, which has a strong influence on its toxicity (e.g., Warheit et al.[80]), and (ii) the accessibility to some properties requiring sophisticated and expensive methods or techniques, which are not standardized and thus often lead to incomparable results across studies.

### 11.3.2.1.2 *Models of Nanoparticle Releases: Also Many Challenges Left*

The general lack of comparable, empirical data has resulted in some research focusing on the development of modeling approaches for quantifying releases of nanoparticles across the nanoproduct life cycle. Table 11.6 provides an overview of these available models, based on a review performed by Gottschalk and Nowack[74] and the authors' own search.

Table 11.6 shows that all currently existing modeling approaches (i) adopt a system-oriented perspective, using material flow analysis (MFA) to typically encompass a whole defined region or market system; (ii) have the implicit purpose of preparing the ground for assessing outdoor exposure, primarily of aquatic ecosystems; and (iii) restrain their scope to selected nanoproducts in a truncated life cycle perspective, with often an exclusive focus on the use stage (exceptions made of Mueller and Nowack[84] and Gottschalk et al.[86,87]). Therefore, although these approaches contribute to provide an overarching overview of releases of nanoparticles to the environment, they do not allow reaching process-specific release data that could be useful inputs for comprehensive LCAs. Also, they do not allow carrying information on the different properties of the released nanoparticles, which may vary through the nanoproduct life cycle.

**TABLE 11.6**

Existing Modeling Approaches for Quantifying Potential Releases of Nanoparticles

| Sources | Object(s) of Study | LC Stages Encompassed | | | Emission Compartments/ Process | Level of Specificity | Technique Used |
|---|---|---|---|---|---|---|---|
| | | Prod. | Use | Disp. | | | |
| Boxall et al.[81] | Products containing metal | × | × | × | Direct emissions to water, air, and soil (e.g., WWTP, runoffs, air deposition) | UK system | MFA |
| Blaser et al.[82] | Ag-embedded textiles and plastics | | × | × | Wastewater treatment plant + direct emissions | EU system | MFA |
| Park et al.[83] | CeO$_2$ in fuel additive | | × | | Fuel combustion | Generic | Existing models for particle emissions |
| Mueller and Nowack[84] | Nano-Ag, nano-TiO$_2$, carbon nanotubes | × | × | × | All compartments (emissions to water, air, and soil) | CH system | MFA |
| O'Brien et al.[85] | Exterior paints (TiO$_2$), food packaging (Ag), fuel additives CeO$_2$ | | × | | Wastewater treatment plant | IR system | Deterministic algorithms |
| Gottschalk et al.[86,87, a] | Nano-TiO$_2$, nano-ZnO, nano-Ag, carbon nanotubes, fullerenes | × | × | × | All compartments (emissions to water, air, and soil) | EU, USA, CH system | Probabilistic MFA |
| Arvidsson et al.[88] | TiO$_2$ products | × | × | × | Wastewater treatment plant + direct emissions | CH system | MFA |

*Source:* Based on Gottschalk, F. and Nowack, B., *J. Environ. Monit.*, 13, 1145, 2011.

a Rely on the same modeling approach.

It can also be noted from these models that the disposal stage, and notably recycling, is not fully represented. Only two studies have addressed recycling but in an incomplete manner, primarily because of the adopted system-oriented perspective. Mueller and Nowack[84] have defined the amount of nanomaterials generated from recycling process as "leaving the system" without further consideration, for example, exported outside the system boundaries (Switzerland). Gottschalk et al.[86,87] have raised the difficulty to quantify the amount of nanomaterials leaving a certain recycling process and has consequently assumed that all particles entering the recycling compartment were eliminated in the model (either combusted or incorporated in new materials). The authors of both studies have advanced that sewage sludge, wastewater, and waste incineration of nanoproducts were the major pathways through which nanoparticles enter the environment. However, with the likelihood of recycling to become a major concern for exposure to nanoparticles in the future (see Section 11.2.4), this demonstrates that further research is still needed to cover the life cycle emissions of nanoparticles in a comprehensive manner.

### 11.3.2.2 Inventory for Nanoproduct-Specific Processes and Potential Releases

The nanoproduct-specific processes, for example, the insertion of the nano-materials in a matrix during the manufacture of the nanoproduct or the grinding of the nanoproduct in view of its recycling, are processes for which little consistent data are currently available (see Section 11.2.4). In addition, the difficulties to quantify nanoparticle releases (see above Section 11.3.2.1) have compelled LCA practitioners to narrow down their ambitions and merely identify "potential" releases in qualitative manner, relying on the fact that the magnitude of the emissions is strongly dependent on (i) the location of the nanomaterials in the product and its structure, and/or (ii) the type of external pressures that the product undergoes during its life cycle.[74,76,89,90] These two major data shortcomings in the settings of complete life cycle inventories are discussed below for each life cycle stage.

*Material extraction* is the life cycle stage that is least affected by the specific issues of nanoparticles as, depending on the type of nanoparticle (e.g., metal oxide, carbon), the specific extraction processes will in most cases correspond to those used in any LCA; no releases of engineered nanoparticles occur at this stage.

*Transport* of nanomaterials or nanoproduct might lead to accidental emissions through leakage or damage of the transport packaging; however, continuous emissions during this stage are unlikely for most products.

*Manufacturing* of nanomaterials (synthesis) can be done through a variety of production pathways, which can be distinguished into top–down (starting from bulk materials) and bottom–up (starting from atomic or molecular level) approaches. These approaches can be further distinguished into wet (using solvents and liquid reagents in lithography or chemical coprecipitation) and dry processes (attrition, thermolysis, laser ablation, vapor deposition, pyrolysis, and plasma arc discharge).[53] Table 11.7 provides an overview of the manufacturing methods for nanomaterials, based on Steinfeldt et al.[30] This implies that rather than having product-specific life cycle inventories it would be more efficient and consistent to have production-pathway-specific inventories for the manufacturing stage, similar to current energy or raw material production inventories. The inventory of the final product manufacture would then be composed of the inventory for the particle production and possible enhancements via surface activation or functionalization plus the integration into the final product.

To achieve this goal for nanomaterial production processes, one promising approach could be to generate gate-to-gate LCI modules following the method described for chemical engineering processes by Jimenez-Gonzalez et al.[91] and Ponder and Overcash.[92] The method consists of (i) selecting the process with consideration of the industrial importance and the access to representative, up-to-date data; (ii) defining the process by its mass flow, the substances it uses, the reactions it involves, and the conditions under which it operates; (iii) determining the mass balance of the system, that is, calculating the inputs and outputs (including losses) for the process; and (iv) identifying the energy requirements and losses of the process. Eventually, the analysis of the system can lead to building a parameterized module, in which inputs and outputs are made dependent on the conditions of operations, for example, the energy-related emissions being correlated to the temperature set in the reaction chamber.

If applied to nanomaterial production, for example, to the techniques displayed in Table 11.7, such approach would bring a number of benefits as it would enable to investigate what process changes could have the greatest impact on raw materials, energy consumption, and emissions. Dealing with immature technologies, this can help to quickly move to more optimized processes. The parameterization of the module would also allow for defining life cycle inventories that are specific to the properties of the manufactured nanomaterials. For example, it could link the energy requirements and process emissions to the grade of the produced nanomaterial, that is, its degree of purity, which is typically imposed by its type of application and very often turn out to be the source of highly increased energy requirements if a high degree is needed (e.g., fullerenes used in organic solar cells[21]). Finally, until reliable measurements can be used, a qualitative or semiqualitative assessment of the potential releases of nanoparticles could be linked to the production intensity within each module, for example, increased risks of releases as a consequence of increased replacements of air filters when the productivity of the process is increased and leads to more waste generation. In their qualitative discussion of the potential for nanoparticle emissions during each of the seven manufacturing pathways, Steinfeldt et al.[30] pointed out that production methods taking place in gaseous media induce a higher potential of nanoparticle releases—see Table 11.7.

**TABLE 11.7**

Characteristics of Nanomaterial Manufacturing Techniques

| Processes | Media | Energy Requirements | Material Conversion | Material Efficiency | Potential for Nanoparticle Releases | | |
|---|---|---|---|---|---|---|---|
| | | | | | Manufacturing Stage—Workplace | Manufacturing Stage—Environment | Use Stage |
| Vapor phase deposition (CVD, PVD) | Gaseous | Very high | Low | High | Very low | Low–medium | Low–medium–high[a] |
| Flame-assisted deposition | Gaseous | Medium | Very high | High | Medium | Low–medium | High |
| Sol–gel process | Fluid or dissolved | Low | Medium–high | High | Low–medium | Low–medium | Low–medium[b] |
| Precipitation | Fluid or dissolved | Low | Medium–high | High | Low–medium | Low–medium | Low–medium[b] |
| Molecular imprinting | Liquid | Low | Medium–high | High | Low–medium | Low–medium | Low |
| Lithography | Solid matter | High | Low–medium | Medium | Low–medium | Low–medium | Low |
| Self-assembled monolayers | Fluid or dissolved | Low | Medium–high | High | Low–medium | Low–medium | Low–medium[c] |

*Source:* Steinfeldt, M. et al., *Nanotechnology and Sustainability*. Discussion Paper of the IOEW 65/04: Institute for Ecological Economy Research: Berlin, Germany, 2004.

[a] Depending on the fixation of the nanomaterials in the nanoproduct: "low" if encapsulated in a fixed coating; "medium" if encapsulated in coating attached to a product; "high" if nanomaterials as powder or tube form.

[b] Depending on the fixation of the nanomaterials in the nanoproduct: "low" if intermediate goods are in liquid form and end products are embedded within a fixed layer; "medium" if nanomaterials are encapsulated within end products with no long-term stability.

[c] Depending on the fixation of the nanomaterials in the nanoproduct: "low" if nanomaterials are encapsulated within a fixed layer; "medium" if nano-materials are encapsulated within end products with no long-term stability or if nanomaterials are encapsulated within a layer attached to a product.

The *use* of nanomaterials and nanoproduct spans a vast range of applications and functions that lead to a similarly large range of emission pathways and quantities depending on usage and handling of the respective product, which cannot be fully covered here. Some examples for typical applications and disposal treatment of nanoproducts and specific issues related to their emissions are discussed in Table 11.8.

The *end-of-life* treatment options for nanoproducts are currently the same as for conventional products—see Table 11.9 for examples of causes of potential nanoparticle releases in waste management systems. However, the dramatic increase in the utilization of nanoproducts inevitably results in an increased generation of nanowaste—although the latter may be delayed in time depending on the nanoproduct lifetimes. At the same time, waste management policies put a strong emphasis on the implementation of recycling and reusing strategies (e.g., the legally binding EU Waste Framework Directive 2008/98/EC). In such context, the recycling of nanowaste may appear as a situation of increasing concern, pertaining to occupational

**TABLE 11.8**

Examples (Nonexhaustive List) of Causes of Potential Releases for Selection of Nanoproducts during Their Use Stage

| Type of Applications | Causes of Potential Releases |
|---|---|
| Paints and coatings (e.g., nano-$TiO_2$ as white pigment, nano-Ag as biocide) | Aging or weathering of the original manufactured nanoparticles due to the influence of rain, wind, atmospheric pollution, UV radiation, and the like might significantly alter their physico–chemical and toxicological properties, as well as influence the emission rate over time.[77] |
| | The application technique might influence the amount, pathway, and state of the particles emitted (e.g., aerosol, suspension) |
| | Various processes related to the paint/coating carrier (e.g., abrasion, washing, renovation, sanding, demolition) may influence emission rates.[93,94] |
| | Nanoparticles might not only be emitted in their pure form but rather as part of a mixture that may or may not interact with the particles (inducing, e.g., adsorption, chemical reactions, alteration of physico–chemical properties) |
| Fuel additives (e.g., $CeO_2$ in diesel added to decrease harmful emissions and increase fuel efficiency) | Nanoparticle characteristics may change significantly during combustion, so that the original particle cannot be assumed to be emitted directly |
| | Exhaust emissions might enter the atmosphere or the surface water via runoff from the road surface |
| Cosmetics (e.g., ZnO in sunscreen) | Emission into surface water due to wash-off during swimming |
| | Emission into surface water via incomplete removal from final effluent due to wash-off during showering |
| Biocides (e.g., Ag– nanosilver applied to packaging, clothing, detergents) | Leakage from products through normal wear and tear (e.g., abrasion,[93] heating/cooling, washing[95]) might lead to a release into surface water via incomplete removal in a sewage treatment plant, or into air via abrasion or other processes |

**TABLE 11.9**

Examples (Nonexhaustive List) of Causes of Potential Releases Associated with Waste Management of Nanoproducts

| Type of Applications | Causes of Potential Releases |
| --- | --- |
| Landfill | Just as for metals, leaching into soil and surface/groundwater might occur with various factors influencing the mobility and state of the nanoparticles released |
| | Bound nanoparticles might be released from their matrix during decomposition of the original product they were applied to, possibly leading to a release into the atmosphere via wind uptake |
| Incineration | Some of the nanoparticles may not be eliminated during the thermal process (e.g., metal and metal oxides) and be potentially released into the atmosphere |
| Recycling | Composting of organic nanomaterials (e.g., nanocellulose). Recycling of CNT-containing batteries.[98] |
| Wastewater treatment | While a fraction of nanoparticles might remain in the final effluent and thus be emitted to surface water, the rest will be in the sewage sludge, which will either be landfilled (leaching to soil or water), incinerated (emitted to air), or spread on land/sea and thus leading to further emissions into the corresponding compartments. However, to date, little is known about the efficiency of wastewater treatment systems regarding nanoparticles.[99] |

exposure to nanoparticles, as also pointed out by Köhler et al.,[72] Abbott and Maynard,[96] or Musee.[97]

### 11.3.2.3 Summary and Perspectives

To follow-up on Table 11.5, further research should thus be directed toward (i) developing inventories for the nanoproduct-specific processes, particularly in the manufacturing stage, where parameterized technology-specific modules are recommended to be built, and (ii) characterizing nanoparticle emissions during the manufacturing, use, and disposal stages. As an illustrative example, a qualitative framework highlighting the specific points to cover for building an inventory for nanosilver T-shirts is presented in Table 11.10.

### 11.3.3 Nano-Specificities for Life Cycle Impact Assessment

#### 11.3.3.1 Life Cycle Impact Assessment Framework for Nanoparticle Toxicity

**Existing LCIA methods and research needs:** According to ISO 14042 (2000), LCIA methods aim to connect each LCI result (emissions and resource extraction) to the corresponding environmental impacts. The LCIA program of the UNEP–SETAC Life Cycle Initiative proposes to first model the cause–effect chain in groups of midpoint categories,[100] according to common mechanisms (e.g., climate change, acidification) or commonly accepted grouping (e.g.,

**TABLE 11.10**

Matrix of Most Needed Inventory Efforts for Nanosilver T-Shirt[a,b]

| | Indirect Processes – Inventory Components | "Nano-Product"-Specific Processes – Inventory Components | Direct Nanoparticle Emissions | |
|---|---|---|---|---|
| | | | Potential Release Sources | Emission Compartment |
| Raw Materials | – | – | NA | NA |
| | Idem conventional T-shirts | Idem conventional T-shirts + existing database | / | / |
| Manufacturing | – | +++ | +++ | +++ |
| | Idem conventional T-shirts | – Parameterized module for flame spray pyrolysis <br> – Parameterized module for plasma polymerization with silver cosputtering | – Manufacturing processes <br> – Transport <br> – Cleaning of equipments (e.g. used filters) | Air, water (WWTP) |
| Use | – | + | +++ | +++ |
| | Idem conventional T-shirts | – Idem conventional T-shirts <br> – Consumer behaviour to evaluate (washing) | – Abrasion during wearing <br> – Abrasion during washing | Air, water (sweat on skin during wearing), water (WWTP) |
| Disposal | – | – | +++ | +++ |
| | Idem conventional T-shirts | Idem conventional T-shirts | – Incineration <br> – Recycling <br> – WWTP | – Air <br> – Air <br> – Water |

[a] The importance of inventory efforts is reflected by the following code in decreasing order: +++ > ++ > + > –. NA: not applicable.

[b] Sources used for completing the table: Mueller et al.[84] and Walser et al.[24]

human toxicity, ecotoxicity). It then relates these categories to four main damage categories—human health, ecosystems, climate change, and resources. Different methods are available, such as CML in Europe and TRACI[101] in the United States concentrating on midpoint levels, as well as ReCiPe[102] and IMPACT2002+[5] that cover both midpoint and damages, and IMPACT World+[103] that extend the IMPACT framework as well as USEtox[7,59] to the whole world. These methods are relatively well developed to cover classic midpoint categories such as global warming, acidification, and ozone depletion linked to indirect inputs for nanomaterial manufacturing. To address the nanoparticle specificities, research should essentially focus on the human toxicity and ecotoxicity impacts of nanoparticles and of their alternatives solutions.

**Proposed framework for ecotoxicity and human toxicity:** To enable the use of expert judgment in case of lack of quantitative information, it is important to express the characterization factors as the product of simple and well-interpretable factors whose order of magnitude can be determined and checked. The USEtox framework[7,59] constitutes a sound basis to combine comparative risks approaches and life cycle toxicity approaches, and corresponds to the latest LCIA methods (Figure 11.1). It is extended here to also include the possibility to account for the fraction of the dose taken up and its distribution inside the body, linking the external to internal dose with pharmacokinetics.

The *human toxicity* impact is calculated as the emission source multiplied by the intake fraction—the fraction of an emission that is taken in by the population (iF, dimensionless)—and by an effect factor (EF, cases per $kg_{in}$), generally based on chronic dose–response information (e.g., ED50—effect dose 50%). The intake fraction is itself the product of the fate factor (FF, d) multiplied by an exposure factor (XP, 1/d) and needs to be determined both for indoor and outdoor emissions. The impact $\vec{n}$, expressed in number of cancer and noncancer cases per year, is therefore given by

$$\vec{n} = \overline{HCF}\,\vec{m} = \overline{EF}\,\overline{iF}\,\vec{m} = \overline{EF}\,\overline{XP}\,\overline{FF}\,\vec{m} \qquad (11.1)$$

where the human characterization factor (HCF) represents the impact per kilogram emitted and is itself equal to the product of the EF multiplied by the iF.

**External to internal dose:** Regarding the lack of chronic dose–response information for different nanoparticle sizes and the recent development in pharmacokinetic modeling, we propose here an extended framework, opening the possibility to model body burden—the mass or concentration inside the body (Figure 11.9) in order to be able to extend *in vivo* measurements obtained for one type of particle to other sizes and surface transformations using *in silico* models. We therefore have alternatively

$$\overline{HCF} = \overline{EC}\,\overline{BB}\,\overline{iF} \qquad (11.2)$$

where $\overline{EC}$ measures the risk associated to a given mass or concentration in the body (or in the target organ) and $\overline{BB} = f_i^{\text{uptake absorbed}}\,\theta_i^b$ is the body burden matrix. BB is a pharmacokinetic matrix representing the increase in mass inside the body per unit intake flow and its subsequent distribution between human organs and tissues. Its diagonal term can be expressed as the product of the fraction of the intake that is taken up and absorbed inside the body ($f_i^{\text{intake absorbed}}$) and possibly transferred to the target organ, multiplied by the residence time of the substance or the particle in different parts of the body or target organ ($\theta_i^b$).

**Ecotoxicological impacts:** The ecological characterization factor (ECF[freshwater]) link an emission to the temporally and spatially integrated

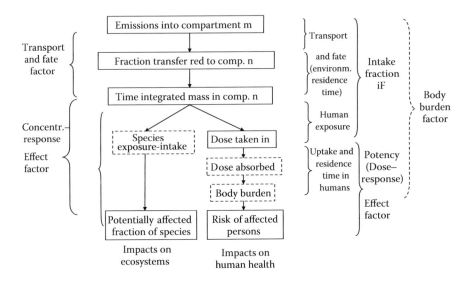

**FIGURE 11.9**
Framework for human toxicity and ecotoxicity of chemicals and nanoparticles. (Extended from Jolliet, O. et al., *Int. J. Life Cycle Assess.*, 11, 137, 2006.)

increase in the affected fraction of species due to an emission into a specific compartment, expressed as PAF $m^3$ $d/kg_{emitted}$. As described by Henderson et al.,[105] the characterization factors can be expressed as the multiplication of four factors. The first three terms describe the transport and exposure of a substance: the fraction transferred from emission compartment $i$ to freshwater ($f_{i,w}$ [-]), the environmental fate factor in freshwater ($FF_{w,w}$ [$kg_{in\ water}/(kg_{emitted}/d) = d$]), and the exposure factor, that is, the dissolved and bioavailable fraction ($XF_w$ [-]). The final term, the effect factor, based on ecotoxicological tests, describes the ecotoxicological response from freshwater ecosystems ($EF_w$ [PAF $m^3/kg_{in\ water}$]):

$$CF_i^{freshwater\ ecotox} = f_{i,w}\ FF_{w,w}\ XF_w\ EF_w \qquad (11.3)$$

### 11.3.3.2 Fate and Exposure to Nanoparticles

**Determination of physico–chemical properties:** Since nanoparticles can widely vary across nanoproducts and therefore vary their behavior in the environment and in the body, it is crucial to have them properly characterized see Chapter 7, present edition, in terms of size distribution, surface chemistry, shape, functionalization, and optical properties. Since these properties might be changed by aging, physical or chemical interaction with other particles, substances, or solids, characterizing these is even more critical as a basis for any evaluation and modeling of their behavior and dose–response effect. According to Oberdörster et al.,[106] biological activity and especially oxidative stress injury[107] appear to be linked to the surface area of the particle. Particle size plays a key role on the translocation and transfer inside the body. For the fate and exposure part, it is unclear if nanomaterial behavior depends on surface or on particle mass or number. Properties playing a key role are solubility, partition properties (hydrophilic/phobic, lipophilic/phobic), and bioconcentration/bioaccumulation factors that can be linked to specific surface groups. Some properties can be calculated based on molecule structure as proposed by Abraham et al.[108] for Buckminster-fullerene leading to a $K_{ow}$ of 12.6, which is at the highest range of PAH organics.[109]

**Fate in the environment:** Little is known about the transport mechanisms and degradation of nanoparticles in the environment and few studies have been published.

In water, aggregation and dissolution of pristine nanoparticles, which might affect their bioavailability and mobility,[110] can be influenced by their size distribution, shape, surface chemistry, and surface charge, but also by the medium's pH, occurrence of organic matter, ionic strength and valence of cations, and the presence of humic substances, which might stabilize suspensions of carbon nanotubes or fullerenes.[111–116] Interaction with biotic or abiotic colloids present in the water column has been reported by Ju-Nam and Lead.[117] Therefore, besides nanoparticle-specific properties, differences in composition between water types (e.g., surface water, marine water, groundwater and wastewater), regarding the properties discussed above, is a critical factor to consider when determining transport and fate of nanoparticles in water.

In soil, nanoparticles are transported via pore water before deposition to the soil matrix takes place. While the transport is mainly driven by the nanoparticles' physical properties, such as size or shape, the deposition depends on the interaction between the particles (van der Waals force, electrostatic force, and steric repulsion), as well as hydrophobic forces between particles and the soil matrix surface.[118,119] These hydrophobic forces are therefore a driving capture mechanism in soil that can be reduced by functionalization, surfactant capping, or other alterations induced over time in the environment. These properties will hence also drive the nanoparticles' mobility in soil,[120,121] and may explain part of the differences observed in their pore water transport efficiency.[122]

The influence of vegetation on fate and transport of nanoparticles is unknown. Zhu et al.[123] demonstrated the potential for nanoparticles to be taken up through the roots and be accumulated in the plant tissue of pumpkins. However, there is not enough evidence yet to conclude about the influence of vegetation on the fate of nanoparticles.

While thus far studies have focused on engineered or pristine nanoparticles, aging or weathering is an important but much neglected factor regarding the behavior of nanoparticles in the environment, as it is likely to alter physical properties such as size, shape, surface charge, or functionalization of nanoparticles. This will therefore change the behavior of the nanoparticles in the environment owing to the observed importance of these properties as discussed in

Section 11.3.3.2. Mueller and Nowack[84] provide an interesting model of multi-media transfer between environmental compartments for nanosilver.

**Human intake fractions:** Specifically, we aim to model the fate and exposure from the emission source to the intake dose nanoparticulate intake fraction, as defined by Bennett et al.,[124] characterizing the fate and exposure of both organics and inorganics, as well as fine particles.[125,126] Taking fullerene as an example, we have built on the work of Maddalena et al.[109] and adapted the IMPACT 2002 multimedia model[127] to the nanoparticle properties proposed by Abraham et al.[108]

Figure 11.10 compares the intake fraction of fullerenes to that of various persistent organic chemicals (POPs). It is interesting to note the predicted reduction in absorption for POPs at high $K_{ow}$, linked to low bioaccumulation in animals[128] and possibly reflected in the low absorption rate for nanomaterials such as fullerenes (2% according to Obersdörster et al.[129]). Such multimedia models can also provide the transfer factors to, and fate factor or residence time in water and soil, as defined in Equation 11.3. For intake fraction emitted indoors, the approach proposed by Wenger et al.[130] enables us to account for adsorption on the indoor surfaces, provided that the substance vapor pressure is given. It should, however, be verified whether the extrapolation between vapor pressure and partition coefficient between air and wall at the wall surface holds for nanoparticles.

**From intake to uptake fraction:** For ultrafine and eventually nanoparticles, Humbert[131] has proposed to determine the uptake fraction, which expresses the ratio of uptake in the respiratory tract (i.e., the deposition in the respiratory tract) to emission rate (in terms of mass, surface area, or number of particles)

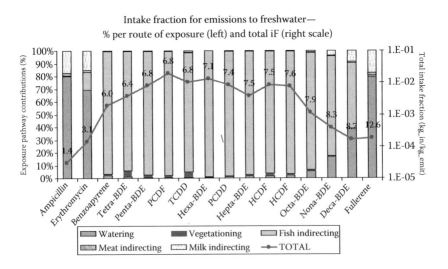

**FIGURE 11.10**
Intake fractions for Buckminster fullerenes compared with organic pollutants. (Adapted from Maddalena, R.L. et al., Hazard assessment and sensitivity analysis for Buckminster fullerene in the environment. *Platform Presentation 681, Proceedings of the SETAC NA 2005 Symposium*, 2005.)

as a function of particulate matter particle size distribution. The modeling used to characterize uptake fraction considers the influence of source-specific particle size distributions, coagulation, differential dry and wet removal mechanisms, population density patterns, and differential deposition in the respiratory tract. Deposition in different zones of the respiratory tract are also defined as a function of particle sizes (Figure 11.11a and b).

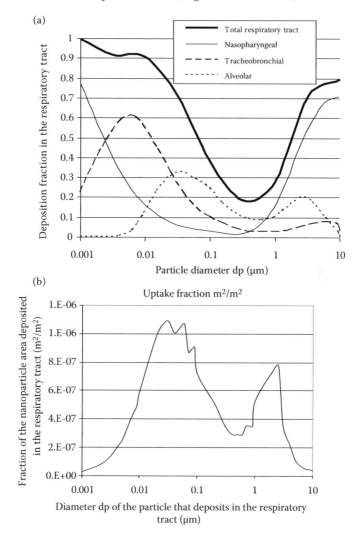

**FIGURE 11.11**
(a) Three zone-specific and total deposition curves in respiratory tract as function of particulate sizes. (Based on Yeh, H.C. et al., *Aerosol Sci. Technol.*, 25, 134, 1996.) (b) Overall uptake fraction accounting for particulate coagulations as determined on surface area basis. (From Humbert, S. Geographically differentiated life-cycle impact assessment of human health. PhD Dissertation. AAT 3402614, 2009.)

### 11.3.3.3 Human Health Dose–Response and Effect Factor

**Dose metrics:** In the absence of specific epidemiological data and with a restricted number of experimental data on the impact of nanoparticle on higher organisms, compared with the large range of different nanoparticles produced, major uncertainties remain regarding their impact on human health.[133] The very same aspects that make these materials so interesting for a vast range of technological applications renders their impact on human health difficult to predict: they may have entirely different behavior compared with the bulk materials they are made from. Oberdörster et al.[134] demonstrated how $TiO_2$, nontoxic in its bulk form, shows toxic effects as a nanoparticle. Choi and Hu[135] studied Ag nanoparticles of different sizes and found that those with diameters <5 nm were more toxic to bacteria not only compared with bulk size Ag but also larger nanoparticular Ag. They also attributed the toxic effects to the generation of reactive oxygen species in cells. Physico–chemical parameters such as size and surface area may be important modifiers of uptake mechanisms, dose, and toxicity (e.g., Wahreit et al.[80] and Roser et al.[136]).

Traditionally, risk and LCA assessments evaluate dose–response relations on the basis of mass concentration or dose, and assess risks by comparing exposure levels to these mass-based doses.[137] Because of the unique properties of some nanometer-scale particles, using mass as the sole basis for determining toxicity has previously resulted in erroneous findings, including equivocal results of toxicological studies on similar materials in different test systems.[138–140] Many of the existing indicators and data are therefore not applicable or representative for their toxicological behavior. Nano-specific metrics such as surface area or particle sizes and number need to be tested and eventually included in dose–response models that currently only account for mass-based exposure.

**Types of endpoints:** On a cellular level, nanoparticles may (i) penetrate cell membranes[141,142]; (ii) penetrate further into mitochondrion and nucleus, potentially inducing toxic effects including DNA damage, oxidative stress, and inflammation on tissue-scale level[143–147]; (iii) cause oxidative damage to cells via promotion of oxyradicals[148]; and (iv) alter the expression of cancer genes[149] and genes involved in cell signaling.[150] Mobility of nanoparticles was observed within higher organisms showing that after inhalation they might be transported via the bloodstream from the lung into other organs such as the heart, brain, or liver where a fraction might be found months after exposure has stopped.[107,141,151,152] Toxic effects such as pulmonary fibrosis and lung tumor formation were observed in rats.[153]

A major issue with many current toxicity studies is the uncertainty about realistic environmental concentrations of nanoparticles. Handy et al.[154] argue that the concentrations applied in the majority of toxicity studies is of unknown environmental relevance. In line with Luoma,[155] the Royal Commission on Environmental Pollution[156] and the European Commission[157] furthermore point out a lack of chronic effects data for nanoparticles, with most studies focusing on acute exposure durations.

Finally, as pointed out by Nowack et al.,[158] most of the tests in laboratory or simulation studies that have been conducted until now are performed on pristine nanomaterials and not on materials from the actual releases from the nanoproducts, which may have different properties due to alterations of transformations occurring during the nanoproduct life cycle.

**Dose–response based on chronic ED50s, NOAEL, and LOAEL:** For a restricted number of well-studied nanoparticles, chronic test on animals are increasingly becoming available (Table 11.11).

For these particles, the approach initially proposed by Crettaz et al.[186] for effect dose of 10% or 50%, its further development by Huijbregts et al.,[187] and its implementation in USEtox,[8] can be used to determine effect factors as follows. Dose–response slopes are based on cancer and noncancer ED50 (effect dose of 50%, which induces a 50% additional risk over background over human lifetime, in kg/lifetime), applying a linear dose–response and effect factor of EF = $0.5/ED_{50h,j}$.

For carcinogenic and noncarcinogenic effects, the $ED_{50h,j}$ adjusted for humans (kg/person/lifetime) is derived from the animal $TD_{50}$ as follows[8]:

$$ED_{50h,j} = \frac{TD_{50a,t,j}\, BW\, LT\, N}{AF_a\, AF_t\, 10^6} \tag{11.4}$$

where $TD_{50a,t,j}$ is the daily dose for animal $a$ (e.g., rat) and time duration $t$ (e.g., subchronic) per kilogram body weight that causes a disease probability of 50% for exposure route $j$ (mg/kg/day); $TD_{50a,t,j}$ is the lowest species-corrected harmonic mean of tumorigenic dose-rate for 50% of animals in a chronic, lifetime cancer test; $AF_a$ is the extrapolation factor for interspecies differences of 4.1 for rats and 11.3 for mice; $AF_t$ is the extrapolation factor for differences in time of exposure, that is, a factor of 2 for subchronic to chronic exposure and a factor of 5 for subacute to chronic exposure[187]; BW is the average body weight of humans (70 kg); LT is the average lifetime of humans (70 years); and N is the number of days per year (365 days/year).

For chemicals with no evidence of carcinogenicity, the $ED_{50}$ can also been estimated from no observed effect level (NOEL) by a NOEL-to-$ED_{50}$ conversion factor of 9. In case only a LOEL is available, a LOEL-to-$ED_{50}$ conversion factor of 2.25 can be applied. New developments for extrapolation of chronic data from acute data are presented leading to a fixed ratio extrapolation of $ED_{50} = LD_{50}/26$, but with a large additional uncertainty characterized by a coefficient of variation of a factor of 46.[8]

**Relating external to internal doses:** Regarding the wide range and size of different nanoparticles produced, it is unrealistic to think that experimental data will become available for each of them, thus the interest to use

**TABLE 11.11**

Existing *In Vivo* Animal Studies on Nanosilver

| NP Size | Exposure Routes | Type of Test | Exposed Animals | Experiment Time | Endpoint Observed | Doses[a] | References |
|---|---|---|---|---|---|---|---|
| 21, 22, 49, 50 nm | Dermal | Subacute | Pig | 14 days | Morphological alterations | 0.34, 3.4, 34 µg/mL | Samberg et al.[159] |
| <100 nm | Dermal | Acute and subchronic | Guinea pigs | 14 days, 13 weeks | Toxicity, biodistribution | 100, 1000, 10,000 µg/mL | Korani et al.[160] |
| 13 nm | Ingestion | Acute | Mice | 4 days | Toxicity, biodistribution, gene expression | 2.5 g | Cha et al.[161] |
| 60 nm | Ingestion | Subchronic | Rats | 29 days | Toxicity, biodistribution, hematology, biochemistry | 30, 300, 1000 mg/kg | Kim et al.[162] |
| 22, 42, 71 nm | Ingestion | Subacute | Mice | 14, 28 days | Toxicity, biodistribution, hematology, biochemistry | 0.25, 0.5, 1 mg/kg | Park et al.[163] |
| 14 nm | Ingestion | Acute and subacute | Rats | 14, 28 days | Toxicity, biodistribution, hematology, biochemistry | 2.25, 4.5, 9 mg/kg bw/day | Hadrup et al.[164] |
| 56 nm | Ingestion | Subchronic | Rats | 91 days | Toxicity, biodistribution, hematology, biochemistry | 30, 125, 500 mg/kg/day | Kim et al.[165] |
| 14 nm | Ingestion | Subchronic | Rats | 29 days | Toxicity, biodistribution | 12.6 mg/kg/day (incl. 1 mg/kg/day of Ag+) | Loeschner et al.[166] |
| 13–15 nm | Inhalation | Subchronic | Rats | 29 days | Toxicity, biodistribution, hematology, biochemistry | 0.5, 3.5, 61 µg/m³ | Ji et al.[167] |
| 22 nm | Inhalation | Subchronic | Mice | 2, 4 weeks | Gene expression, morphology | 4271 µg/m³ | Lee et al.[168] |
| 18–19 nm | Inhalation | Subchronic | Rats | 13 weeks | Toxicity, biodistribution, hematology, biochemistry | 49, 133, 515 µg/m³ | Sung et al.[169,170] |
| 15 nm | Inhalation | Acute | Rats | 6 h, 30 h, 4.25 days, 7.25 days | Biodistribution | 133 µg/m³ | Takenaka et al.[171] |
| 12–15 nm | Inhalation | Subchronic | Rats | 28 days | Nasal respiratory mucosa | 0.5, 3.5, 61 µg/m³ | Hyun et al.[172] |
| 18 nm | Inhalation | Subchronic | Rats | 91 days | Genotoxicity | 49, 133, 515 µg/m³ | Kim et al.[173] |

| Size | Exposure route | Exposure duration | Species | Time points | Endpoint | Dose | Reference |
|---|---|---|---|---|---|---|---|
| 14–15 nm | Inhalation | Subchronic/chronic | Rats | 12, 16, 24 weeks | Toxicity, biodistribution | 49, 117, 381 µg/m³ | Song et al.[174] |
| 5 nm | Inhalation | Subacute | Mice | 12 days, 36 days | Toxicity, dosimetry | 3.3 mg/m³ | Stebounova et al.[175] |
| 18–20 nm | Inhalation | Acute | Rats | 2 weeks | Mortality, pulmonary function | 76, 135, 750 µg/m³ | Sung et al.[176] |
| ca. 60 nm[b] | Intratracheal instillation | Acute | Rats | 6 h | Platelets | 0, 10, 50, 100, 250 µg/mL | Jun et al.[177] |
| NA (aggregate: 244 nm) | Intratracheal instillation | Subacute | Mice | 1, 7, 14, 28 days | Toxicity, genotoxicity | 125, 250, 500 µg/kg | Park et al.[178] |
| 29 nm | I.p. injection | Acute | Mice | 24 h | Gene expression | 100, 500, 1000 mg/kg | Rahman et al.[179] |
| 10–15 nm | I.v. injection | Acute | Mice | 25 min | Hematology, mortality | 0, 4, 6, 8 mg/kg bw | Shrivastava et al.[180] |
| 15–40 nm | I.v. injection | Subchronic | Rats | 32 days | Hematology, biochemistry, biodistribution | 0, 4, 10, 20, 40 mg/kg | Tiwari et al.[181] |
| ca. 50 nm | I.v. injection | Acute | Mice | 4 days | Biodistribution in pregnant mice | 0, 1.2, 2.2 mg Ag/kg | Austin et al.[182] |
| 50–100 nm | S.c. injection | Subacute | Rats | 2, 4, 8, 12, 18, 24 weeks | Accumulation in the brain and blood–brain barrier effects | 62.8 mg/kg | Tang et al.[183] |
| 13 nm | Implantation | Acute | Mice | 13 days (after transfer) | Blastocyst development | 0, 25, 50 µM | Li et al.[184] |
| <100 nm[b] | Implantation | Subchronic/chronic | Rats | 7, 14, 30, 90, 180 days | Local inflammation | NA | Chen et al.[185] |

*Source:* Based on studies published in the scientific literature by April 2012. The studies addressing the use of nanosilver-containing dressings were excluded. A number of studies used the same experiments to investigate different endpoints (e.g., hence same doses).

*Note:* NA, data not available.

[a] Doses are only indicated in mass unit (although not shown here, surface area and number of particle concentrations are also reported in some studies).

[b] Weak or lacking documentation in the reported studies.

physiologically based pharmacokinetic models for two complementary functions: (i) to extrapolate *in vivo* results obtained for a given nanoparticle to particles of the same kind but of different sizes or with different surfaces and (ii) to relate the biological concentration and internal doses tested in *in vitro* experiments and in high-throughput screening toxicity testing to external doses in terms of intake or uptake. Thus far, physiologically based toxicokinetic (PBTK) models have typically been developed for specific individual chemicals, with little attempt to generalize to key physico–chemical properties associated with nanoparticles. However, toxicokinetic data and models are beginning to emerge for nanoparticles, reflecting mechanisms at different scales: Wilhelm et al.[188] and Luciani et al.[189] present a model of endocytosis of negatively charged iron oxide superparamagnetic nanoparticles described as a two-step process: a Langmuir adsorption for the binding of anionic magnetic nanoparticles onto the cell surface followed by a saturable cell internalization mechanism. Semmler et al.[190] provide experimental clearance kinetics of inhaled ultrafine insoluble iridium particles from the rat lung, including transient translocation into secondary organs. Lin et al.[152] provide a first PBTK for quantum dots based on experimentally derived blood-to-tissue distribution ratios. Wenger et al.[191] have shown that the residence time and biodistribution of nanopolymers in the body was directly related to particle size (Figure 11.12).

Since accumulation of nanoparticles in tissues and especially in the liver appears to be linked to macrophage uptake, Li et al.[190] has developed and

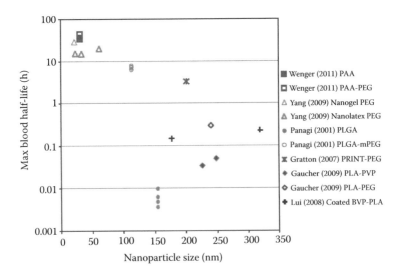

**FIGURE 11.12**

Comparison of maximum half-lives in blood with results of five other experiments on pegylated (empty symbols) and nonpegylated (filled symbols) polymeric nanoparticles. (From Wenger, Y. et al., *Toxicol. Appl. Pharmacol.*, 251, 181, 2011.)

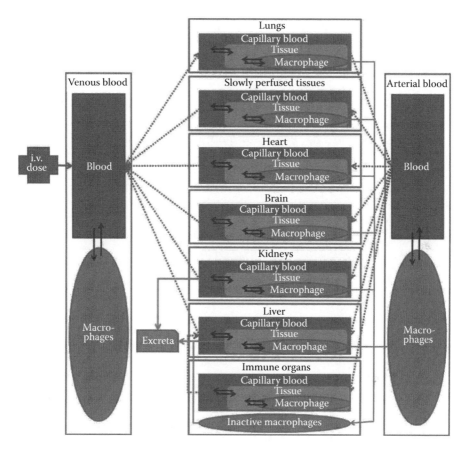

**FIGURE 11.13**
General framework of the PBPK model for nanoparticles. (From Li, D., Emond, C., Johanson, G., Jolliet, O. PBPK modeling of polyacrylamide nanoparticle biodistribution in rats. *International Society of Exposure Science 21st Annual Meeting*, Oct 23–27, 2011, Baltimore, and *Society of Toxicology 51st Annual Meeting*, Mar 11–15, 2012, San Francisco.)

validated an extended PBTK model that embeds macrophage subcompartments within each PBTK model compartment to better reflect biodistribution and capture mechanisms (Figure 11.13). The first results from Li et al.[192] suggest that the uptake rate by macrophages will decrease by up to 20-fold as the size of nanoparticles increases from 30 to 300 nm, while the uptake capacity for mass increases up to 6-fold.

### 11.3.3.4 Ecotoxicological Impacts

Historically, the characterization modeling of freshwater ecotoxicity has used the reciprocal of the predicted no effect concentration (PNEC) as the effect factor. While the conservative nature of the PNEC concept suits the purpose of chemical risk assessment, recent expert workshops[103,193,194] have recommended that the purpose of LCIA is served better with more robust and less conservative effect parameters. For the concentration at which 50% of the species are affected, the $HC_{50}$ was found suitable.[195–199] It is calculated as the geometric mean of all the $EC_{50}$ values of the species measured and shows the potentially affected fraction of species exposed above their chronic $EC_{50}$ value. Using $HC_{50}$ in LCA enables a more robust derivation of freshwater ecotoxicological effect factors because it is less dependent on the species tested than the PNEC or on safety factors.

In keeping with the recommendations to use a more robust effect parameter, an effect-based chronic PAF approach has been retained as best practice for comparative assessment, leading to the adoption of the following definition of freshwater ecotoxicological effect factor (EF) in USEtox:

$$EF = \frac{0.5}{HC50_{EC50}} \tag{11.5}$$

Species selection for calculation of $HC_{50}$ values should in general aim for the highest physiological variability, for as many species as possible, representing as many taxonomic groups as possible. Information on most commonly used nanoparticles and on their basic constituents are becoming available in the literature, the first ecotoxicological tests on common species having been recently made available. For instance, Lovern al.[200] observed a significant acute toxicity in *Daphnia magna* when associated with $TiO_2$ or $C_{60}$-fullerenes. Haasch et al.[201] showed that the toxicity of the latter can be influenced by the solvent used to solubilize it. At this time, exposure data are becoming increasingly available and published.[202,203] It is therefore very likely that it will be feasible to complement the USEtox $HC_{50}$ database of close to 1000 chemicals (merge of five databases[196]) with $HC_{50}$ values for the most commonly studied nanoparticles.

### 11.3.4 Nanospecific Interpretation

**Understanding and quantifying main uncertainties:** In the rapidly evolving nanoproduct field, understanding uncertainties and the limitations in the LCA studies due to missing life cycle stages or impact categories is crucial to properly inform decision making. However, very few of the case studies provide assessment of uncertainties. Moreover, uncertainties in LCA are often focused on the sole inventory, whereas large variations between methods and data also occur in the LCIA step.

It is therefore important for every nano-LCA to provide estimates of uncertainty and variability of results for nanoproducts and to put them in perspective compared with the variability across all chemical substances and to the uncertainty associated with the conventional products. Several methods are available to quantify uncertainty. *Sensitivity studies* can be carried out by, for example, looking at variation in impacts when varying each input variable between its lower and upper confidence limits. This enables the practitioner to identify the most influential parameters for the considered nanoproducts and to help focus data search on the most relevant data. *Uncertainty propagation* can be carried out using more or less transparent and numerically intensive methods. Hong et al.[10] propose a parsimonious Taylor Series expansion approach based on lognormal distributions that apply well to the type of calculations used to assess nanoparticle impacts, with zero-bounded multiplicative factors. It enables the analyst to easily determine the contribution of every parameter to the overall uncertainty. Monte-Carlo approaches can handle a wider range of distributions[204,205] but has often been limited to uncertainty propagation in the sole inventory, thus the need to have uncertainty in impact assessment explicitly defined by LCIA developers, users applying them to nanoproducts, and to have this LCIA uncertainty contribution integrated in the mostly used LCA software.

**Interpreting uncertainty in the nano-LCA context and for sound decision making:** As emphasized by Rosenbaum et al.,[7] uncertainty on chemical characterization factors (their impact per kilogram emitted) is relatively high, within a factor of 100–1000 for human health and 10–100 for freshwater ecotoxicity. Such a precision of 2 to 3 orders of magnitude is, however, significantly lower than the roughly 10 to 12 orders of magnitude variation between the impacts of the different chemicals.

The inventories and impact characterization factors calculated for nanoproducts and nanoemissions must therefore be used in a way that reflects the large variation of 10 orders of magnitude between chemical characterization factors as well as the 3 orders of magnitude uncertainty on the individual factors. This means that contributions of 1%, 5%, or 90% to the total human toxicity score are essentially equal but significantly larger than those of a conventional chemical contributing to less than one per thousand or less than one per million of the total score. In practice, this means that for LCA practitioners, these toxicity factors are very useful to identify the 10 most important toxics pertinent for their nano-applications. The life cycle toxicity scores thus enable the identification of all chemicals contributing more than, for example, one thousandth to the total score. In most applications, this will allow the practitioner to identify whether direct nanoparticle emissions may be relevant compared with the 10 chemicals to look at in priority, and perhaps, more importantly, to disregard 400 other substances whose impacts are not significant for the considered application. For the nanosilver T-shirt, it will be interesting to identify the order of magnitude of impacts related to nanosilver emissions during washing compared with detergent impacts, especially if the number of washing cycle per functional unit is reduced due to the antibacterial effect of nanosilver.

## 11.4 Conclusion

This review of LCA applied to nanoproducts provides several important insights:

- The LCA framework is well suited to study the benefits and impacts of nanotechnologies and nanoproducts since it is a function-based approach that matches the specific functionalities of the considered nanomaterials. These specificities make clear that there is no intrinsic environmental performance of a nanomaterial, but that the life cycle performances need to be assessed in the context of a given nanoproduct.

- In practice up to this point in time, the scope of many LCAs has left out very important issues. Many studies have limited their scopes to mere life cycle energy assessments, and the potential impact assessments have often been constrained to just investigating global warming. These indicators are, however, not sufficient to prevent environmental problem shifting in a decision-making context. In addition, although recent studies indicate that quantitative approaches are being developed, the direct exposure of consumers and workers to nanoparticles during all the nanoproduct life cycle stages have only been addressed qualitatively.

- Contrary to the preconceived idea that nanoproducts is a data-poor environment, compared with other materials and other new chemicals, the field of nanomaterials and nanoproducts is rapidly becoming a data-rich environment. Measurements of direct nanoparticle releases are becoming increasingly available. It is, for example, one of the unique fields in which a large number of subchronic *in vivo* toxicity tests are nowadays performed in multiple laboratories worldwide. This growing realm of data now needs to be used and applied to broaden the scope of LCA to cover most important direct and indirect emissions as well as related impacts.

- The science is ready for providing screening toxicity characterization factors based on *in vivo* no observed adverse effect level (NOAEL) for human health and hazard concentration of 50% ($HC_{50}$ of $EC_{50}$) for the ecosystem impacts of most studied nanoparticle types. Partitioning in the environment and bioconcentration and bioaccumulation in the food chain need to be further studied, especially considering aging and agglomerates of nanoparticles.

- The wide diversity of nanoparticle sizes and types advocates for developing modular approaches that can be then customized to the specific properties, function, and use of the considered nanoproduct. For the inventory side, this advocates for applying the modular approach proposed for the modeling of chemical plants to the main nanomaterial pathways. For impact assessment, it involves the use of physiologically based pharmacokinetic models to interpolate results on well-studied nanoparticles to different sizes and surface transformations.

• Screening factors need to be accompanied by uncertainty estimates, at least for the main multiplicative factors determining both the inventory emissions and the characterization factor. The inventories and impact characterization factors calculated for nanoproducts and nanoemissions must therefore be used in a way that reflects the large variation of 10 orders of magnitude between chemical characterization factors as well as the 3 orders of magnitude uncertainty on the individual factors. It basically enables at this stage to screen whether direct impacts of nanoparticles are negligible, comparable, or larger than indirect impacts linked to, for example, fine particulate emissions linked to energy production.

# References

1. Jolliet, O.; Small, M.J. Integrated Environmental Assessment-Part IV Human Health Risk Assessment. *J. Ind. Ecol.* 2010, 14, 188–191.
2. Shaked, S. and Jolliet, O. Global life cycle impacts of consumer products, In *Encyclopedia of Environmental Health*, Volume 2; Nriagu, J.O., ed.; Elsevier: Burlington, MA, 2011, pp. 1002–1014.
3. International Organization for Standardization ISO 14040 International Standard. In *Environmental Management—Life Cycle Assessment—Principles and Framework*. Geneva, Switzerland, 2006.
4. Frischknecht, R.; Jungbluth, N.; Althaus, H.; Doka, G.; Dones, R.; Heck, T.; Hellweg, S. et al. The EcoInvent database: Overview and methodological framework. *Int. J. Life Cycle Assess.* 2005, 10, 3–9.
5. Jolliet, O.; Margni, M.; Charles, R.; Humbert, S.; Payet, J.; Rebitzer, G.; Rosenbaum, R. IMPACT 2002+: A new life cycle impact assessment methodology. *Int. J. Life Cycle Assess.* 2003, 8, 324–330.
6. Hauschild, M.Z.; Goedkoop, M.; Guinée, J.; Heijungs, R.; Huijbregts, M.; Jolliet, O.; Margni, M. et al. Identifying best existing practice for characterization modelling in life cycle impact assessment. *Int. J. Life Cycle Assess.* 2013, 18, 683–697.
7. Rosenbaum, R.K.; Bachmann, T.M.; Gold, L.S.; Huijbregts, M.A.J.; Jolliet, O.; Juraske, R.; Koehler, A. et al. USEtox—The UNEP-SETAC toxicity model: Recommended characterisation factors for human toxicity and freshwater ecotoxicity in life cycle impact assessment. *Int. J. Life Cycle Assess.* 2008, 13, 532–546.
8. Rosenbaum, R.K.; Huijbregts, M.A.J.; Henderson, A.D.; Margni, M.; McKone, T.E.; van de Meent, D.; Hauschild, M.Z.; Shaked, S.; Li, D.S.; Gold, L.S.; Jolliet, O. USEtox human exposure and toxicity factors for comparative assessment of toxic emissions in life cycle analysis: Sensitivity to key chemical properties. *Int. J. Life Cycle Assess.* 2011, 16, 710–727.

9. Huijbregts, M.A.J.; Norris, G.; Bretz, R.; Ciroth, A.; Maurice, B.; von Bahr, B.; Weidema, B.; de Beaufort, A.S.H. Framework for modelling data uncertainty in life cycle inventories. *Int. J. Life Cycle Assess.* **2001**, *6*, 127–132.

10. Hong, J.; Shaked, S.; Rosenbaum, R.K.; Jolliet, O. Analytical uncertainty propagation in life cycle inventory and impact assessment: Application to an automobile front panel. *Int. J. Life Cycle Assess.* **2010**, *15*, 499–510.

11. Jolliet, O.; Cotting, K.; Drexler, C.; Farago, S. Life-cycle analysis of biodegradable packing materials compared with polystyrene chips: The case of popcorn. *Agric. Ecosyst. Environ.* **1994**, *49*, 253–266.

12. Klöpffer, W.; Curran, M.A.; Frankl, P.; Heijungs, R.; Köhler, A.; Olsen, S.I. *Nanotechnology and Life Cycle Assessment—A Systems Approach to Nanotechnology and the Environment*, Woodrow Wilson International Center for Scholars—Project on Emerging Nanotechnologies, Washington DC, **2007**.

13. International Organization for Standardization ISO 14044 International Standard. In *Environmental Management—Life Cycle Assessment—Requirements and Guidelines*. ISO, Geneva, Switzerland, **2006**.

14. Khanna, V.; Bakshi, B.R.; Lee, L.J. Carbon nanofiber production: Life cycle energy consumption and environmental impact. *J. Ind. Ecol.* **2008**, *12*, 394–410.

15. Khanna, V. and Bakshi, B.R. Carbon nanofiber polymer composites: Evaluation of life cycle energy use. *Environ. Sci. Technol.* **2009**, *43*, 2078–2084.

16. Merugula, L.A.; Khanna, V.; Bakshi, B.R. Comparative life cycle assessment: Reinforcing wind turbine blades with carbon nanofibers. Proceedings of the 2010 *IEEE International Symposium on Sustainable Systems and Technology* (Arlington, VA; 17–19 May 2010). **2010**, 1–6.

17. Healy, M.L.; Dahlben, L.J.; Isaacs, J.A. Environmental assessment of single-walled carbon nanotube processes. *J. Ind. Ecol.* **2008**, *12*, 376–393.

18. Wender, B.A. and Seager, T.P. Towards prospective life cycle assessment: Single wall carbon nanotubes for lithium-ion batteries. *Proceedings of the 2011 IEEE International Symposium on Sustainable Systems and Technology* (Chicago, IL; 16–18 May 2011). **2011**, 1–4.

19. Kushnir, D. and Sanden, B.A. Energy requirements of carbon nanoparticle production. *J. Ind. Ecol.* **2008**, *12*, 360–375.

20. Anctil, A.; Babbitt, C.; Landi, B.; Raffaelle, R.P. Life-cycle assessment of organic solar cell technologies. *Conference Record of the IEEE Photovoltaic Specialists Conference* **2010**, 742–747.

21. Anctil, A.; Babbitt, C.W.; Raffaelle, R.P.; Landi, B.J. Material and energy intensity of fullerene production. *Environ. Sci. Technol.* **2011**, *45*, 2353–2359.

22. Grubb, G.F. and Bakshi, B.R. Life cycle of titanium dioxide nanoparticle production impact of emissions and use of resources. *J. Ind. Ecol.* **2011**, *15*, 81–95.

23. Kuck, A.; Steinfeldt, M.; Prenzel, K.; Swiderek, P.; von Gleich, A.; Thoming, J. Green nanoparticle production using micro reactor technology. *J. Phys. Conf. Ser.* **2011**, *204*, 1–10.

24. Walser, T.; Demou, E.; Lang, D.J.; Hellweg, S. Prospective environmental life cycle assessment of nanosilver T-shirts. *Environ. Sci. Technol.* **2011**, *45*, 4570–4578.

25. Roes, A.L.; Marsili, E.; Nieuwlaar, E.; Patel, M.K. Environmental and cost assessment of a polypropylene nanocomposite. *J. Polym. Environ.* **2007**, *15*, 212–226.

26. Joshi, S. and Joshi, S. Can nanotechnology improve the sustainability of bio-based products? The case of layered silicate biopolymer nanocomposites. *J. Ind. Ecol.* **2008**, *12*, 474–489.

27. Dhingra, R.; Naidu, S.; Upreti, G.; Sawhney, R. Sustainable nanotechnology: Through green methods and life-cycle thinking. *Sustainability (Switzerland)* **2010**, *2*, 182–197.

28. Bauer, C.; Buchgeister, J.; Hischier, R.; Poganietz, W.R.; Schebek, L.; Warsen, J. Towards a framework for life cycle thinking in the assessment of nanotechnology. *J. Clean. Prod.* **2008**, *16*, 910–926.

29. Eckelman, M.J.; Mauter, M.S.; Isaacs, J.A.; Elimelech, M. New perspectives on nanomaterial aquatic ecotoxicity: Production impacts exceed direct exposure impacts for carbon nanotubes. *Environ. Sci. Technol.* **2012**, *46*, 2902–2910.

30. Steinfeldt, M.; Petschow, U.; Haum, R.; von Gleich, A. *Nanotechnology and Sustainability.* Discussion Paper of the IOEW 65/04; Institute for Ecological Economy Research: Berlin, Germany, **2004**.

31. von Gleich, A.; Steinfeldt, M.; Petschow, U. A suggested three-tiered approach to assessing the implications of nanotechnology and influencing its development. *J. Clean. Prod.* **2008**, *16*, 899–909.

32. Singh, A.; Lou, H.H.; Pike, R.W.; Agboola, A.; Li, X.; Hopper, J.R.; Yaws, C.L. Environmental impact assessment for potential continuous processes for the production of carbon nanotubes. *Am. J. Environ. Sci. (USA)* **2008**, *4*, 522–534.

33. Dahlben, L.J. and Isaacs, J.A. Environmental assessment of manufacturing with carbon nanotubes. *IEEE International Symposium on Sustainable Systems and Technologies*, **2009**, 45–49.

34. Steinfeldt, M. Environmental relief effects of nanotechnologies—Factor 10 or only incremental increase of efficiency. *Third International Conference on Eco-Efficiency 2010, 9 June 2010*, Egmond aan Zee, The Netherlands, **2010**.

35. Ganter, M.J.; Seager, T.P.; Schauerman, C.M.; Landi, B.J.; Raffaelle, R.P. A Life-cycle energy analysis of single wall carbon nanotubes produced through laser vaporization. *IEEE International Symposium on Sustainable Systems and Technologies* **2009**, 36–39.

36. Garcia-Valverde, R.; Cherni, J.A.; Urbina, A. Life cycle analysis of organic photovoltaic technologies. *Prog. Photovolt. Res. Appl.* **2010**, *18*, 535–558.

37. Meyer, D.E.; Curran, M.A.; Gonzalez, M.A. An examination of silver nanoparticles in socks using screening-level life cycle assessment. *J. Nanopart. Res.* **2011**, *13*, 147–156.

38. Emmott, C.J.M.; Urbina, A.; Nelson, J. Environmental and economic assessment of ITO-free electrodes for organic solar cells. *Solar Energy Mater. Solar Cells* **2012**, *97*, 14–21.

39. Lloyd, S.M. and Lave, L.B. Life cycle economic and environmental implications of using nanocomposites in automobiles. *Environ. Sci. Technol.* **2003**, *37*, 3458–3466.

40. Roes, A.L.; Tabak, L.B.; Shen, L.; Nieuwlaar, E.; Patel, M.K. Influence of using nanoobjects as filler on functionality-based energy use of nanocomposites. *J. Nanopart. Res.* **2010**, *12*, 2011–2028.

41. Sengul, H. and Theis, T.L. An environmental impact assessment of quantum dot photovoltaics (QDPV) from raw material acquisition through use. *J. Clean. Prod.* **2011**, *19*, 21–31.

42. Kim, H.C. and Fthenakis, V.M. Comparative life-cycle energy payback analysis of multi-junction a-SiGe and nanocrystalline/a-Si modules. *Prog. Photovolt. Res. Appl.* **2011**, *19*, 228–239.

43. Fthenakis, V.; Kim, H.C.; Gualtero, S.; Bourtsalas, A. Nanomaterials in PV manufacture: Some life cycle environmental and health considerations. *Conference Record of the IEEE Photovoltaic Specialists Conference* **2009**, 1068–1073.
44. Roes, A.L.; Alsema, E.A.; Blok, K.; Patel, M.K. Ex-ante environmental and economic evaluation of polymer photovoltaics. *Prog. Photovoltaics* **2009**, *17*, 372–393.
45. Greijer, H.; Karlson, L.; Lindquist, S.; Hagfeldt, A. Environmental aspects of electricity generation from a nanocrystalline dye sensitized solar cell system. *Renew. Energy* **2001**, *23*, 27–39.
46. Osterwalder, N.; Capello, C.; Hungerbohler, K.; Stark, W.J. Energy consumption during nanoparticle production: How economic is dry synthesis? *J. Nanopart. Res.* **2006**, *8*, 1–9.
47. Espinosa, N.; Garcia-Valverde, R.; Krebs, F.C. Life-cycle analysis of product integrated polymer solar cells. *Energy Environ. Sci.* **2011**, *4*, 1547–1557.
48. Espinosa, N.; Garcia-Valverde, R.; Urbina, A.; Krebs, F.C. A life cycle analysis of polymer solar cell modules prepared using roll-to-roll methods under ambient conditions. *Solar Energy Mater. Solar Cells* **2011**, *95*, 1293–1302.
49. Lloyd, S.M.; Lave, L.B.; Matthews, H.S. Life cycle benefits of using nanotechnology to stabilize platinum-group metal particles in automotive catalysts. *Environ. Sci. Technol.* **2005**, *39*, 1384–1392.
50. Moign, A.; Vardelle, A.; Themelis, N.J.; Legoux, J.G. Life cycle assessment of using powder and liquid precursors in plasma spraying: The case of yttria-stabilized zirconia. *Surf. Coat. Technol.* **2010**, *205*, 668–673.
51. Krishnan, N.; Boyd, S.; Dornfeld, D.; Somani, A.; Raoux, S.; Clark, D. A hybrid life cycle inventory of nano-scale semiconductor manufacturing. *Environ. Sci. Technol.* **2008**, *42*, 3069–3075.
52. Wen, D. Nanofuel as a potential secondary energy carrier. *Energy Environ. Sci.* **2010**, *3*, 591–600.
53. Meyer, D.E.; Curran, M.A.; Gonzalez, M.A. An examination of existing data for the industrial manufacture and use of nanocomponents and their role in the life cycle impact of nanoproducts. *Environ. Sci. Technol.* **2009**, *43*, 1256–1263.
54. Gavankar, S.; Suh, S.; Keller, A.F. Life cycle assessment at nanoscale: Review and recommendations. *Int. J. Life Cycle Assess.* **2012**, *17*, 295–303.
55. Steinfeldt, M. A method of prospective technological assessment of nanotechnological techniques, In *Towards Life Cycle Sustainability Management*; Finkbeiner, M., ed.; Springer: The Netherlands, **2011**, pp. 131–140.
56. Upadhyayula, V.K.K.; Meyer, D.E.; Curran, M.A.; Gonzalez, M.A. Life cycle assessment as a tool to enhance the environmental performance of carbon nanotube products: A review. *J. Clean. Prod.* **2012**, *26*, 37–47.
57. Olsen, S.I. and Miseljic, M. Assessing potential nanoparticle release during nanocomposite shredding using direct-reading instruments, In *Symposium "Safety Issues of Nanomaterials Along Their Life Cycle," May 4–5, 2011*, Barcelona, Spain, **2011**.
58. Hischier, R. and Walser, T. Life cycle assessment of engineered nanomaterials: State of the art and strategies to overcome existing gaps. *Sci. Total Environ.* **2012**, *425*, 271–282.
59. Hauschild, M.Z.; Huijbregts, M.; Jolliet, O.; Macleod, M.; Margni, M.; Rosenbaum, R.K.; van de Meent, D.; McKone, T.E. Building a model based on scientific consensus for life cycle impact assessment of chemicals: The search for harmony and parsimony. *Environ. Sci. Technol.* **2008**, *42*, 7032–7037.

60. Dreyer, L.; Hauschild, M.; Schierbeck, J. A framework for social life cycle impact assessment. *Int. J. Life Cycle Assess.* **2006**, *11*, 88.
61. Pant, R.; Van Hoof, G.; Schowanek, D.; Feijtel, T.C.J.; de Koning, A.; Hauschild, M.; Pennington, D.W.; Olsen, S.I.; Rosenbaum, R. Comparison between three different LCIA methods for aquatic ecotoxicity and a product environmental risk assessment—Insights from a detergent case study within OMNIITOX. *Int. J. Life Cycle Assess.* **2004**, *9*, 295–306.
62. Pizzol, M.; Christensen, P.; Schmidt, J.; Thomsen, M. Impacts of metals on human health: A comparison between nine different methodologies for Life Cycle Impact Assessment (LCIA). *J. Clean. Prod.* **2011**, *19*, 646–656.
63. Pizzol, M.; Christensen, P.; Schmidt, J.; Thomsen, M. Eco-toxicological impact of metals on the aquatic and terrestrial ecosystem: a comparison between eight different methodologies for Life Cycle Impact Assessment (LCIA). *J. Clean. Prod.* **2011**, *19*, 687–698.
64. Huijbregts, M.A.J.; Rombouts, L.J.A.; Hellweg, S.; Frischknecht, R.; Hendriks, A.J.; Van, d.M.; Ragas, A.M.J.; Reijnders, L.; Struijs, J. Is cumulative fossil energy demand a useful indicator for the environmental performance of products? *Environ. Sci. Technol.* **2006**, *40*, 641–648.
65. Huijbregts, M.A.J.; Hellweg, S.; Frischknecht, R.; Hendriks, H.W.M.; Hungerbuhler, K.; Hendriks, A.J. Cumulative energy demand as predictor for the environmental burden of commodity production. *Environ. Sci. Technol.* **2010**, *44*, 2189–2196.
66. Laurent, A.; Olsen, S.I.; Hauschild, M.Z. Limitations of carbon footprint as indicator of environmental sustainability. *Environ. Sci. Technol.* **2012**, *46*, 4100–4108.
67. Maynard, A.D. and Aitken, R.J. Assessing exposure to airborne nanomaterials: Current abilities and future requirements. *Nanotoxicology* **2007**, *1*, 26–41.
68. Stone, V.; Hankin, S.; Aitken, R.; Aschberger, K.; Baun, A.; Christensen, F.; Fernandes, T. et al. *Engineered Nanoparticles: Review of Health and Environmental Safety (ENRHES)*. Available at http://ihcp.jrc.ec.europa.eu/whats-new/enhres-final-report, **2010**.
69. MINChar Physicochemical Parameters List. *Recommended Minimum Physical and Chemical Parameters for Characterizing Nanomaterials on Toxicology Studies*. Woodrow Wilson International Center for Scholars: Washington, DC, **2008**.
70. Landsiedel, R.; Ma-Hock, L.; Kroll, A.; Hahn, D.; Schnekenburger, J.; Wiench, K.; Wohlleben, W. Testing metal-oxide nanomaterials for human safety. *Adv. Mater.* **2010**, *22*, 2601–2627.
71. Oberdörster, G. Safety assessment for nanotechnology and nanomedicine: Concepts of nanotoxicology. *J. Intern. Med.* **2010**, *267*, 89–105.
72. Köhler, A.R.; Som, C.; Helland, A.; Gottschalk, F. Studying the potential release of carbon nanotubes throughout the application life cycle. *J. Clean. Prod.* **2008**, *16*, 927–937.
73. SCENIHR (Scientific Committee on Emerging and Newly Identified Health Risks). *Risk Assessment of Products of Nanotechnologies*. Available from: http://ec.europa.eu/health/ph_risk/committees/04_scenihr/docs/scenihr_o_023.pdf;European Commission Health and Consumer Protection Directorate-General, Directorate C—Public Health and Risk Assessment. Brussels, Belgium, **2009**.
74. Gottschalk, F. and Nowack, B. The release of engineered nanomaterials to the environment. *J. Environ. Monit.* **2011**, *13*, 1145–1155.

75. Brouwer, D. Exposure to manufactured nanoparticles in different workplaces. *Toxicology* **2010**, *269*, 120–127.
76. Kuhlbusch, T.A.J.; Asbach, C.; Fissan, H.; Gohler, D.; Stintz, M. Nanoparticle exposure at nanotechnology workplaces: A review. *Part. Fibre Toxicol.* **2011**, *8*, 22–39.
77. Kaegi, R.; Ulrich, A.; Sinnet, B.; Vonbank, R.; Wichser, A.; Zuleeg, S.; Simmler, H. et al. Synthetic TiO$_2$ nanoparticle emission from exterior facades into the aquatic environment. *Environ. Pollut.* **2008**, *156*, 233–239.
78. Fleury, D.; Bomfim, J.A.S.; Vignes, A.; Girard, C.; Metz, S.; Munoz, F.; R'Mili, B.; Ustache, A.; Guiot, A.; Bouillard, J.X. Identification of the main exposure scenarios in the production of CNT-polymer nanocomposites by melt-moulding process. *J. Clean. Prod.* **2011**, 1–15.
79. Raynor, P.C.; Cebula, J.I.; Spangenberger, J.S.; Olson, B.A.; Dasch, J.M.; D'Arcy, J.B. Assessing potential nanoparticle release during nanocomposite shredding using direct-reading instruments. *J. Occup. Environ. Hyg.* **2012**, *9*, 1–13.
80. Warheit, D.B.; Webb, T.R.; Reed, K.L.; Frerichs, S.; Sayes, C.M. Pulmonary toxicity study in rats with three forms of ultrafine-TiO$_2$ particles: Differential responses related to surface properties. *Toxicology* **2007**, *230*, 90–104.
81. Boxall, A.B.A.; Chaudhry, Q.; Sinclair, C.; Jones, A.D.; Aitken, R.; Jefferson, B.; Watts, C. Current and future predicted environmental exposure to engineered nanoparticles. Central Science Laboratory: Sand Hutton, UK, **2007**.
82. Blaser, S.A.; Scheringer, M.; MacLeod, M.; Hungerbuhler, K. Estimation of cumulative aquatic exposure and risk due to silver: Contribution of nano-functionalized plastics and textiles. *Sci. Total Environ.* **2008**, *390*, 396–409.
83. Park, B.; Donaldson, K.; Duffin, R.; Tran, L.; Kelly, F.; Mudway, I.; Morin, J. et al. Hazard and risk assessment of a nanoparticulate cerium oxide-based diesel fuel additive—A case study. *Inhal. Toxicol.* **2008**, *20*, 547–566.
84. Mueller, N.C. and Nowack, B. Exposure modeling of engineered nanoparticles in the environment. *Environ. Sci. Technol.* **2008**, *42*, 4447–4453.
85. O'Brien, N. and Cummins, E. Nano-scale pollutants: Fate in Irish surface and drinking water regulatory systems. *Hum. Ecol. Risk Assess.* **2010**, *16*, 847–872.
86. Gottschalk, F.; Sonderer, T.; Scholz, R.W.; Nowack, B. Modeled environmental concentrations of engineered nanomaterials (TiO$_2$, ZnO, Ag, CNT, fullerenes) for different regions. *Environ. Sci. Technol.* **2009**, *43*, 9216–9222.
87. Gottschalk, F.; Sonderer, T.; Scholz, R.W.; Nowack, B. Possibilities and limitations of modeling environmental exposure to engineered nanomaterials by probabilistic material flow analysis. *Environ. Toxicol. Chem.* **2010**, *29*, 1036–1048.
88. Arvidsson, R.; Molander, S.; Sanden, B.A.; Hassellov, M. Challenges in exposure modeling of nanoparticles in aquatic environments. *Hum. Ecol. Risk Assess.* **2011**, *17*, 245–262.
89. Hansen, S.F.; Michelson, E.S.; Kamper, A.; Borling, P.; Stuer-Lauridsen, F.; Baun, A. Categorization framework to aid exposure assessment of nanomaterials in consumer products. *Ecotoxicology* **2008**, *17*, 438–447.
90. Kohler, A.R.; Som, C.; Helland, A.; Gottschalk, F. Studying the potential release of carbon nanotubes throughout the application life cycle. *J. Clean. Prod.* **2008**, *16*, 927–937.
91. Jimenez-Gonzalez, C.; Kim, S.; Overcash, M.R. Methodology for developing gate-to-gate life cycle inventory information. *Int. J. Life Cycle Assess.* **2000**, *5*, 153–160.

92. Ponder, C. and Overcash, M. Cradle-to-gate life cycle inventory of vancomycin hydrochloride. *Sci. Total Environ.* **2010**, *408*, 1331–1337.
93. Vorbau, M.; Hillemann, L.; Stintz, M. Method for the characterization of the abrasion induced nanoparticle release into air from surface coatings. *J. Aerosol Sci.* **2009**, *40*, 209–217.
94. Koponen, I.K.; Jensen, K.A.; Schneider, T. Comparison of dust released from sanding conventional and nanoparticle-doped wall and wood coatings. *J. Expo. Sci. Environ. Epidemiol.* **2011**, *21*, 408–418.
95. Benn, T.M. and Westerhoff, P. Nanoparticle silver released into water from commercially available sock fabrics. *Environ. Sci. Technol.* **2008**, *42*, 4133–4139.
96. Abbott, L.C. and Maynard, A.D. Exposure assessment approaches for engineered nanomaterials. *Risk Anal.* **2010**, *30*, 1634–1644.
97. Musee, N. Nanotechnology risk assessment from a waste management perspective: Are the current tools adequate? *Hum. Exp. Toxicol.* **2011**, *30*, 820–835.
98. Olapiriyakul, S. and Caudill, R.J. Thermodynamic analysis to assess the environmental impact of end-of-life recovery processing for nanotechnology products. *Environ. Sci. Technol.* **2009**, *43*, 8140–8146.
99. Chang, M.R.; Lee, D.J.; Lai, J.Y. Nanoparticles in wastewater from a science-based industrial park—Coagulation using polyaluminum chloride. *J. Environ. Manage.* **2007**, *85*, 1009–1014.
100. Jolliet, O.; Muller-Wenk, R.; Bare, J.; Brent, A.; Goedkoop, M.; Heijungs, R.; Itsubo, N. et al. The LCIA midpoint-damage framework of the UNEP/SETAC life cycle initiative. *Int. J. Life Cycle Assess.* **2004**, *9*, 394–404.
101. Bare, J.C.; Bare, J.C.; Norris, G.A.; Pennington, D.W.; McKone, T. TRACI: The tool for the reduction and assessment of chemical and other environmental impacts. *J. Ind. Ecol.* **2003**, *6*, 49–78.
102. Goedkoop, M.; Heijungs, R.; Huijbregts, M.A.J.; De Schryver, A.; Struijs, J.; van Zelm, R. *ReCiPe 2008. A Life Cycle Impact Assessment Method which Comprises Harmonised Category Indicators at the Midpoint and the Endpoint Level.* First edition; Ministry of Housing, Spatial Planning and the Environment, The Netherlands, **2009**.
103. Bulle, C.; Jolliet, O.; Humbert, S.; Rosenbaum, R.; Margni, M. IMPACT World +: A new global regionalized life cycle impact assessment method. Proceedings of the International Conference on Ecobalance, P-111, Yokohama, Japan, November **2012**.
104. Jolliet, O.; Rosenbaum, R.; Chapmann, P.M.; McKone, T.; Margni, M.; Scheringer, M.; van Straalen, N.; Wania, F. Establishing a framework for life cycle toxicity assessment: Findings of the Lausanne review workshop. *Int. J. Life Cycle Assess.* **2006**, *11*, 137–140.
105. Henderson, A.; Hauschild, M.Z.; Van de Meent, D.; Huijbregts, M.A.J.; Larsen, H.F.; Margni, M.; McKone, T.E.; Payet, J.; Rosenbaum, R.K.; Jolliet, O. USEtox fate and ecotoxicity factors for comparative assessment of toxic emissions in LCA. *Int. J. Life Cycle Assess.* **2011**, *16*, 701–709.
106. Oberdörster, G.; Oberdörster, E.; Oberdöster, J. Nanotoxicology: An emerging discipline evolving from studies of ultrafine particles. *Environ. Health Perspect.* **2005**, *113*, 823–839.
107. Nel, A.; Xia, T.; Mädler, L.; Li, N. Toxic potential of materials at the nanolevel. *Science* **2006**, *311*, 622–627.

108. Abraham, M.H.; Green, C.E.; Acree Jr., W.E. Correlation and prediction of the solubility of Buckminster-fullerene in organic solvents; estimation of some physicochemical properties. *J. Chem. Soc. Perkin Trans.* **2000**, *2*, 281–286.
109. Maddalena, R.L.; MacLeod, M.J.; McKone, T.E. and Sohn, M.D. Hazard assessment and sensitivity analysis for Buckminster fullerene in the environment. *Platform Presentation 681, Proceedings of the SETAC NA 2005 Symposium,* **2005**.
110. Nowack, B. and Bucheli, T.D. Occurrence, behavior and effects of nanoparticles in the environment. *Environ. Pollut.* **2007**, *150*, 5–22.
111. Baalousha, M.; Manciulea, A.; Cumberland, S.; Kendall, K.; Lead, J.R. Aggregation and surface properties of iron oxide nanoparticles: Influence of pH and natural organic matter. *Environ. Toxicol. Chem.* **2008**, *27*, 1875–1882.
112. Diegoli, S.; Manciulea, A.L.; Begum, S.; Jones, I.P.; Lead, J.R.; Preece, J.A. Interaction between manufactured gold nanoparticles and naturally occurring organic macromolecules. *Sci. Total Environ.* **2008**, *402*, 51–61.
113. Hyung, H.; Fortner, J.D.; Hughes, J.B.; Kim, J. Natural organic matter stabilizes carbon nanotubes in the aqueous phase. *Environ. Sci. Technol.* **2007**, *41*, 179–184.
114. Hyung, H. and Kim, J. Natural organic matter (NOM) adsorption to multiwalled carbon nanotubes: Effect of NOM characteristics and water quality parameters. *Environ. Sci. Technol.* **2008**, *42*, 4416–4421.
115. Chen, K.L. and Elimelech, M. Influence of humic acid on the aggregation kinetics of fullerene (C60) nanoparticles in monovalent and divalent electrolyte solutions. *J. Colloid Interface Sci.* **2007**, *309*, 126–134.
116. Labille, J.; Brant, J.; Villieras, F.; Pelletier, M.; Thill, A.; Masion, A.; Wiesner, M; Rose, J.; Bottero, J.Y. Affinity of C60 fullerenes with water. *Fuller. Nanotub. Carbon Nanostruct. (USA)* **2006**, *14*, 307–314.
117. Ju-Nam, Y. and Lead, J.R. Manufactured nanoparticles: An overview of their chemistry, interactions and potential environmental implications. *Sci. Total Environ.* **2008**, *400*, 396–414.
118. Kretzschmar, R.; Borkovec, M.; Grolimund, D.; Elimelech, M. Mobile subsurface colloids and their role in contaminant transport. *Adv. Agron.* **1999**, *66*, 121–194.
119. Ryan, J.N. and Elimelech, M. Colloid mobilization and transport in groundwater. *Colloids Surf. A Physicochem. Eng. Asp.* **1996**, *107*, 1–56.
120. Franchi, A. and O'Melia, C.R. Effects of natural organic matter and solution chemistry on the deposition and reentrainment of colloids in porous media. *Environ. Sci. Technol.* **2003**, *37*, 1122–1129.
121. Espinasse, B.; Hotze, E.M.; Wiesner, M.R. Transport and retention of colloidal aggregates of C-60 in porous media: Effects of organic macromolecules, ionic composition, and preparation method. *Environ. Sci. Technol.* **2007**, *41*, 7396–7402.
122. Lecoanet, H.F.; Bottero, J.; Wiesner, M.R. Laboratory assessment of the mobility of nanomaterials in porous media. *Environ. Sci. Technol.* **2004**, *38*, 5164–5169.
123. Zhu, H.; Han, J.; Xiao, J.Q.; Jin, Y. Uptake, translocation, and accumulation of manufactured iron oxide nanoparticles by pumpkin plants. *J. Environ. Monit.* **2008**, *10*, 713–717.
124. Bennett, D.H.; McKone, T.E.; Evans, J.S.; Nazaroff, W.W.; Margni, M.D.; Jolliet, O.; Smith, K.R. Defining intake fraction. *Environ. Sci. Technol.* **2002**, *36*, 206A–211A.
125. Evans, J.S.; Wolff, S.K.; Phonboon, K.; Levy, J.I.; Smith, K.R. Exposure efficiency: An idea whose time has come? *Chemosphere* **2002**, *49*, 1075–1091.

126. Levy, J.I.; Wilson, A.M.; Evans, J.S.; Spengler, J.D. Estimation of primary and secondary particulate matter intake fractions for power plants in Georgia. *Environ. Sci. Technol.* **2003**, *37*, 5528–5536.

127. Pennington, D.W.; Margni, M.; Ammann, C.; Jolliet, O. Multimedia fate and human intake modeling: spatial versus nonspatial insights for chemical emissions in Western Europe. *Environ. Sci. Technol.* **2005**, *39*, 1119–1128.

128. Rosenbaum, R.K.; McKone, T.E.; Jolliet, O. CKow: A dynamic model for chemical transfer to meat and milk. *Environ. Sci. Technol.* **2009**, *43*, 8191–8198.

129. Oberdorster, E. Manufactured nanomaterials (fullerenes, C60) induce oxidative stress in the brain of juvenile largemouth bass. *Environ. Health Perspect.* **2004**, *112*, 1058–1062.

130. Wenger, Y.; Li, D.S.; Jolliet, O. Indoor intake fraction considering surface sorption of air organic compounds for life cycle assessment. *Int. J. Life Cycle Assess.* **2012**, *17*, 919–931.

131. Humbert, S. Geographically differentiated life-cycle impact assessment of human health. PhD Dissertation. AAT, University of Berkeley, CA, 3402614, **2009**.

132. Yeh, H.C.; Cuddihy, R.G.; Phalen, R.F.; Chang, I.Y. Comparisons of calculated respiratory tract deposition of particles based on the proposed NCRP model and the new model. *Aerosol Sci. Technol.* **1996**, *25*, 134–140.

133. Hoet, P. and Boczkowski, J. What's new in nanotoxicology? Brief review of the 2007 literature. *Nanotoxicology* **2008**, *2*, 171–182.

134. Oberdörster, G.; Maynard, A.; Donaldson, K.; Castranova, V.; Fitzpatrick, J.; Ausman, K.; Carter, J. et al. Principles for characterizing the potential human health effects from exposure to nanomaterials: Elements of a screening strategy. *Part. Fibre Toxicol.* **2005**, *2*, 8.

135. Choi, O. and Hu, Z. Size dependent and reactive oxygen species related nanosilver toxicity to nitrifying bacteria. *Environ. Sci. Technol.* **2008**, *42*, 4583–4588.

136. Roser, M.; Fischer, D.; Kissel, T. Surface-modified biodegradable albumin nano- and microspheres. II: Effect of surface charges on *in vitro* phagocytosis and biodistribution in rats. *Eur. J. Pharm. Biopharm.* **1998**, *46*, 255–263.

137. US Environmental Protection Agency Guidelines for Carcinogen Risk Assessment. *EPA/630/P-03/001B*, US EPA: Washington, DC, **2005**.

138. Aggarwal, P.; Hall, J.B.; McLeland, C.B.; Dobrovolskaia, M.A.; McNeil, S.E. Nanoparticle interaction with plasma proteins as it relates to particle biodistribution, biocompatibility and therapeutic efficacy. *Adv. Drug Deliv. Rev.* **2009**, *61*, 428–437.

139. Brown, D.M.; Wilson, M.R.; MacNee, W.; Stone, V.; Donaldson, K. Size-dependent proinflammatory effects of ultrafine polystyrene particles: A role for surface area and oxidative stress in the enhanced activity of ultrafines. *Toxicol. Appl. Pharmacol.* **2001**, *175*, 191–199.

140. Zhu, M.; Feng, W.; Wang, Y.; Wang, B.; Wang, M.; Ouyang, H.; Zhao, Y.; Chai, Z. Particokinetics and extrapulmonary translocation of intratracheally instilled ferric oxide nanoparticles in rats and the potential health risk assessment. *Toxicol. Sci.* **2009**, *107*, 342–351.

141. Unfried, K.; Albrecht, C.; Klotz, L.; Von Mikecz, A.; Grether-Beck, S.; Schins, R.P.F. Cellular responses to nanoparticles: Target structures and mechanisms. *Nanotoxicology* **2007**, *1*, 52–71.

142. Geiser, M.; Rothen-Rutishauser, B.; Kapp, N.; Schuerch, S.; Kreyling, W.; Schulz, H.; Semmler, M.; Hof, V.I.; Heyder, J.; Gehr, P. Ultrafine particles cross cellular membranes by nonphagocytic mechanisms in lungs and in cultured cells. *Environ. Health Perspect.* **2005**, *113*, 1555–1560.

143. AshaRani, P.V.; Valiyaveettil, S.; AshaRani, P.V.; Mun, G.L.K.; Hande, M.P. Cytotoxicity and genotoxicity of silver nanoparticles in human cells. *ACS Nano* **2009**, *3*, 279–290.

144. Ahamed, M.; Karns, M.; Goodson, M.; Rowe, J.; Hussain, S.M.; Schlager, J.J.; Hong, Y. DNA damage response to different surface chemistry of silver nanoparticles in mammalian cells. *Toxicol. Appl. Pharmacol.* **2008**, *233*, 404–410.

145. Yang, H.; Liu, C.; Yang, D.; Zhang, H.; Xi, Z. Comparative study of cytotoxicity, oxidative stress and genotoxicity induced by four typical nanomaterials: The role of particle size, shape and composition. *J. Appl. Toxicol.* **2009**, *29*, 69–78.

146. Xu, A.; Chai, Y.; Nohmi, T.; Hei, T.K. Genotoxic responses to titanium dioxide nanoparticles and fullerene in gpt delta transgenic MEF cells. *Part. Fibre Toxicol.* **2009**, *6*, 3.

147. Raun Jacobsen, N.; Møller, P.; Alstrup Jensen, K.; Vogel, U.B.; Ladefoged, O.; Loft, S.; Wallin, H.; Division of Toxicology and Risk Assessment, National Food Institute, Technical University of Denmark. Lung inflammation and genotoxicity following pulmonary exposure to nanoparticles in ApoE$^{-/-}$ mice. *Part. Fibre Toxicol.* **2009**, *6*, 2.

148. Xia, T.; Kovochich, M.; Brant, J.; Hotze, M.; Sempf, J.; Oberley, T.; Sioutas, C.; Yeh, J.I.; Wiesner, M.R.; Nel, A.E. Comparison of the abilities of ambient and manufactured nanoparticles to induce cellular toxicity according to an oxidative stress paradigm. *Nano Lett. (USA)* **2006**, *6*, 1794–1807.

149. Omidi, Y.; Hollins, A.J.; Benboubetra, M.; Drayton, R.; Benter, I.F.; Akhtar, S. Toxicogenomics of non-viral vectors for gene therapy: A microarray study of lipofectin- and oligofectamine-induced gene expression changes in human epithelial cells. *J. Drug Target.* **2003**, *11*, 311–323.

150. Regnstrom, K.; Ragnarsson, E.G.E.; Fryknas, M.; Koping-Hoggard, M.; Artursson, P. Gene expression profiles in mouse lung tissue after administration of two cationic polymers used for nonviral gene delivery. *Pharm. Res.* **2006**, *23*, 475–482.

151. Kreyling, W.G.; Semmler-Behnke, M.; Möller, W. Health implications of nanoparticles. *J. Nanopart. Res.* **2006**, *8*, 543–562.

152. Lin, P.; Chen, J.; Chang, L.W.; Wu, J.; Redding, L.; Chang, H.; Yeh, T. et al. Computational and ultrastructural toxicology of a nanoparticle, Quantum Dot 705, in mice. *Environ. Sci. Technol.* **2008**, *42*, 6264–6270.

153. Wang, J.J.; Sanderson, B.J.S.; Wang, H. Cyto- and genotoxicity of ultrafine TiO$_2$ particles in cultured human lymphoblastoid cells. *Mutat. Res.* **2007**, *628*, 99–106.

154. Handy, R.D.; Owen, R.; Valsami-Jones, E. The ecotoxicology of nanoparticles and nanomaterials: Current status, knowledge gaps, challenges, and future needs. *Ecotoxicology* **2008**, *17*, 315–325.

155. Luoma, S.N. *Silver Nanotechnologies in the Environment: Old Problem or New Challenge?* The Pew Charitable Trusts, Project on emerging nanotechnologies, Washington DC, **2008**.

156. Royal Commission on Environmental Pollution. *Novel Materials in the Environment: The Case of Nanotechnology*; Office of Public Sector Information, **2008**, p. 146.

157. European Commission. *Towards a European Strategy for Nanotechnology*; European Commission: Brussels, Belgium, **2004**.

158. Nowack, B.; Ranville, J.F.; Diamond, S.; Gallego-Urrea, J.; Metcalfe, C.; Rose, J.; Horne, N.; Koelmans, A.A.; Klaine, S.J. Potential scenarios for nanomaterial release and subsequent alteration in the environment. *Environ. Toxicol. Chem.* **2012**, *31*, 50–59.

159. Samberg, M.E.; Oldenburg, S.J.; Monteiro-Riviere, N. Evaluation of silver nanoparticle toxicity in skin *in vivo* and keratinocytes in vitro. *Environ. Health Perspect.* **2010**, *118*, 407–413.

160. Korani, M.; Rezayat, S.M.; Gilani, K.; Arbabi Bidgoli, S.; Adeli, S. Acute and subchronic dermal toxicity of nanosilver in guinea pig. *Int. J. Nanomed.* **2011**, *6*, 855–862.

161. Cha, K.; Hong, H.; Choi, Y.; Lee, M.J.; Park, J.H.; Chae, H.; Ryu, G.; Myung, H. Comparison of acute responses of mice livers to short-term exposure to nano-sized or micro-sized silver particles. *Biotechnol. Lett.* **2008**, *30*, 1893–1899.

162. Kim, Y.S.; Kim, J.S.; Cho, H.S.; Rha, D.S.; Kim, J.M.; Park, J.D.; Choi, B.S. et al. Twenty-eight-day oral toxicity, genotoxicity, and gender-related tissue distribution of silver nanoparticles in Sprague–Dawley rats. *Inhal. Toxicol.* **2008**, *20*, 575–583.

163. Park, E.; Bae, E.; Yi, J.; Kim, Y.; Choi, K.; Lee, S.H.; Yoon, J.; Lee, B.C.; Park, K. Repeated-dose toxicity and inflammatory responses in mice by oral administration of silver nanoparticles. *Environ. Toxicol. Pharmacol.* **2010**, *30*, 162–168.

164. Hadrup, N.; Loeschner, K.; Bergstrom, A.; Wilcks, A.; Gao, X.; Vogel, U.; Frandsen, H.L.; Larsen, E.H.; Lam, H.R.; Mortensen, A. Subacute oral toxicity investigation of nanoparticulate and ionic silver in rats. *Arch. Toxicol.* **2012**, *86*, 543–551.

165. Kim, Y.S.; Song, M.Y.; Park, J.D.; Song, K.S.; Ryu, H.R.; Chung, Y.H.; Chang, H.K. et al. Subchronic oral toxicity of silver nanoparticles. *Part. Fibre Toxicol.* **2010**, *7*, 20.

166. Loeschner, K.; Hadrup, N.; Qvortrup, K.; Larsen, A.; Gao, X.; Vogel, U.; Mortensen, A. et al. Distribution of silver in rats following 28 days of repeated oral exposure to silver nanoparticles or silver acetate. *Part. Fibre Toxicol.* **2011**, *8*, 18.

167. Ji, J.H.; Jung, J.H.; Kim, S.S. Twenty-eight-day inhalation toxicity study of silver nanoparticles in Sprague–Dawley rats. *Inhal. Toxicol.* **2007**, *19*, 857–871.

168. Lee, H.; Choi, Y.; Jung, E.; Yin, H.; Kwon, J.; Kim, J.; Im, H. et al. Genomics-based screening of differentially expressed genes in the brains of mice exposed to silver nanoparticles via inhalation. *J. Nanopart. Res.* **2010**, *12*, 1567–1578.

169. Sung, J.H.; Ji, J.H.; Yoon, J.U.; Kim, D.S.; Song, M.Y.; Jeong, J.; Han, B.S. et al. Lung function changes in Sprague–Dawley rats after prolonged inhalation exposure to silver nanoparticles. *Inhal. Toxicol.* **2008**, *20*, 567–574.

170. Sung, J.H.; Ji, J.H.; Park, J.D.; Yoon, J.U.; Kim, D.S.; Jeon, K.S.; Song, M.Y. et al. Subchronic inhalation toxicity of silver nanoparticles. *Toxicol. Sci.* **2009**, *108*, 452–461.

171. Takenaka, S.; Karg, E.; Roth, C.; Schulz, H.; Ziesenis, A.; Heinzmann, U.; Schramel, P.; Heyder, J. Pulmonary and systemic distribution of inhaled ultrafine silver particles in rats. *Environ. Health Perspect.* **2001**, *109*, 547–551.

172. Hyun, J.; Lee, B.S.; Ryu, H.Y.; Sung, J.H.; Chung, K.H.; Yu, I.J. Effects of repeated silver nanoparticles exposure on the histological structure and mucins of nasal respiratory mucosa in rats. *Toxicol. Lett.* **2008**, *182*, 24–28.

173. Kim, H.R.; Kim, M.J.; Lee, S.Y.; Oh, S.M.; Chung, K.H. Genotoxic effects of silver nanoparticles stimulated by oxidative stress in human normal bronchial epithelial (BEAS-2B) cells. *Mutat. Res.* **2011**, *726*, 129–135.

174. Song, K.S.; Sung, J.H.; Ji, J.H.; Lee, J.H.; Lee, J.S.; Ryu, H.R.; Lee, J.K. et al. Recovery from silver-nanoparticle-exposure-induced lung inflammation and lung function changes in Sprague Dawley rats. *Nanotoxicology* **2013**, *7*, 169–180.

175. Stebounova, L.V.; Adamcakova-Dodd, A.; Kim, J.S.; Park, H.; O'Shaughnessy, P.T.; Grassian, V.H.; Thorne, P.S. Nanosilver induces minimal lung toxicity or inflammation in a subacute murine inhalation model. *Part. Fibre Toxicol.* **2011**, *8*, 5.

176. Sung, J.H.; Ji, J.H.; Song, K.S.; Lee, J.H.; Choi, K.H.; Lee, S.H.; Yu, I.J. Acute inhalation toxicity of silver nanoparticles. *Toxicol. Ind. Health* **2011**, *27*, 149–154.

177. Jun, E.; Lim, K.; Kim, K.; Bae, O.; Noh, J.; Chung, K.; Chung, J. Silver nanoparticles enhance thrombus formation through increased platelet aggregation and procoagulant activity. *Nanotoxicology* **2011**, *5*, 157–167.

178. Park, E.; Choi, K.; Park, K. Induction of inflammatory responses and gene expression by intratracheal instillation of silver nanoparticles in mice. *Arch. Pharm. Res.* **2011**, *34*, 299–307.

179. Rahman, M.F.; Wang, J.; Patterson, T.A.; Saini, U.T.; Robinson, B.L.; Newport, G.D.; Murdock, R.C.; Schlager, J.J.; Hussain, S.M.; Ali, S.F. Expression of genes related to oxidative stress in the mouse brain after exposure to silver-25 nanoparticles. *Toxicol. Lett.* **2009**, *187*, 15–21.

180. Shrivastava, S.; Bera, T.; Singh, S.K.; Singh, G.; Ramachandrarao, P.; Dash, D. Characterization of antiplatelet properties of silver nanoparticles. *ACS Nano* **2009**, *3*, 1357–1364.

181. Tiwari, D.K.; Jin, T.; Behari, J. Dose-dependent in-vivo toxicity assessment of silver nanoparticle in Wistar rats. *Toxicol. Mech. Methods* **2011**, *21*, 13–24.

182. Austin, C.A.; Umbreit, T.H.; Brown, K.M.; Barber, D.S.; Dair, B.J.; Francke-Carroll, S.; Feswick, A. et al. Distribution of silver nanoparticles in pregnant mice and developing embryos. *Nanotoxicology* **2012**, *6*, 912–922

183. Tang, J.; Xiong, L.; Wang, S.; Wang, J.; Liu, L.; Li, J.; Wan, Z.; Xi, T. Influence of silver nanoparticles on neurons and blood–brain barrier via subcutaneous injection in rats. *Appl. Surf. Sci.* **2008**, *255*, 502–504.

184. Li, P.; Kuo, T.; Chang, J.; Yeh, J.; Chan, W. Induction of cytotoxicity and apoptosis in mouse blastocysts by silver nanoparticles. *Toxicol. Lett.* **2010**, *197*, 82–87.

185. Chen, D.; Xi, T.; Bai, J. Biological effects induced by nanosilver particles: *In vivo* study. *Biomed. Mater.* **2007**, *2*, S126–S128.

186. Crettaz, P.; Pennington, D.; Rhomberg, L.; Brand, K.; Jolliet, O. Assessing human health response in life cycle assessment using ED10s and DALYs: Part 1—Cancer effects. *Risk Anal.* **2002**, *22*, 931–946.

187. Huijbregts, M.A.J.; Rombouts, L.J.A.; Ragas, A.M.J.; van de Meent, D. Human-toxicological effect and damage factors of carcinogenic and noncarcinogenic chemicals for life cycle impact assessment. *Integr. Environ. Assess. Manag.* **2005**, *1*, 181–244.

188. Wilhelm, C.; Gazeau, F.; Bacri, J.C.; Roger, J.; Pons, J.N. Interaction of anionic superparamagnetic nanoparticles with cells: Kinetic analyses of membrane adsorption and subsequent internalization. *Langmuir* **2002**, *18*, 8148–8155.

189. Luciani, N.; Gazeau, F.; Wilhelm, C. Reactivity of the monocyte/macrophage system to superparamagnetic anionic nanoparticles. *J. Mater. Chem.* **2009**, *19*, 6373–6380.

190. Semmler, M.; Seitz, J.; Erbe, F.; Mayer, P.; Heyder, J.; Oberdorster, G.; Kreyling, W.G. Long-term clearance kinetics of inhaled ultrafine insoluble iridium particles from the rat lung, including transient translocation into secondary organs. *Inhal. Toxicol.* **2004**, *16*, 453–460.

191. Wenger, Y.; Schneider, R.J., II; Reddy, G.R.; Kopelman, R.; Jolliet, O.; Philbert, M.A. Tissue distribution and pharmacokinetics of stable polyacrylamide nanoparticles following intravenous injection in the rat. *Toxicol. Appl. Pharmacol.* **2011**, *251*, 181–190.

192. Li, D.; Emond, C.; Johanson, G.; Jolliet, O. PBPK modeling of polyacrylamide nanoparticle biodistribution in rats. *International Society of Exposure Science 21st Annual Meeting*, Oct 23–27, 2011, Baltimore, and *Society of Toxicology 51st Annual Meeting*, Mar 11–15, 2012, San Francisco.

193. Diamond, M.L.; Gandhi, N.; Adams, W.J.; Atherton, J.; Bhavsar, S.P.; Bulle, C.; Campbell, P.G.C. et al. The clearwater consensus: The estimation of metal hazard in fresh water. *Int. J. Life Cycle Assess.* **2010**, *15*, 143–147.

194. Ligthart, T.; Aboussouan, L.; van de Meent, D.; Schönnenbeck, M.; Hauschild, M.; Delbeke, K.; Struijs, J. et al. Declaration of Apeldoorn on LCIA of non-ferrous metals. Abstract by Sonnemann G. *Int. J. Life Cycle Assess.* **2004**, *9*, 334.

195. Larsen, H.F. and Hauschild, M. Evaluation of ecotoxicity effect indicators for use in LCIA. *Int. J. Life Cycle Assess.* *12*, **2007**, 24–33.

196. Pennington, D.W.; Payet, J.; Hauschild, M. Life-cycle assessment—Aquatic ecotoxicological indicators in life-cycle assessment. *Environ. Toxicol. Chem. 23*, **2004**, 1796.

197. Pennington, D.W.; Margni, M.; Payet, J.; Jolliet, O. Risk and regulatory hazard-based toxicological effect indicators in life-cycle assessment (LCA). *Hum. Ecol. Risk Assess.* **2006**, *12*, 450–475.

198. Payet, J. Assessing toxic impacts on aquatic ecosystems in life cycle assessment (LCA). *Dissertation No 3112*. Ecole Polytechnique Fédérate de Lausanne, Switzerland, **2004**.

199. Payet, J. and Jolliet, O. Comparative assessment of the toxic impact of metals on aquatic ecosystems: The AMI method, In *Life Cycle Assessment of Metals: Issues and Research Directions*; Dubreuil, A., ed.; SETAC Press: Pensacola, FL, **2004**, pp. 188–191.

200. Lovern, S.B.; Klaper, R.D.; Strickler, J.R. The Influence of nanoparticles on behavior: the diminutive diet of Daphnia. *SETAC North America 26th Annual Meeting*, Baltimore, **2005**.

201. Haasch, M.L.; McClellan-Green, P.; Oberdorster, E. Nanotoxicology in aquatic species: Acute toxicity and effects on biotransformation. *SETAC North America 26th Annual Meeting*, Baltimore, **2005**.

202. Lovern, S.B. and Klaper, R. Daphnia magna mortality when exposed to titanium dioxide and fullerene (C-60) nanoparticles. *Environ. Toxicol. Chem.* **2006**, *25*, 1132–1137.

203. Bar-Ilan, O.; Albrecht, R.M.; Fako, V.E.; Furgeson, D.Y. Toxicity assessments of multisized gold and silver nanoparticles in zebrafish embryos. *Small* **2009**, *5*, 1897–1910.

204. Ciroth, A.; Fleischer, G.; Steinbach, J. Uncertainty calculation in life cycle assessments—A combined model of simulation and approximation. *Int. J. Life Cycle Assess.* **2004**, *9*, 216–226.

205. Heijungs, R.; Suh, S.; Kleijn, R. Numerical approaches to life cycle interpretation—The case of the Ecoinvent'96 database. *Int. J. Life Cycle Assess.* **2005**, *10*, 103–112.

# Section VII

# Ethical, Legal, and Social Implications of Bionanotechnology

# 12

## Anticipating Ethical, Legal, and Social Aspects of Emerging Technology Gaps in Innovation Chain: The Case of Body Area Networks

**Alireza Parandian**

## CONTENTS

## 12.1 Introduction

Several advancements in different scientific and technological disciplines (e.g., nanotechnology, biotechnology, and information and communications technology [ICT]) appear to be promising for enabling an increasing number of medical technologies and devices appropriate for home and mobile applications. The trend to develop such medical technologies is stimulated by the recent developments in the dynamics of supply and demand of the health-care sector. In this study, we will focus on one selected case, that of Body Area Networks (BAN) in health care (see Jones et al. 2007). The concept of BAN was first coined by Zimmerman (1999) at the Massachusetts Institute of Technology and IBM under the topic of Personal Area Networks (PAN) and has been further developed by other groups at Philips (van Dam et al. 2001) and by the MobiHealth team at the University of Twente and Fraunhofer (Jones et al. 2001). Although there might be a general consensus on the significance of this concept for improving health practices in various domains, the level of its actual impact is still undefined particularly in respect to its long-term implications. Therefore, this chapter will address the anticipation of aspects that will have an effect on the successful societal embedding of BAN technologies into the health-care system. To this end, we use the philosophy of constructive technology assessment and will utilize its tools to anticipate on ethical, legal, and societal implications of the concept of BAN in health-care settings.

Figure 12.1 is a diagram that has been drawn on the basis of a visionary program at the Holst Centre in the Netherlands, called the Human++ program (Gyselinckx et al. 2006). The diagram illustrates a simplified example of such advanced BAN architecture. It represents a patient or a client with a number of sensors attached, worn, or implanted in the body. The sensor nodes are envisioned to be autonomous and extremely miniaturized and capable of transmitting data wirelessly. Data from the sensors are then wirelessly transmitted to a processing unit before being transmitted (wirelessly) to a central monitoring server via a network.

Body area networks in health care must be seen as part of a broader vision, that of Ambient Intelligence, "a future environment that is aware of our presence and responsive to our needs" (Aarts and Roovers 2003). "Ambient" extends from the external environment to the internal environment. Related to health care, miniaturization of chips, computer devices, and sensors promise to enable cheap, light, wearable, and even implantable autonomous systems for continuous monitoring of vital health signs. BAN form a particular, and promising, approach (Jones et al. 2007; Penders et al. 2007; Gyselinckx et al. 2008). The resulting opportunities for use in health care are broad, but one important focus is the shift from monitoring patients in health-care facilities and hospitals, to their daily environment. Of course, this requires further technological and social innovation, already in the systems to receive and

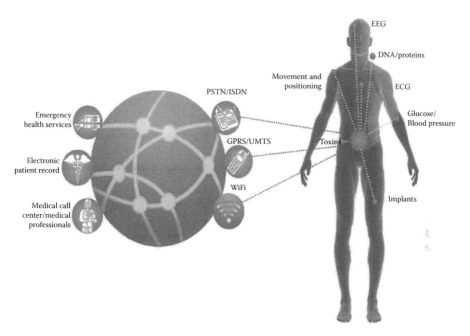

**FIGURE 12.1**
Scheme drawn and adapted from Imec's Human++. (From www.imec.be.)

handle all the signals. What we see happening is, in a sense, an alliance between actors pushing imminent and projected changes in health care, and actors offering promises about functionalities of new technologies. There are lots of open issues, at the side of health care as well as of new technologies and the coevolution of the two.

The other important consideration is that the present "alliance" (at least in the Netherlands) focuses almost exclusively on wonderful new opportunities, and might well overlook other aspects and dynamics. That is why approaches introducing further interactions and interventions are important to broaden perspectives of the various stakeholders and allow them to develop better strategies. In particular, present and new roles and responsibilities should be addressed because these can hamper developments but also offer openings. For instance, if a private company offers home-care monitoring, what quality assurance is possible? What will be the role of the government and regulatory actors in ensuring quality and availability of care and ensuring the safety of patients? What liability issues will emerge, for instance if a patient comes to harm because of miscommunication or failure of device, or when an actual emergency situation is not part of the present software? Another cluster of issues relates to reimbursement: who will carry the costs of the new systems (their putting into place and the actual monitoring)? The structure of the health insurance system is important here, and it is not clear how present changes in the system (toward privatization) will evolve and stabilize. In addition, there is the issue of electronic patient records (EPRs) and how these will be used.

## 12.2 Understanding and Managing Societal Embedding

Understanding and managing the societal embedment of potential break-through technologies is attractive to look at in early stages of technological development (Rip et al. 1995). The main motivation for this early analysis is because the state of affairs is more compliant and susceptible to change at this stage. Promises and expectations are imperative entrance points for analysis in early stages of technology development. Promises have the form of compact stories about the potential role of the findings (technologi-cal options) in a future world where they should function in. These are in fact diffuse scenarios and can be traced and judged on their consistency and plausibility. Constructive technology assessment provides the tools to make such assessment on the basis of the conceptualization of innovation process as coevolution of technological and societal change. Therefore, anticipation on ethical, legal, and societal aspects represents an opportunity to address gaps in the innovation chain. To this end, constructive technology assess-ment puts emphasis on anticipation informed by dynamics of emergence combined with broadening the technology design processes by bringing together and reflecting on multiple stakeholder perspectives (Schot and Rip 1997). Thereby, it is recognized that eventual impacts are always the result of interactions among various groups such as technology developers, users, governments, NGOs, and others.

### 12.2.1 Diagnosis of Gaps in Innovation Chain: Case of Body Area Networks

Road mapping has been widely recognized as a fruitful method to coor-dinate action in order to create alignment for creating intentional tech-nological paths. However, owing to lack of obvious drivers, many of the developments needed for the development of BAN technologies (specifi-cally the "More than Moore" domain) cannot be road mapped (van Hoof 2006). Instead, for most of More than Moore* technologies, visionary appli-cation drivers are used that can provide guidance in development and

---

* More than Moore (MtM) explores a new area of micro/nanoelectronics, which reaches beyond the boundaries of conventional semiconductor technologies and applications. Creating and integrating various nondigital functionality to semiconductor products, MtM focuses on cre-ating high-value micro/nanoelectronics systems, motivating new technological possibilities and unlimited application potential (Zhang et al. 2006).

allow extraction of technological needs in time. These are then considered as milestones and requirements that have to be met in repeated stages. The Human++ program of Holst Centre (Gyselinckx et al. 2008) provides an example of such visionary application programs. Their vision describes a future world with a large number of visionary devices for medical, sport, and entertainment applications, which make use of sensors and actuator systems in and around the body. In a more general context, such miniaturized network devices might find wider applications in complete different sectors to meet different purposes and needs (generic BAN), that is, agriculture, process automation, and automobile industry. While this is the case, the underlying hardware platforms necessary for such applications will be to a great extent alike. Therefore, visionary applications for each sector provide guidance in defining the underlying technical requirements for the different components, such as sensors and actuators, signal processing, power generation/storage, and wireless communications. Architectural innovation will then be needed to realize such applications (van Hoof 2006). Promises, in this situation, in terms of visionary applications (such as Human++), are used by technology developers to drive technical requirements, that is, for power generation purposes (to guide the developments). In a broader context, such prospective projections travel further and are circulated to others than just technical actors. The picture with envisioned applications (see Figure 1 in Gyselinckx et al. 2006) is then picked up by others as a real proposition and materializes a future world where such applications are used, thus linking up with the broader promises of Ambient intelligence.

Although these future worlds are communicated as real propositions, there is a lack of understanding of their eventual impact on society. Consequently, essential requirements (techno-institutional ones) for such technologies to become embedded in society are not fed back to the developers of technology, which might hamper societal embedding of products in later stages. This is because stakeholders and other actors use such a future representation to position themselves and others, and allocate roles and responsibilities to other stakeholders, which might be contradictory from different perspectives. Subsequently, little effort is made to feed back requirements, which eventually shape the alignments necessary for the social embedding of the products to be made.

This gap has been generally recognized before in the literature (Deuten et al. 1997; Rip and Te Kulve 2008) and has been explained by the fact that "enactors" (those directly involved in research and development of technologies) (Garud and Ahlstrom 1997) work with a concentric perspective. Deuten et al. (1997) explain that in the development of new products, product managers often view the environment as concentric layers around the new product, starting with the business environment and ending with the wider society. They suggest three parts of the environment that product (listed below) developers seem to consider with a concentric bias.

1. Technology environment: actors continuously interacting on technological issues and milestones of development (scientists and different actors in the industry)
2. Regulatory environment: standard setting regulatory bodies, and
   local, national, and international regulation environment
3. Wider society: consumer organizations, environmental groups, public opinion leaders, media, and independent scientists

It is evident that eventually alignments with all layers are necessary for
societal embedding to take place. Yet managers fail to deal with them in a
sequential manner. In contrast, what often happens is that clarifying functional aspects of the product are addressed first before addressing broader
(societal) aspects.

To recapitulate, there might be a general agreement on the significance
of technologies, but the world that is expected to adopt such products to
be developed has a comparing and selecting position (Garud and Ahlstrom
1997). Besides, promises are used to bridge the gaps along the innovation
chain as the infrastructure for their realization does not exist. As the promise travels to society in the early stages of development, different stakeholders speculate on the future arrangement of actors and their own position in
particular within that future scenario. For instance, a researcher in academia
link up to such goals with a broader interest to attract resources, produce new
knowledge, and acquire reputation and credibility within their specialized
field. Governments stimulate developments that promise economic prospect
while at the same time having to account for effective and safe medical systems for the general public. Industrial actors and medical device manufacturers recognize the opportunity of new health markets and embrace these
trends to develop and strengthen their resilient position in these emerging
markets to enhance prosperity. Furthermore, there are different perspectives
advocated about the organization of care practices by the medical community in general, patient organizations, and health-care insurance companies.
Disagreements on prospective roles and responsibilities based on expectations might eventually hamper societal embedment of the envisioned products to be developed. This emphasizes the need for an approach that aims to
anticipate on broader aspects in early stages of technology development than
just focusing on the technological functionalities.

Our approach recognizes that the take-up of what is available and (partial) materialization of technological options coevolves with the changes in
the health-care sector, and the role and responsibilities of different actors
involved. Emphasizing that the societal embedment of the BAN concept in
health care is also very much dependent on its social context (cf. how actors
in practice accept changes to their roles, tasks, responsibilities, and mutual
relationships), it is also necessary to consider the care arrangements within
which the BAN concept operates and include that in our prospective analysis.

## 12.3 Anticipating Issues Surrounding Possible New Health Practice

Body area networks are seen as real options to solve challenges (aging society, increasing number of chronic illnesses, etc.) that lie ahead in the long run in the health-care sector. The introduction of such technological interventions causes the care situation and its context to be altered. Such changes might further bring about unforeseen consequences related to the way care processes are structured, the way people interact and pursue their professional obligations. In this paragraph, the aim is to anticipate on these issues in the context of the emergence and uptake of BAN technologies in health care. To fulfill this goal, it was necessary to trace how different actors expect future health-care settings to change, what should be in place, which requirements have to be fulfilled, and what consequences can be expected if the technological concepts of BAN are to be socially embedded in the health-care setting of the Netherlands. Our entrance point has been to collect and evaluate the expectations of relevant actors along the innovation value chain (Den Boer et al. 2009). To this end, we have performed semistructured interviews with 36 direct stakeholders from different backgrounds to collect their perspectives on the necessary changes that have to take place and evaluate the evolution of actions, roles, and responsibilities of different actors and the effect on the entire system from different perspectives. The number of interviews conducted for this study and the background of respondents are indicated in Figure 12.2. Table 12.1 summarizes our interview results and describes the role different actors in the health-care value chain envisioned to play with

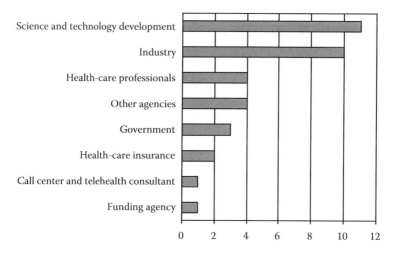

**FIGURE 12.2**
Number of interviews conducted for this study and background of respondents.

**TABLE 12.1**

Interview Results: Summary of Role and Main Concerns Envisioned by Different Actors with Regard to Social Embedding Process of Visionary BAN Applications in Health Care

| Actor | | Description |
|---|---|---|
| Science | Envisioned role | Envision a role in solving scientific and technological issues to enable further advancement of BAN technologies (miniaturizing sensors and actuators, battery technologies, interoperability issues, and developing reliable measurement methods). Technical scientists mainly focus on improving specific parts of the BAN concept (e.g., sensor reliability and functioning, battery and energy efficiency, signal processing, and efficient and secure ways of data transfer). They are not likely to fulfill the role to prove effects on quality of life or care through clinical testing. Such a role is mainly envisioned for scientists active in medical universities. Early interaction between these actors is viewed to have positive effect on the societal embedding. |
| | Main concerns | Technical barriers such as reliability of the BAN systems, interoperability of devices, battery life and energy efficiency, or even autonomy, information security issues, information management, and compliance with legacy systems, are issues of main concern. |
| | | Have very limited resources available to clinical testing of applications. Large investments and samples population is required to meet health-care regulatory requirements. |
| Large companies | Envisioned role | Large companies envision the role of developing and producing BAN devices to serve large and emerging health markets (cf. monitoring chronically ill patients). Large and smaller companies do not view technical issues as main barriers for societal embedding; rather the organizational complexity in health-care system of the Netherlands and the highly regulated health-care sector is viewed as difficult to breakthrough. |
| | Main concerns | Technical barriers such as reliability of the BAN systems, interoperability of devices, battery life and energy efficiency, or even autonomy, information security issues, information management, and compliance with legacy systems, are issues of main concern. |
| | | Large companies have to focus on volume of products sold and therefore they will have to focus on maximizing profits. There are concerns that BAN services might remain a niche product in health care. In contrast, the wellness market is viewed as a huge opportunity. |
| | | Concern about the heavy investment requirements for clinical tests while the outset to the future adoption of the BAN technologies remains obscure (this causes waiting games to emerge). |
| | | Concern about the ambiguity of who will eventually purchase the BAN products. A problem owner has to be identified in the case of each visionary application so as to create more clarity on this issue. Concerns relate also to the complexity of the health-care sector (highly regulated sector in the Netherlands). |

| | | |
|---|---|---|
| | | Concerns about underdeveloped/lack of infrastructure or national platform on which BAN technologies can function (EPRs are facing huge implementation issues in the Netherlands). Since BAN technologies are in initial developmental stages, there is no definitive standard (on interoperability of devices). Competition among the rival developers and commercial interests to make their standard as industry standard play a role and put much pressure on early cooperation among the industry players. Much more coordination and alignment work inside the medical device industry is necessary to deal with standardization issues. Concerns about possible gray zones in regulation regarding the transfer (cf. wireless transfer) of health-related data. |
| Technology-oriented SMEs | Envisioned role | Envision the role of innovative R&D and serving of niche markets in health care. |
| | Main concerns | Technical barriers such as reliability of the BAN systems, interoperability of devices, battery life and energy efficiency, or even autonomy, information security issues, information management, and compliance with legacy systems, are issues of main concern. Have very limited resources available to clinical testing of applications. Large investments and samples population is required to meet health-care regulatory requirements. Concerns about lack of clear business cases that attend hidden agenda of all actors involved. Linked to this is the concern about the ambiguity of who will eventually purchase the BAN products. A problem owner has to be identified in the case of each visionary application so as to create more clarity on this issue. Concerns relate also to the complexity of the health-care sector (highly regulated sector in the Netherlands). Concerns about lack of standards of interoperability but also regarding data storage and handing systems. |
| Government | Envisioned role | Envisions a proactive role in stimulating and supporting innovations that enable efficiency in health care. Initiating ethical debates and policy development where necessary (cf. wireless transfer of medical data and modes of security). Also envisions the role of providing a safe infrastructure for storage and exchange of medical information (cf. EPR and a national storage point through NICTIZ). |
| | Main concerns | Concerns about rising health-care costs due to demographic changes, such as aging society and increasing rate of chronic illnesses. Scarcity of health resources and medical professionals. Concerns about the information provision to the users on new technologies. |

*(continued)*

**TABLE 12.1 (Continued)**

Interview Results: Summary of Role and Main Concerns Envisioned by Different Actors with Regard to Social Embedding Process of Visionary BAN Applications in Health Care

| Actor | | Description |
|---|---|---|
| | Main concerns | Concern about the mismatch between demand and supply in the medical devices sector. The development of medical technologies is mainly driven by technology push strategies from the view of government and more interaction with the users is required to enable the societal embedding of medical devices like BAN. There is need to articulate the concerns of society and if necessary to implement new regulations to deal with the concerns about ethical aspects that may arise to hamper societal embedding of BAN technologies (cf. privacy concerns). |
| | | Concern about the level of organizational changes required to make new technologies like BAN societal embedded. This requires lots of effort to create alignments and coordinate incentives of different actors and may take a long time to realize. |
| | | Concerns about equal access to BAN applications in the society. |
| Health-care professionals | Envisioned role | Envision using BAN applications if these are evidence based and bring added value to their daily activities and their patients. Also envision the role of gateway through which devices have to be chosen and further information provision to patients. |
| | Main concerns | From the health-care professionals' perspective, health-care processes cannot be taken over by technologies measuring factual data alone; there are different factors that have to be taken into account when making medical judgments. They are concerned that this might undermine the whole care aspect of the medical profession, causing negative impact on the patient. On the basis of this, they call for early involvement in assessment of usefulness of different visionary applications. |
| | | Concerns about uncertainty regarding the way of handling of false alarms. This could be generated by BAN-monitoring devices, which in turn might put extra workload on the health-care system. |
| | | Concerns about private parties becoming involved in delivering health-care services with BAN applications. Private parties may be driven by commercial stakes, and this might affect the quality of health care. |
| | | Concerns about lack of proper reimbursement policies, which may have serious effects on the societal embedding of BAN technologies. For example, there are concerns about possible changes to current business models (as many of the envisioned BAN applications might reduce the number of visits to medical institutions and at the same time requires health-care professionals to bear certain responsibilities.). In general, there are concerns at the side of medical professionals about possible hidden agendas of health-care insurance companies to introduce new business models on the basis of the data that can be generated by BAN technologies. |

| | |
|---|---|
| | Concerns that new applications of BAN may require major changes in roles and responsibilities of actors in the health-care chain. In case this may lead to more complexity in the health-care system, this will reduce chances of adoption by medical professionals. |
| | Concerns about lack of experience and expertise in handling and decision making based on large amount of raw data. Concerns about lack of clear protocols describing the roles and responsibilities of health-care professionals and other external parties involved in the services. Legal and liability problems arising due to misinterpretation is another concern of the medical professionals linked to the previous. |
| | For hospitals, a major concern is related to processing data and storing information generated by BAN devices. Since hospital databases across the country have no definitive/common structure of information storage and processing, that may lead to practical problems. |
| Patient-oriented organizations | |
| Envisioned role | Envision a role to stimulate the use of proven application. As representative of users also a supportive role in the debate on ethical issues to prevent unwanted consequences for the users. Also a bridging role between users (patients) and industry to incorporate user preferences and values. |
| Main concerns | Concerns about user-friendliness of BAN devices being developed. Related to this is the lack of knowledge of the users to use and operate devices. |
| | Concern about the mismatch between demand and supply in the medical devices sector. The development of medical technologies is mainly driven by technology push strategies from the view of government and more interaction with the users is required to enable the societal embedding of medical devices like BAN. There is need to articulate the concerns of society and if necessary to implement new regulations to deal with the concerns about ethical aspects that may arise to hamper societal embedding of BAN technologies (cf. privacy concerns). Although it is not directly mentioned, patient organizations are concerned about possible future strategies of health-care insurance companies to introduce new business models on the basis of the data that can be generated by BAN technologies. |
| Health-care insurance companies | |
| Envisioned role | Envision a role to stimulate efficiency in health care and recognize the fact that this is only possible through cooperation between the triangle of health-care professionals, health-care insurance companies, and the patients or representative patient organizations. Envision a limited role to stimulate pilot and experimental projects to prove effectiveness of BAN applications. Large investments in innovation would put pressure on the costs of insurance companies. Owing to regulatory issues and the competition in the Dutch health-care insurance system on the basis of price of insurance policies, it is not simple to increase prices of health-care insurance policies. |

*(continued)*

**TABLE 12.1 (Continued)**

Interview Results: Summary of Role and Main Concerns Envisioned by Different Actors with Regard to Social Embedding Process of Visionary BAN Applications in Health Care

| Actor | | Description |
|---|---|---|
| | Main concerns | Market share is one of the largest concerns all health-care insurance companies in the Netherlands face in a price/premium-sensitive market environment. This restricts health-care insurance companies from taking initiatives that threaten them to raise their premiums (cf. invest in new innovations). At the same time, there are huge concerns about the spiraling costs in health-care mainly due to shifting demographics. |
| | | Concerns about the effectiveness of BAN devices in practice. Lack of sufficient evidence that new innovations like the BAN concept will drive down the costs of the health-care system. Huge time and resources have to be spent in clinical trials to collect such evidence. |
| | | Concerns about lack of trust of patients and health-care providers in incentives of health-care insurance companies. Creation of more transparency through interactions with other actors in the health-care chain is crucial in the future to improve the image of health-care insurance companies. |
| Tele-health centers | Envisioned role | Envision a role of data hub between patients and medical professionals by providing information security and management. |
| | Main concerns | Concerns about lack of concrete protocols describing roles and responsibilities of different parties regarding the access, reliability of information. |
| | | Concerns related to lack of standards related to processing data and storing information generated by BAN devices. Since the hospital databases across the country have no definitive/common structure of information storage and processing, that may lead to practical problems. |
| Domotica and home automation consultancies | Envisioned role | Envision a role to provide and install the necessary equipment at patients home. |
| | Main concerns | Concerns about lack of communication between industry and health-care providers and consultancies to articulate roles and responsibilities. |
| Network providers | Envisioned role | Envision the role of providing the physical network infrastructure and other IT services to implement reliable services in health care. |
| | Main concerns | Concerns about the complexities and liability issues in case of mistakes or malfunctioning of the systems. |

regard to the societal embedding process of BAN application in health care. Table 12.1 also summarizes the main concerns different actors anticipated on regarding the societal embedding process of BAN. We will present our main findings first by shortly reflecting on different important stakeholders and their positions in the field and then in sequential steps we will elaborate on various relevant issues through looking at changes that will result from introduction of BAN in terms of location of the health-care setting, arrangement of health-care services, and funding mechanisms. On the basis of this, we will highlight some of the key issues that need urgent consideration.

### 12.3.1 Key Factors Influencing Social Embedding of Body Area Networks

There is clear distinction to be made about the mechanisms that influence the successful social embedment of products and services that are related to health care compared with other goods and services that are traded on the consumer markets. One of the important reasons underlying this distinction is the consumption behavior of users related to health-care products. Instead of being determined by cost-and-benefit tradeoffs, the acceptance or adoption of health-care-related products and services is very much determined by contextual factors (such factors may include user characteristic or actor characteristics as well as the inherent characteristics of technologies). Another important factor is uncertainty. Namely, the health conditions of individuals is highly uncertain and different individuals are hardly aware of when they might become ill while they are also not always aware of state of their health. The use of services and facilities to safeguard health condition or treat certain illnesses is therefore an uncertain factor. Moreover, citizens and patients are not always capable of assessing their state of health because they lack the knowledge necessary to form a precise judgment. At the same time, there is a knowledge deficit at the side of users (or patients) to evaluate what is available in the medical market and decide on what exactly fits their situation.

Government policy can play a crucial role in regulating the market dynamics of health care, including positioning and strategic behavior of different professional groups. Interest groups can also have an important role, and therefore the timely involvement of stakeholder groups is important to understand desired directions for further development. For instance, it is important to understand how the introduction of medical applications might influence the status of health-care professionals and their economical incentives. Health-care insurance companies play a major role in the financial structure of health care through reimbursement schemes. Their strategic and economical incentives play a crucial role in the social embedding process of medical and health-care-related products. Health-care providers form a gateway between the industry and their patients, and therefore can exert great influence in promoting the applications that would also benefit their own practice, status, and economic position. (Note that medical professionals can also endorse negative propaganda to hamper the diffusion process of new products, cf. as was attempted in the case of genetic self-test in the Netherlands.) Further technical issues, such as reliability and interoperability, are issues that are important considerations for medical professionals and nonprofessional users. Moreover, the provision of good information with regard to usage and benefits of applications together with user-friendly design are factors that stimulate users to use certain technologies in specific situations, and thus require users (sometimes their representatives such as professional patient organizations) to be involved in the development process.

Finally, a factor that may seem commonplace at first sight is the availability of infrastructure. For the applications of BAN, the existence of a database system where data can be securely stored and viewed by different professionals is necessary. The EPR could provide such platform. However, until now, the introduction of the EPR in the Netherlands has been faced with great barriers. Our interview with the representatives of NICTIZ* (the institution that is responsible for the implementation of EPR in the Netherlands) and all other major stakeholders active in this field has made it evident that without a basic EPR, it becomes difficult to guarantee that relevant stakeholders such as patients themselves and health-care providers will have adequate access to all relevant information that is required at point of care. The data that are generated through monitoring activities has to be coherently stored and be available along with other medical information to be meaningful for all relevant parties. The chairman of the Dutch tele-health workgroup on cardiovascular diseases confirms this conclusion in a professional ICT health care magazine, where he tersely stated, "Tele-health without EPD is no Tele-health" (Flim 2008).

### 12.3.2  Changing Health-Care Sector and Position of Different Stakeholders

Specific to the Netherlands, since January 2006, the health-care sector has witnessed relatively radical reforms. This has caused the central role of the state in the enduring operation of the health-care system has been replaced by private health suppliers. Health-care insurances were privatized, and the government's responsibility since then mainly concerns the accessibility and quality issues of health care. These changes have opened new opportunities for actors in the field to organize their businesses in a more pragmatic way. For instance, health-care insurers in the new system have received more

---

* NICTIZ was founded in 2002 by organizations representing the Dutch health care and IT sectors. NICTIZ is funded by the Ministry of Health, Welfare and Sports of the Netherlands. It is principally focused on two initiatives: to develop an Electronic Health Record and to build a national secure electronic communication infrastructure for the health-care sector.

room to distinguish their services through provision of supplementary policies and services. Such mechanism should contribute to the competitiveness in the market and at the same time facilitate an enhanced quality of care in general (Bomhoff 2002). This is deemed necessary to deal with demographic and epidemiologic changes (aging society, increasing number of chronically ill) that are occurring. In this context, the issue of patient empowerment also plays an important role especially for citizens (or patients) who are dealing with chronic diseases and for the elderly who want to remain living independently for as long as possible. Such demand is recognized by the medical devices industry as they have to assess society's needs and adjust to the norms and values of the public; however, at the same time, they have to comply with legal contexts, regulations, and rules.

Meanwhile, the situation has caused health-care professionals to increasingly operate efficiently and negotiate for reimbursement for services that they find necessary for their patients. On the other hand, while governmental supervision on the health-care system is moving to the background and other actors in the health-care market find more room to safeguard their own stakes, they will attempt to incorporate their own interests in the services to be offered to the customers. One possible impact to be considered then is that as more weight is given to the individual needs for provision of health care, the control over collective interests such as equal access to high-quality care and affordability of health care might decrease. Another possibility that is suggested is the adjustment of health-care policies to the state of health of patients as a plausible market mechanism (reward mechanism) to encourage efficiency and quality (KPN 2006).

The health-care professionals that were interviewed in this study have collectively raised the concern with regard to the way medical devices and services are envisioned to be offered to patients. Their concern is based on the argument that citizens (and patients) are not always capable of making the right choices with regard to what kind of care and services they need. This does not only have to do with knowledge and availability of information about a specific procedure, but also the fact that there is a difference between healthy individuals and ill patients in their ability to consider the pros and cons of specific diagnostic or treatment service. Moreover, it was argued by health-care professionals that information that is provided to patients by private parties might be biased because there are commercial interests involved. Finally, it was emphasized that considerations and choices of health-care professionals with regard to what is appropriate for the patient has to be balanced in many different dimensions and is dependent on the context and individual situations.

In this brief section, we have shown that there are specific issues to be addressed with regard to social embedding of BAN and the position and perspectives of different actors play a crucial role in shaping that process. Therefore, we will first look at the major stakeholders and their positions with regard to the introduction of BAN applications in a broad sense. This will open up the opportunity to devote attention to specific issues in the following sections.

### 12.3.2.1 Medical Device Industry

The rapidly growing market of health-care and wellness products is an essential opportunity for the industry to be exploited in the coming years. Health economy is globally recognized as one of the major sources of innovation (Amara et al. 2003). The demand for health care is inevitably rising and the requirements to enhance health-care products and services become more demanding in time. Generally, one can say that such pressure has been the driving force behind the enormous enhancements in medical technologies and great enhancement of quality of interventions in health care in the past decades.

The vision of ambient intelligence in turn has created new opportunities for the industry to exploit in the coming years. Namely, the challenge of delivering personalized health-care products that are well tailored to individual needs. Industrial strategies are mainly focused on the creation of a new branch of consumer market where consumers can choose and buy their own health-related equipment. However, it is still a question as to what extent such activities can be profitable without cooperation of medical specialists and health-care insurance companies, especially in the health-care setting of the Netherlands. Cooperation with health insurance companies can have a large impact on the scale of diffusion of products and services that the industry is developing. Economies of scale can be the result of close cooperation with health-care insurances in case they would be interested in purchasing products and services. Our interviews with major health-care insurance companies in the Netherlands reveal that such cooperation is based on the incentive to make insurance policies more attractive in terms of delivering better services to enhance quality of care/life (as a competitive advantage to their clients). Furthermore, health-care insurance companies have argued that collaboration in pilot settings is a fruitful way to determine whether technologies can fulfill the promises about contribution to efficiency and quality of life. However, such collaboration is also faced with question marks when it comes to the information that is generated about a patient through possible applications of BAN. The context in which medical information is used can raise privacy issues and can carry potential risks of public controversy if abuse of information becomes evident. Such an effect is difficult to foresee, particularly because of the special character of the health-care industry, its services, and the added value these bring to the patients. In situations where an individual's life is in threat, adoption of technology and medical procedures and their further direct and indirect consequences are easily accepted by patients (Parandian 2006). The context in which the BAN technologies are delivered are important and patients can make trade-off decisions with regard to their privacy for the sake of more comfort and certainty about their health state.

### 12.3.2.2 Health-Care Insurances

Since 2006, the difference between public and private health insurance has been abolished in the Netherlands (Healthcare IT Management 2007). Every adult citizen is obliged to purchase the basic health-care insurance policy. This service is available to all Dutch citizens, and the content of different services covered in this policy is regulated by the government. This ensures access to adequate health-care services for all Dutch citizens. For supplementary services, health-care insurance companies have a free hand in putting together services, what it should cost, and to whom it is provided.

With the rise of technological possibilities (such as the BAN concept) and the opportunities it promises to increase efficiency in health care (in terms of costs and quality of life), the incentive for the health-care insurances to invest in such technologies is growing. A possible role envisioned for the health-care insurance companies is the provision (or investing in and the setup of) of health-care services connected to BAN technologies (or tele-health in general). In fact, some health-care insurance companies in the Netherlands are already experimenting with tele-health technology pilot settings (cf. Motiva Project). Call centers and medical consultancy services connected to health-care professionals are a necessary foundation of such technologies where continuous data uptake, storage, monitoring, and analysis can take place. According to the medical professionals we have interviewed, health-care insurance companies have incentives to invest in such service centers because the information generated there can open new opportunities to implement control mechanisms. Different strategies can be obtained by health-care insurances in the future, such as the reward system. On the one hand, patients might be offered to benefit from discounts in exchange of loss of privacy, and on the other hand they would hand over control over their lifestyle because they give away control through provision of their medical data. The pressure to control the spiraling costs of health care together with the new technological possibilities might also open up new opportunities for health-care insurances to develop strategies toward an output-driven financial infrastructure for health care. In other words, this will provide health-care insurance companies a much better control over their long-term financial investments and expenditures.

There are different expectations with regard to the possibility of use of information management systems in health care through which the quality of care provision can be monitored and steered if necessary. The possibilities to compare the quality of services of health-care professionals, institutions, and facilities through analysis of a set of indicators are progressively growing. The argument is that comparative analysis will increase awareness on quality issues for health-care institutions, increase competitiveness, and thereby maintain the quality of care at high standards (KPN 2006). From a societal perspective, a more critical elaboration is needed on the selection of criteria on the basis of which such comparisons are made. Furthermore, there should be a debate on what kind of information can be used for internal evaluations and which could be used for external benchmarking. This is important to consider because strategies that basically use calibrating methods for comparison might drive health care to orient toward average scores.

### 12.3.2.3 Health-Care Providers

Health-care professionals have an important position and role to play with regard to the emergence and societal embedding of the BAN concept and its applications in health care. The responsibility of health-care professionals in delivering adequate health care to their patients is quite complex, and there are many factors that determine such decision-making processes. Therefore, the knowledge and experience of these professionals play an important role in the setup and tailoring of services to patient needs. Furthermore, health-care professionals recognize their supportive role to inform patients about the use of specific technologies and supporting patients to choose products that fit their norms and values.

All stakeholders that have been interviewed for this study have collectively agreed that the introduction of BAN technologies will have an impact on the complexity of roles and responsibilities of health-care professionals. This is linked to the fact that care processes will not only be related to one professional but a chain of different professionals. The responsibilities are not only exclusive to how patient information exchange is handled, but also responsibilities relating to good information provision and the direct responsibility for the health state of the patient. In fact, Oudshoorn (2007) suggests that adoption of tele-medical technologies (cf. ambulatory EEG recorder) is highly dependent on a well-organized and well-staffed tele-medical center. Oudshoorn's empirical study shows the importance of the invisible work that is done by the nurses and other professionals in the chain and therefore suggests that the agency of patients themselves is not a motivational factor, but should be extended to the level of sociotechnical networks in which health-care services are embedded. Another issue that seems to be crucial to the health-care professionals is the requirement of using evidence-based devices. The work of health-care professionals is highly sensitive and therefore it is necessary that any conclusion reached or advice given by them is justifiable. At the same time, cultural changes have led to an increasing trend among patients to question the decisions of health professionals and seek legal action in case of mistakes. This has created the need for health-care providers to be able to demonstrate that their decisions or advice given to patients are based on relevant and valid information.

### 12.3.2.4 Government

A solid information provision and the right to high-quality care is the basic requirement that the government safeguards with regard to new products and services. The argument is that patients should be able to make informed choices with regard to technology adoption and its consequences (cf. impact on privacy of the patient). Another issue that the government is concerned with is related to equal access to technologies. An issue that needs further consideration by policy makers is the legal framework according to which the health-care or wellness services (including applications of BAN) are offered on the market. How should the quality of these services be assessed and who should be allowed to offer such services? For instance, if a private company offers home-care monitoring, what quality assurance is possible? Lack of legal framework and guidelines in this respect can have dramatic impacts not only for the social embedment of these technologies but also for the users of the technology in case widespread diffusion takes place.

Our interview with representatives of the Ministry of Health, Welfare and Sports in the Netherlands suggests that the main issue from an ethical point of view that needs to be addressed concerns information provision and safeguarding the right of the patients to be well informed about the pros and cons of technology adoption. Such information provision is essential for the decision-making process of the patient in terms of maintaining their personal norms and values. Related to this, of course, is the issue of freedom of choice. Thus, when the patient refuses to use specific applications or technologies on the basis of their norms and values, this should not have further consequences for the right of the patient for access to high-quality care. Furthermore, the quality of care should be preserved at all times and that will remain the main responsibility of the government. Therefore, alternatives have to be considered and patients should always be provided with alternative choices.

### 12.3.3 Anticipating Ethical, Legal, and Social Aspects

In the previous paragraphs, we have explained the transformational forces that are at interplay among various stakeholders in the field of health care. We have argued that these forces along with the new promises of ambient intelligence, and in particular the concept of BAN, play an important role in facing future challenges and shaping the system to provide the necessary solutions. Although these new solutions are promising, they also bring along challenges. Provision of health-care services to patients at mobile locations according medical standards can cause changes to the situation of the patients, care providers, and other involved stakeholders. For BAN, technological issues are being addressed in a variety of settings; however, to be successfully embedded in the practice of health care, other challenges have to be addressed that lie beyond technological issues and are more related to the ethical, social, and relational contexts.

#### 12.3.3.1 *Blurring Boundary between Health-Care and Wellness Services*

An important issue that needs further consideration is that strategies for implementation and integration of BAN concept will be dependent on the specific application that will be used and the domain within which it has to be embedded. The blurring boundaries between the purposes of different applications are problematic for quality control and reimbursement issues and therefore needs further consideration. In this regard, Hatcher and Heetebry (2004) argue that while the convergence of the various technologies and fields is causing a revolt of innovative technologies into the health-care practice, it is at the same time causing a paradigm shift that is blurring the boundaries between public health, acute care, and preventative health. This has implications for the way social and ethical impact of the applications are assessed. Furthermore, it has been argued by health-care professionals in our interviews that the symptoms associated with different illnesses often converge; therefore, health-care processes cannot be taken over by technologies measuring factual data alone because this might undermine the whole care aspect of the medical profession, causing a negative impact on the patient. The blurring boundary between health-care and wellness-related applications of the BAN concept also raises questions to the way these technologies are assessed. Namely, the desire for a more efficient, organized health-care process is a societal issue and is based on the normative argument that while the society as whole invests in health care, it is expected that the society will become healthier as a result. However, at a time when the responsibility for the health state of individuals is pushed more and more toward the individuals themselves, and technologies are being developed to support persons taking such responsibility, the question has to be raised whether the issue is about becoming healthier or are technologies being developed to also contribute to the wellness and lifestyles of patients? This has a consequence for the assessment norms that are applied to technologies, for example, to approve reimbursement policies. In other words, the normative frame in which technologies are being assessed should be adjusted to their general purpose and the context of use of technologies that are being developed.

### 12.3.3.2 Different Applications and Quality Control of Services

One entrance point to finding requirements is the market introduction (in a broad sense) of services enabled by the BAN concept. While there are existing regulations such as various medical device directives (e.g., Medical Device Directive 93/42/EEG), new applications of BAN in some cases can be seen as medical services (e.g., monitoring of patients with increased risk of heart failure) rather than just devices, and the quality and the management of the service in itself is important to consider. This is challenging because many of these so-called e-Health services are yet under development and might adopt many different forms and sizes. Other applications, for instance, related to lifestyle management and preventive care, can also be provided by private parties, such as sport consulting firms, which can provide preventive advises on the basis of monitoring the performances of their clients. The motivation to, and success of, market introduction is linked to capturing a share of the health-care market: in general, to have a business model that allows a return on investment (in a broad sense) and acquiring a reputation for good service delivery. Some cooperation with health-care professionals will be necessary because of their role in defining the indications of good service. However, there are uncertainties with regard to whether the applications of BAN should be embedded into clinical practice (and perhaps insurance provision). Our investigation and interviews with the medical professionals in the Netherlands suggest that the use of mobile health applications should be well thought out, and medical professionals have to be included in the service provision to meet requirements with regard to efficiency, patient safety, and quality. They further articulated that the evaluation of functioning of technologies in the health-care setting does not only relate to technical characteristics of devices; much more fundamental in the medical professionals' view is whether these applications contribute to the quality of care provided to the patients and its impact on the welfare and health state of the patients. Therefore, the medical professionals we have interviewed called for a more critical consideration and raised the question of whether the various envisioned applications of BAN that enable lifestyle monitoring fit into the general health and welfare policy. For this question to be answered, effort is needed to make such measurement devices evidence based from a clinical standpoint, and connections to those different strategies have to be developed for coaching and guidance of individuals from their health-care professionals. Health-care professionals argue that this is important because if such applications are openly available via the consumer markets, people would be using such applications without a prior understanding of the usefulness of the resulting data.

### 12.3.3.3 Context of Use of BAN Applications and Responsibilities

As mentioned before, the context in which applications of BAN will be used will also have impact on the implementation in the health-care setting. One productive distinction can be made between patients that require short-term monitoring, or long-term monitoring from remote locations (outside the hospital). Early discharge from the hospital is expected to enhance the efficiency of health care and improve quality because patients are allowed to recover at their own living environment where they feel more comfortable. In this context, our interviewees at the hospital have mentioned that in case short-term monitoring of the patient is required, the hospital often provides the necessary equipment. Information provision to the patient is then key to ensuring that the patient is well instructed and has the skills that are necessary for handling the equipment. Further articulation of their tasks and responsibilities is important. It is also essential that roles and responsibilities are well articulated in protocols. It is also envisioned that a monitoring center either in the hospital or an independent one to which the care process of the hospital is connected has to be capable of dealing with data collection and calamities. Considering this, a productive way of educating/training medical professionals is required so they are fully competent and capable of operating different equipment and interpreting the data generated by that equipment. In a health-care system, such as that in the Netherlands where there is a division of labor between the first, second, and third line of care, clear agreements (protocols) are needed between consultants at the hospital and general practitioners (GPs) and social care providers if shifts in responsibilities and arrangement in care process are to take place.

For patients with chronic disorders and high-risk patients for whom continuous monitoring can contribute to early diagnosis or better treatment management (e.g., through monitoring the effect of certain drugs on the condition of the patient), it is not yet clear who will be responsible for the provision of the monitoring equipment. This has to be assessed for each application. Monitoring and treatment of different disorders (e.g., chronic illnesses such as diabetes and heart failure) rely on a good working relationship between the hospital, home-care service, pharmacists, and GPs. Such chain arrangements of care do not easily fit into the existing funding schemes of health-care insurances, and thus cause considerable bureaucratic problems that might hamper diffusion of innovation. In addition, the communication and coordination of actions between different professionals has to be articulated in standard protocols that require early interaction between health-care professionals and the medical device industry.

### 12.3.3.4 Burden of Responsibilities for User

For many of the visionary applications to be enabled by the BAN concept (see Jones et al. 2007 and Holst Centre 2007 for some visionary applications applied to health-care settings), the tasks, roles, and responsibilities of patients will inevitably change compared with the health-care monitoring setting being applied today. The vision that encompasses monitoring and care provision on mobile locations offers different new possibilities and opportunities to enhance user independence. It is further envisioned that applications of BAN contribute to patient empowerment (in terms of enabling users to take responsibility and control over their own care) and integration of the user in society because they are not expected to spend much time in the medical institutions anymore. Yet, a question has to be raised about patient compliance. The patient will eventually have to use the technology in a proper manner to achieve results. If mistakes happen, for instance because the user was not in a condition to react or just because of miscommunication, the eventual impact may be irreversible. A problem that pertains is that determining such mistakes is not easy after the fact because there are many technologies and actors involved, which is why clear norms need to be applied to the procedures for use of these technologies.

The distinction between different applications and categories of patients mentioned in the previous section is also important to consider here. We will take the two examples of patients who need to be discharged from the hospital early and need to be monitored for irregularities, and the chronically ill patients who would use such technologies to monitor their vital signs so that the professionals can get a more clear picture of their health dynamics to make better diagnosis decisions and to make more adequate decisions for the management of treatment trajectory.

The first category of patients, generally, will have to develop new skills to cope with the technology that they wear and operate. For instance, patients would be required to learn new skills for measuring their blood glucose, or hearing the heart sounds of their unborn baby, or, for epilepsy patients, knowing what they have to do when they receive an alarm before having an attack. These situations require the user of the technologies to accept new responsibilities. One example of such responsibility is that the user should be in a position where data can be transferred via wireless signals. The user should also make sure that the mobile gateway unit, which might be their mobile phone, functions well and transfers the data timely, and finally they have to be able to understand what they have to do if something goes wrong. The role of informing the user on these responsibilities is often on the shoulder of the medical professionals. However, in our interviews, medical professionals suggest that this can be a very time-consuming task in the case of patients who need to use the technology for a limited period after certain medical interventions. In contrast, chronically ill patients are most often well informed about their illnesses and can cope with using assistive technologies in an easier manner because they will be using these technologies for the longer run. Still, consultation with medical professionals about different possible technological solutions and what might fit the individual situation better is an important issue to be considered if efficient solutions are to be delivered.

The issue of trust and dependency of the user to the application is also an element to be considered. One of our interviewees who was involved in the evaluation of a pilot project on BAN for monitoring cardiovascular patients, mentioned that after the pilot study, some of the patients with heart disorders who were given mobile monitoring devices were not willing to take distance from the equipment at the end of the pilot trajectory because it gave them a certain feeling of confidence, safety, and security.

At the moment, there are also different endeavors to develop and provide technologies (that enable monitoring of vital signs on a remote location) also outside the setting of health-care supervision that include lifestyle management services. The health-care professionals interviewed in this study have shown concerns about how services in this setting are defined. They argued that provision of medical services should not have profitability as its basic goals but rather provision of a high-quality service, which is based on adequate indication and analysis of facts and professional medical insight. Thus, if such services are delivered through private companies, then commercial interests will become important, which might undermine the focus on high-quality health-care for the patient. A possible negative impact of such a construct anticipated from the view of one medical professional was the risk that commercial parties select the patients who do not require lots of attention and leave the patients that require more intensive attention to the public sector. Furthermore, it was argued that medical professionals have the exclusive knowledge and experience that is required to judge the situation and determine the norms and quality of care that needs to be delivered and therefore should always function as a gateway.

Another important concern that was collectively raised by the medical professionals relates to the risk of "medicalization" of worried healthy people. It was argued that without relevant indication, the usability of monitoring devices is pointless and can even cause unnecessary anxiety with regard to the health state. The issue of increasing concern that patients and citizens are not always capable of making the right choices with regard to what kind of care/services they need leaves an open policy question to be addressed for the future of health-care reforms. Should the government take necessary actions to protect citizens against taking wrong decisions, or in light of the increasing shift of responsibility to citizens, just allow them to make independent choices?

### 12.3.3.5 Quality and Safety Aspects

Safety and quality of care are important factors that shape the acceptance of technologies by different actors. In our investigation, almost all actors interviewed believe that the safety and quality of care are fundamental requirements to the acceptance of health-care technologies in general and becomes particularly important when transition takes place toward an arrangement that involves monitoring on distance. Problems can arise, for example, because of lack of protocols and agreements, instructions for users, or recording system failures. Such issues should be investigated well before introduction, and responsibilities should be allocated and accepted by all parties involved. Related to this, the limited role of technology in training and teamwork skills of the medical professionals is problematic. The care process in terms of planning and communication can be enhanced by means of the technologies that are being developed; however, its success is dependent on the concurrent development with teamwork processes and organizational factors as part of the operational structure. Such factors are important because a noteworthy amount of work that leads to the success of technologies is embedded in the teamwork and invisible work carried out behind delivering that care (Oudshoorn 2007). Also, it should be noticed that the design of health-care services that require multidisciplinary cooperation in the health-care chain should consider the business models of the different professionals, and funding schemes have to be developed so that all parties involved do get a fare share of income.

An important feature that plays an integral role in the advancement of BAN concept and its applications in health care is the capability of the systems to become context aware (see Aarts and Roovers 2003). This means that advances in technology will enable the information infrastructure of the BAN device to recognize and react to the real-world context of the user/ patient, including the identity of the user, its physical location, and if necessary also the activities that are being undertaken by the user. As these monitoring devices become more responsive, more responsibilities are delegated and incorporated to the technology. All forms of remote care involve the replacement of clinical and nursing observations by sensor-generated readings and wireless data exchange. In many forms, the technology also has an incorporated interpretation function. One example is the envisioned application of BAN for monitoring epilepsy patients (Holst Centre 2007). The BAN application in this case will incorporate sensor nodes integrated in wearables such as hats or caps. The sensors will be capable to communicate wirelessly with a mobile gateway unit, which can be the mobile phone of the patient. The data that are sent (e.g., EEG) are interpreted via software in a way to anticipate on a possible seizure in advance. This way the patient can be alarmed in time and instructions can be sent to prepare the patient for the attack (cf. to search for a safe place). This application has its added value in creating more freedom and independence, and should bring more comfort to the life of an epilepsy patient. However, the reliability of the software program that interprets data should be guaranteed. What happens if a seizure goes undetected owing to some kind of system failure and the patient comes into a tragic accident? The lack of legal framework and guidelines in this respect can have dramatic impacts in case an accident happens.

### 12.3.3.6 Issue of Responsibility and Availability in Multiactor e-Health Platforms

Related to the issue of safety and responsibility, it should be mentioned that future envisioned e-health platforms will not be exclusively delivered by the traditional actors in the health-care chain, such as the medical devices industry, hospitals, GPs, and health-care insurance companies. Many other industries such as the mobile network providers, health and wellness consultancies, and even cable companies, housing institutions, and companies specialized in installing home automation equipment see opportunities to be involved in delivering services. As the future scene in the health-care industry becomes more crowded, the roles and responsibilities that have to be fulfilled and allocated to different actors become highly complex to manage and as a result quality control might become more difficult to realize. All interviewees have highlighted the utmost importance of developing protocols and clear descriptions of responsibilities before services can be delivered. Because the field of BAN is only emerging, the issues of responsibilities and legal obligations are not clearly defined. This causes many actors to remain in a "waiting game," or not move away from pilot settings. An eventual outcome might be that such projects only remain in pilot settings and at best become available in regional settings. In this sense, access to mobile health services might remain limited to certain regions. Unequal access is an issue that is difficult to avoid, but if not anticipated on, can have negative impacts. Our interviewees from health care and health-care insurance background anticipated that BAN might remain limited to niches because not enough patients can subscribe to ensure profitability in the long run. The problem of scale of implementation is difficult to deal with and will remain an issue so long as monitoring equipment is not widely used and is not eligible for reimbursement. The majority of the stakeholders we have interviewed mentioned that patient organizations can play a vital role in the development processes and active cooperation with the medical device industries. The arguments that were put forward were twofold. First, it was argued that patient organizations have access to incredible amount of knowledge and experience with regard to patient needs in specific contexts. This in turn can contribute to the design process. Second, it was argued that patient organizations have the power to promote proven medical applications via their channels to patients.

### 12.3.3.7 *Privacy and Security Aspects of Medical Data*

Various publications have appeared that warn about security and privacy aspects related to the vision of ambient intelligence, the most prominent of which is the series of publications by the IST advisory group (ISTAG) on safeguards that needs to be considered in the design of different technological applications in a world of ambient intelligence (ISTAG 2001). This has caused privacy issues to appear seriously on research agendas to deploy various safeguards and privacy-enhancing mechanisms in the development of various applications, including those of BAN. Thus, privacy is certainly an issue that needs further elaboration with regard to applications of BAN, especially in health-care settings. The question of access to medical data by different stakeholders is important to consider. The first consideration is that for privacy reasons, it is generally required that medical data of patients be transferred in a secure manner. Furthermore, the transfer of data needs to take place reliably to enable correct interpretation by health-care professionals. Our interviews with different experts involved in the MobiHealth project (see Jones et al. 2007) in the Netherlands suggest that there are still some technical challenges involved in developing such a secure infrastructure (cf. energy consumption and availability of reliable bandwidth resources). For a subject like privacy protection, cooperation and involvement of all stakeholders is considered significant. However, it is the large number of involved stakeholders that makes the process of coordination complex to manage. Access to medical records by unauthorized parties can have serious consequences for individuals; however, as more responsibilities are allocated along the health-care chain, it becomes more difficult to restrict access by different parties. Serious impacts like theft of identity information and utilizing it for criminal purposes or strategic reasons (think of employers being interested in the medical records of their employees or applicants) can cause serious problems for individuals in society.

Besides safe transfer of medical data, at the same time health insurance companies have particular interest in data generated by monitoring technologies because it can potentially give them more control over their long-term expenditures and over patient behavior and lifestyles and their compliance to medical advice. In our interviews, it has been anticipated that in light of cutting health-care costs, one possibility is that health-care insurance companies will become interested in the data in return for reimbursement options (as a new business model). More specific, two options have been mentioned during our interviews. One possibility was related to rewarding patients for their healthy lifestyles and compliancy with medical advice in return for access to their medical data. These business models might have benefits in terms of empowering the society to become more aware of their responsibilities for their own health, thereby tackling the roots of costs of health care (also by promoting preventive health care); however, at the same time, it also means that the risk of violating the privacy of individuals is increasing. This situation can become controversial, for example, if individuals refuse using these technologies in the long term.

The other strategy mentioned in the interviews was related to rewarding medical professionals for their performance results (payment on the basis of result). There is already more transparency required from health-care institutions in the Netherlands (KPN 2006). It is argued that such transparency will enhance the quality of care delivered by several health-care institutions that are functioning in this sector. In effect, this might contribute to the competitive drive of these institutions in the market. However, shifting reimbursement strategies toward result-based payment can have serious negative impacts. For instance, one of our interviewee's in the health-care sector mentioned that such strategies might affect the business models of health-care professionals to shift weighing commercial incentives stronger than humanitarian incentives while delivering their services. This undermines the whole notion of equal access to health care and can have serious consequences for society.

Another issue related to compliance with medical advice. The envisioned applications of BAN are usually intended to monitor vital physiological signs, assuming that the context is according to normal conditions of living and in compliance with specific medical advice. However, it should be considered that the main target groups, such as seniors and patients with chronic illnesses, do not necessarily live healthy lifestyles all the time. The capability of BAN applications to monitor and identify unhealthy lifestyle or behavior then becomes intrusive. The interesting question to be posed here are as follows: If detected by the monitoring system, should people be held responsible for their noncompliance to certain advice? Can people also refuse to use these technologies in the long term? Or is it desirable if professionals or health-care insurance companies label the individual as noncompliant and refuse health-care support? These questions need to be considered in public and policy debates, which are ongoing anyhow.

### 12.3.3.8 Modes of Reimbursement

In the Netherlands, health-care insurance companies are obliged to provide a statutory basic health-care policy to all Dutch citizens, the content of which is determined under the supervision of the Dutch Health Care Insurance Board (CVZ).* For medical services to be taken up in the basic health-care insurance policy, the CVZ will look at several issues such as the urgency in need, the effectiveness in terms of fulfilling the promise (evidence-based), and the cost-effectiveness (in terms of balance between costs and benefits). For the applications of BAN being developed for monitoring purposes, it is unclear how urgent and effective such applications are and will be. Our interviews suggest that actors in the innovation chain of the health-care collectively agree that there is a clear need for more and stronger cooperation between medical education institutes with scientific and industrial community to determine the usability and effectiveness of different envisioned applications of BAN already in early stages of development. The main argument that was mentioned frequently in our interviews was that early cooperation between health-care professionals and scientific/industrial community who are developing such applications can lead to a better assessment of the evidence for the functioning and benefits of specific devices.

Early cooperation between the medical community (e.g., academic institutions for primary health care) and the medical devices industry could also function as a productive strategy to ensure funding schemes in the future. Added value in terms of quality of life is an important requirement in reimbursement decision making. Almost all our interviewees who were involved in the development of BAN concepts mentioned to face challenges with regard to proving the added value of devices in terms of quality of life. In our interviews with medical education institutes, it became clear that there are various methods available on the table to tackle such challenges. However, due to limited interaction, such methods were never applied. This point makes the early cooperation with medical institutions to be considered seriously. The argument is that if devices have been proven to work on the basis of medical studies, the medical community and the industry can then approach health-care insurers to adopt these technologies in their policies. Adopting proven services would bring added value to the clients of

---

* The CVZ coordinates the implementation and funding of the Cure Insurance Act (Zvw) and the Exceptional Medical Expenses Act (AWBZ). The CVZ adopts an independent position: in between policy and practice on the one hand, and in between the central government and the health insurers, care providers, and citizens on the other (http://www.cvz.nl/english).

health-care insurances through which they can strengthen their competitive advantage within the health-care insurance market to attract more clients.

Finally, early cooperation can then be effective in highlighting the incentives for the adoption of technologies, and the added value in clinical processes becomes clearer to the professional users. In this manner, specific user values can also be considered in the design process of new applications of BAN.

The involvement of medical education institutions can also be valuable in terms of early cooperation in protocol development and standardization processes that are imperative to the social embedding of technologies in the clinical setting. Thus, a choice has to be made by the actors involved in development processes of BAN applications: wait until development has reached a state of maturation and then try to link up with interested techno-savvy medical professionals and provide shattered courses (relying on professionals to link up with the promises in later stages of development), or to engage in early cooperation with basic and specialized medical education institutes, and instead of offering shattered educational programs, establish a concerted effort to integrate these developments in medical education, and also collaborate in research to highlight key issues for the professionals.

## 12.4 Conclusion

In this chapter, we have taken up the challenge of anticipating on broader aspects that are relevant for the social embedment of the BAN concept in the health-care sector of the Netherlands. We have presented our analysis of possible social, ethical, and legal impacts of BAN applications on the basis of literature research and interviews with relevant actors along the value chain. This has further enabled us to draw on various social, political, and ethical implications, which might affect alignments at different levels.

The main message this chapter conveys is that early consideration of various social, ethical, and legal issues is imperative to the quality of the innovation process and social embedding of its eventual products in a specific context. What happens usually is that, on the one hand, scientists continuously develop new knowledge and resources. In the early stages, expectations clearly present the value of technologies under development. Promises and expectations become inflated to attract attention (Figure 12.3). On the other hand, firms, industrial actors, and policy makers are confronted by promises (sometimes this results in excitement but often also in concerns) and have to decide what to do about them (Figure 12.3). Quality control of expectations is crucial here because misjudging expectations might have great implications later in the innovation process.

This is because actors, in reaching their endeavors, tend to project linear maps of the future and often in the enthusiasm about the new idea they

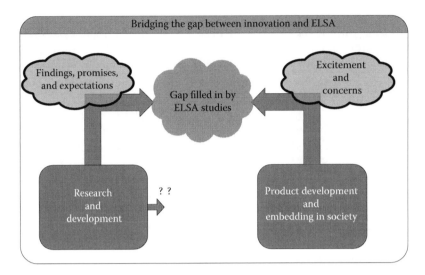

**FIGURE 12.3**
Bridging the gap between innovation and ethical, legal, and social aspects (ELSA).

forget to take other requirements, for instance, how to manage the social embedding of technologies, into account. The technical and legal infrastructure that has to be put in place, the ethical questions that must be addressed, and the wider public acceptance of a technology are most often left to the end of the innovation process where the situation has become rigid and flexibility for change has been reduced.

Identification of social, ethical, and legal aspects in early stages as presented in this chapter can provide a platform for further discussion for scientists, policymakers, managers, and other stakeholders. Early interaction can lead to further articulation of key (techno-institutional) design requirements that can guide an optimal social-embedding process of the applications of BAN. Our claim is that taking broader sets of actors and aspects into account in the early stages will enable more informed strategic assessments and decisions. This in turn enables making more reflexive choices. This is important because until existing and emerging issues cannot be addressed in the affirmative, the clear implication will be uncertainty, waiting games, and barriers to further embedment processes.

## References

Aarts E and Roovers R. IC design challenges for ambient intelligence, in *Proceedings of the Design, Automation and Test IEEE Computer Society in Europe Conference and Exhibition*, IEEE 1530–1591/2003, 2003.

Amara R et al. *Health and Health Care 2010: The Forecast, the Challenge*, Second edition, Grosel C, Hamilton M, Koyano J, and Eastwood S (eds.), Prepared by the Institute for the Future, Princeton, NJ, 2003.

Bomhoff EJ. Meer Markt in de Gezondheidszorg, Mogelijkheden en Beperkingen. Background Study by the Dutch Health Council, 2002.

Den Boer D, Rip A, and Speller S. Scripting possible futures of nanotechnologies: A methodology which enhances reflexivity. *Technology in Society* 31(3), 295–304, 2009.

Deuten J, Rip A, and Jelsma J. Societal embedding and product creation management. *Technology Analysis and Strategic Management* 9, 131–148, 1997.

Flim C. De bakens moeten worden verzet, in *ICT-zorg*, 8th year edition, Nr. 4, July–August 2007, pp. 14–15, 2008.

Garud R and Ahlstrom D. Technology assessment: A socio-cognitive perspective. *Journal of Engineering and Technology Management* 14, 25–48, 1997.

Gyselinckx B et al. *Human++: Autonomous Wireless Sensors for Body Area Networks*, IMEC Belgium, 2008.

Gyselinckx B et al. HUMAN++: Emerging technology for body area networks, in *IEEE, IFIP International Conference*, 2006, ISBN: 3-901882-19-7.

Hatcher M and Heetebry I. Information technology in the future of healthcare. *Journal of Medical Systems Issue* 28(6), 673–688, 2004.

Healthcare IT Management. *Country Focus: The Netherlands*, 2(1), 42 p., Spring 2007, ISSN: 1782-8406. www.hitm.eu.

Holst Centre. *Roads Into the Future*. Fletterman, A. (Composition). First edition. Holst Centre, 2007.

ISTAG Scenarios. *Scenarios for Ambient Intelligence in 2010*, Edited by IPTS-ISTAG (Ducatel K et al. (eds.)), IPTS, Seville, 2001.

Jones VM, Bults R, Konstantas D, and Vierhout P. Body area networks for healthcare, in *Proceedings Wireless World Research Forum Meeting*, Stockholm, September 17–18, 2001.

Jones VM, van Halteren A, Konstantas D, Widya L, and Bults R. An application of augmented MDA for the extended healthcare enterprise, *International Journal of Business Process Integration and Management, (IJBPIM)*, ISSN (Print): 1741-8763, ISSN (Online): 1741-8771, Inderscience Publishers (www.inderscience.com), Editor-in-Chief: Frank Leymann, University of Stuttgart, Germany, Liang-Jie (LJ) Zhang, IBM T.J. Watson Research Center, USA, 2(3), 215–229, October 21, 2007, DOI: 10.1504/IJBPIM.2007.015496, http://dx.doi.org/10.1504/IJBPIM.2007.015496.

KPN. Sneller Beter Innovatie en ICT in Curatieve Zorg. Zorg Voor Innovatie!, Eindrapportage KPN, 2006.

Oudshoorn N. Diagnosis at a distance: The invisible work of patients and healthcare professionals in cardiac telemonitoring technology. *Sociology of Health and Illness* 30(2), 272–288, 2007.

Parandian A. Nanotechnology in healthcare. Master thesis (January 2006). Delft University of Technology (Section: Technology Dynamics and Sustainable Development), Delft, 65 p., 2006.

Penders J, Gyselinckx B, Vullers R, Rousseaux O, Berekovic M, De Nil M, van Hoof C, Ryckaert J, Yazicioglu RF, Fiorini P, and Leonov V. VLSI-SoC: Research trends in VLSI and systems on chip, in De Micheli G, Mir S, and Reis R (eds.). *IFIP International Federation for Information Processing*, Volume 249, Springer, Boston, pp. 377–397, 2007.

Rip A and Te Kulve H. Constructive technology assessment and socio-technical scenarios, in Fisher E et al. (eds.). *Yearbook of Nanotechnology in Society*, Volume 1,
Dordrecht: Springer, 2008.

Rip A, Misa T, and Schot J. *Managing Technology in Society: The Approach of Constructive
Technology Assessment*, Pinter, London, 1995.

Schot JW and Rip A. The past and the future of constructive technology assessment.
*Technological Forecasting and Social Change* 54(2–3), 251–268, 1997, ISSN 00401625.

van Hoof C. More than Moore and heterogeneous integration, in Doorn M (ed.).
*Converging Technologies*, Study Centre for Technological Trends, The Hague, STT
Netherlands, 200 p., 2006.

Zhang GQ, Graef M, and van Roosmalen F. The rationale and paradigm of "More
than Moore," in *IEEE Proceedings. 56th Electronic Components and Technology
Conference*, 2006, ISBN: 1-4244-0152-6.

Zimmerman TG. Wireless networked devices: A new paradigm for computing and
communication. *IBM Systems Journal* 38(4), 1999.

# 13

# Capability Approach to Nanotechnology for Sustainable Development*

Ineke Malsch

## CONTENTS

---

* This has also been published as Chapter 5 in the author's PhD thesis "Ethics and Nano-technology; Responsible development of nanotechnology at global level in the 21st century," Radboud University, October 4, 2011, www.nanoarchive.org/11110.

## 13.1 Introduction

In this chapter, the capability approach as proposed by Martha Nussbaum and Amartya Sen is used for analyzing government strategies for nanotechnology development in a number of Latin American countries, including Brazil, Mexico, and Argentina. The intention is to contribute to deeper insights on sustainable development of nanotechnology beyond the often-cited Millennium Development Goals (MDG) of the United Nations (UN General Assembly 2000).

In the current debate on nanotechnology for sustainable development, the UN MDG play a key role in selecting relevant nanotechnologies and applications that may contribute to halving poverty in the world by 2015. Such applications include nanofood, sustainable energy, water purification and desalination, environmental technologies, and nanomedicine (e.g., Mnyusiwalla et al. 2003; Salamanca-Buentello et al. 2005; Meridian Institute, 2004, 2007; Malsch 2005). This discussion of nanotechnology for the poor is complemented by a broader debate on strategic implications of nanotechnology and its applications for the socioeconomic development of less developed countries. In this debate on the nano-divide,* issues like these have been discussed by the Meridian Institute, the ETC group, and Foladori and Invernissi:

- Implications of nanotechnology for resource efficiency and the world market for commodities
- Intellectual property rights of nanotechnology-based inventions
- The balance between who reaps the benefits and who carries the risks

The current debate on nanotechnology for development has been summarized by Malsch (2008b).

In the area of political philosophy, Amartya Sen (1985, 1999, 2009), Nussbaum and Sen (1993) and Martha Nussbaum (2006) have developed the capability approach as a conceptual framework for evaluating how governments contribute to human wellbeing. The capability approach is based on John Rawls' Theory of Justice (1999). In this chapter, the conceptual framework will be introduced by discussing relevant elements of Rawls' theory and the contributions and adaptations made by Sen and Nussbaum. Nussbaum (2006) divides the capability approach into 10 capabilities: life; bodily health; bodily integrity; senses, imagination, and thought; emotions; practical reason; affiliation; other species; play; and control over one's environment.

The capability approach has been applied in political philosophy and economics. Anand and colleagues (2008) have developed indicators to measure

---

* The nano-divide is a technology gap between countries or individuals with access to nanotechnology and those without it.

capabilities in order to assess the socioeconomic policy of countries. The capability approach is also applied in the Human Development Index (HDI), used by the UN Development Programme (UNDP) for ranking countries on their "achievement in attaining a long and healthy life, access to knowledge; and a decent standard of living" (UNDP 2006).

In the present chapter, the capability approach will be applied to evaluate nano science, technology, and innovation (ST&I) policies in or in cooperation with developing countries and emerging economies. Are current national nanotechnology programs expected to contribute to better distributive justice as proposed by Martha Nussbaum? This adaptation of the capability approach is expected to enable a longer time horizon and a more encompassing assessment of the potential long-term implications of nanotechnology for sustainable development.

## 13.2 Theory of Justice and Capability Approach

### 13.2.1 Theory of Justice according to John Rawls

In 1971, the American philosopher John Rawls (1921–2002) first published his comprehensive theory of justice. The revision published in 1999 incorporates a response to comments and criticism. Rawls' theory of justice is grounded in the utilitarian ethical tradition, which he criticizes from the perspective of social contract thinking. Utilitarian ethics can be characterized by the aim "the greatest good for the greatest number of people." Rawls is concerned with the question of how a fair distribution of common goods among individuals can be argued in a theory of social distributive justice. Social contract thinkers like Locke, Rousseau, and Kant propose that the institutions of a just state should be based on a theoretical social contract among the citizens of that state. Society is interpreted as a form of cooperation to mutual advantage of the citizens. To build up his theory of justice, Rawls assumes an original position in which all individual citizens involved in the contract have no information on their social position, whether they are rich or poor, which talents and resources are available to them, or in which age they live. This information is hidden from them by a "veil of ignorance." In this original position, it is assumed that the contracting parties will adopt two principles of justice:

1. Principle of Equal Liberty: Each person is to have an equal right to the most extensive scheme of equal basic liberties compatible with a similar scheme of liberties for others.

2. Difference Principle: Social and economical inequalities are to be arranged so that

a. They are to be of the greatest benefit of the least-advantaged members of society, consistent with the just savings principle

b. Offices and positions must be open to all under conditions of fair equality of opportunity (Rawls 1999).

First rule of priority (priority of liberty): The principles of justice are to be ranked in a lexical order; hence, the fundamental liberties can only be restricted for the sake of liberty. Rawls distinguishes two cases:

1. A reduced liberty should strengthen the total system of liberties shared by all.
2. A less than equal liberty must be acceptable for those with a reduced freedom.

Second rule of priority (priority of justice over efficiency and welfare): The second principle of justice is lexically before the principle of efficiency and of maximizing the sum of advantages, and the principle of equal opportunities is before the difference principle. There are two cases:

1. An inequality of opportunities must improve the opportunities of the persons with less opportunities.
2. An excessive savings quote must in general reduce the burden of the ones bearing these costs (Rawls 2009, p. 321).

It is assumed that all contracting parties have physical needs and psychological faculties within the normal range, excluding issues of health-care and intellectual abilities (Rawls 2009, p. 133). Rawls does not postulate independent criteria for choosing a concept of justice but considers it necessary that the contracting individuals choose the optimal concept of justice in the original position in which they are covered by the veil of ignorance. The theory of justice as fairness also presupposes that the contracting parties are in circumstances of justice, where there are limited resources to be distributed and conflicts of interest between the contracting parties (Rawls 2009, pp. 162–163).

A number of boundary conditions for the concept of right are distinguished. A concept of right is a collection of principles general in form and universal in application, which must be recognized publicly as the highest authority for ranking the conflicting claims of moral persons. Principles of justice are determined on the basis of their special role and the object they are applicable to (Rawls 2009, p. 167).

### 13.2.2 Idea of Justice according to Amartya Sen

Amartya Sen is an Indian economist and winner of the Nobel Prize for Economics in 1998, who builds upon Rawls' theory of justice in a critical way. His main criticism is that Rawls' theory prescribes an ideal just society, and is not suitable for ranking different imperfect systems on their relative justice. Sen's idea of justice aims to do just that. He stresses the role of public reasoning in different cultural traditions (Western as well as non-Western), in determining how a particular society can become less unjust. Whereas Rawls proposes to let the people who will live in a particular society close a social contract under the veil of ignorance, Sen favors an impartial observer who can judge fairness of a society from a position of positional objectivity. This is necessary to overcome parochialism and address questions of global justice (Sen 2009).

In Sen's concept, divergent views on what is the more just solution in a particular case are allowed. Contrary to conventional economic theory, rationality is not limited to furthering one's own personal interests. People who want to promote the common good or the interests of other people can also be considered to maximize these interests in an economically rational way. The materials of justice are not public goods, as Rawls states, but capabilities of individual persons that should be developed in a just societal arrangement.

Sen's Idea of Justice is a comparative system for ranking different actual societies on being more or less just according to different preferences. These preferences cannot all be ranked in one single closed ordering with one single optimum. Instead, it is possible to use the system for comparing two particular societies on their comparative justness in accordance with a particular set of preferences. The identification of redressable injustice is central to Sen's theory of injustice, starting from an intuitive sense of justice. In addition, there is a need for a formal theory of justice to enable reasoning about our intuition and critically examining the intuition and what we can do to overcome the perceived injustice. What kind of reasoning is appropriate for ethical and political concepts like (in)justice? An impartial observer is allowed to comment on the justness of a particular society, rather than limiting this to the people who will live in that society. There is a clear role for rationality and reasonableness (Sen 2009).

Grounds for judgments of justice could be freedoms, capabilities, resources, happiness, or wellbeing. Sen's idea of justice assumes a connection between justice and democracy. It is not enough to establish just institutions, but we must examine how these institutions and people's behavior influence other people's lives. The focus should be on the lives people are able to lead and on their freedoms. Democracy is defined as government by discussion. It also encompasses the capacity to enrich reasoned engagement through enhancing informational ability and the feasibility of interactions. It is not just about institutions but also about enabling people to be heard. At the global level, democracy can be seen as the possibility and reach of public reasoning. Advancing global democracy and justice is an understandable ambition and can inspire concrete actions (Sen 2009).

Sen's concept of justice is placed in the tradition of Western enlightenment, but similar ideas can be found in non-Western traditions. One example is the

Indian concept of institutional and behavioral justice, *niti,* versus the concept of justness of the actual lives people lead, *nyaya*. There are two enlightenment traditions. First, social contract thinking concentrates on the institutions of justice. Second, the comparative tradition compares different ways of life, influenced by institutions and actual behavior of others, social interactions, etc. The social choice theory developed by Condorcet (1785) and Arrow (1951) belongs to the comparative tradition. Both traditions rely to a great extent on (practical) reason. Sen believes that good public reasoning for more justice should help overcome bad parochial reasoning. He maintains that there is not one single best way because different positions can be equally reasonably defended.

In earlier writings, Amartya Sen has developed the capability approach, together with Martha Nussbaum. He builds on this in formulating his Idea of Justice. Nussbaum's conceptualization of the capability approach is more elaborate than Sen's. Therefore, only Nussbaum's formulation and discussion of the implications of the capability approach for global justice will be presented below.

### 13.2.3 Philosophical Basis of Martha Nussbaum's Capability Approach

In *Frontiers of Justice* (2006), the American philosopher Martha Nussbaum builds upon theories of justice in the tradition of social contract thinking, mainly Rawls' theory. She explicitly discusses the concepts proposed by other philosophers than Rawls, which she uses in her own capability approach. In this section, the contributions of these other philosophers will be sketched in order to enable a better understanding of Nussbaum's theory outlined below.

In general, social contract theories assume an original natural position in which all humans are free, equal, and independent. These individuals will only agree to limits to their freedom in a mutual social contract intended to achieve the benefits of communal life, including comfort, safety and peace, and protection of their property rights (Locke, Second Treatise of Government, quoted in Nussbaum 2006, p. 23). David Hume introduces the idea of "circumstances of justice," developed further by Rawls. Incidentally, Hume is not a social contract thinker, but this idea is more fitting to Rawls' theory of justice than similar concepts from social contract thinkers (Nussbaum 2006, p. 25).

In Nussbaum's capability approach, she focuses on those who have not been involved in designing the social contract, including women, disabled persons, people in poor countries, and nonhuman animals.* In this regard, she disagrees with Rawls, according to whom people can only have access to justice if they are in the right circumstances of justice (free, equal, and independent). Rawls considers mutual benefit as the aim of societal cooperation and assumes that contracting parties are driven by their own interests. Nussbaum, on the other hand, points out that other relevant theories assume

---

* Nussbaum considers human beings to be rational animals, a concept borrowed from Aristotle.

different motivations for cooperating, including those of Grotius, Hobbes, and Locke. In the seventeenth century, Hugo Grotius developed a vision on the interdependence of nations. He argues that moral norms impose restrictions to the actions of all nations and individuals in the international society. Human rights of individuals may justify intervention in the internal affairs of other states. Determination of ownership of goods requires detailed examination because this depends on needfulness of the poor in one state and surplus in another state (Nussbaum 2006, p. 31).

Nussbaum wants to revive the natural law approach of the foundations of international affairs of Hugo Grotius. This natural law approach also offers a framework for considering internal affairs. In *De jure belli ac pacis*, Grotius (1625) founds the principles of international relations on human dignity and sociability in the tradition of the Greek and Roman STOA (Seneca and Cicero). Even though Grotius connects these aspects with a particular metaphysical theory of human nature, his approach can also form the basis of a political concept of the person that can be accepted by people with another vision on metaphysics and religion. Human dignity and sociability form the basis for certain specific rights and are necessary conditions for a humane life. Grotius focuses on the space between states, where there is no sovereign. This space is still morally ordered and some very specific principles shape human interactions in it. These principles inspired his interpretation of the "Ius ad Bellum" and the "Ius in Bello": starting a war is only justified in response to an unjustified act of aggression. Preventive war is prohibited as it is a way to use humans as instruments for the interest of others. During the war, strict rules have to be obeyed: no excessive or cruel punishment, no killing of civilians, minimal damage to property, and prompt restitution of property and sovereignty in ending a war. Interestingly, Grotius' theory starts with an outcome: the fundamental rights of people that must be respected in the name of justice. If these rights are respected, a society is minimally justified. This theory is based on an intuitive notion of human dignity, and explicitly not on mutual benefits (Nussbaum 2006, pp. 44–45).

Thomas Hobbes' *Leviathan* (1651) holds that there are natural moral laws that call for "justice, equality, fairness, charity and doing to others as we want others to do to us." These natural moral laws cannot form the basis of a stable political order because they are "in contradiction with our natural passions that lead us towards partisanship, pride, revenge, etc." Natural sociability can be observed among ants but not among humans. The natural state is a state of war. All humans are equal in capabilities and means in this natural state. In this state, our passions stimulate us to make peace so as to live securely to some extent. This social contract does not lead to justice. Hobbes does not have a clear vision on justice. In some places it can only be enforced, whereas elsewhere natural principles of justice exist but are ineffective, given our natural passions. The social contract generates the fundamental principles for a political society, as a mutual agreement to hand over political rights. Hobbes includes the contracting parties as well as those on whose behalf the contract is made, but excludes animals. Hobbes considers a state form with a sovereign who has been handed over all powers as the only attractive form of contract, enforcing security by imposing fear of punishment. Anywhere outside the realm of such sovereigns is characterized by a state of war (e.g., in international relations) (Nussbaum 2006, pp. 46–48).

John Locke's theory of the social contract contains several ideas used in Nussbaum's capability approach. In the natural state, people are free, equal, and independent. They are free in the sense that nobody rules over another person and that each has the right to govern oneself. They are equal in the sense that nobody has the right to rule over another person and that any jurisdiction is mutual. They are independent in the sense that all people have the right to further their own interests, without hierarchical relations. People have similar physical and mental capabilities that are connected to moral rights. Equal capabilities are sufficient grounds for a general status of each person to be considered a goal in oneself, rather than as a means to another end. Such equal capabilities also are a necessary precondition, because animals, lacking the same capabilities, can be used as means to an end according to Locke. Nussbaum does not include this in her theory. Locke distinguishes binding moral obligations in his natural state, including the obligation to maintain oneself and others, not to take another's life, and to abstain from damaging another's freedom, health, or property. The principle of moral equality leads to the obligation to charity and good will. A social contract is not a precondition for moral reciprocity. Humans also have a natural dignity because they are created by God. They are entitled to a dignified life, but are also needful and not able to realize such a life on one's own. They have a natural tendency to look for community and fraternity with others in political communities. Locke combines elements of a natural law theory that are similar to Grotius' ideas. However, Locke has also formulated the founding idea for the social contract. Even though the natural state is not necessarily a state of war, nothing outside a political society can prevent this natural state from falling into a state of war. Mutual benefit is the main goal for which the contracting parties agree to accept the authority of laws and institutions. Nussbaum builds upon the natural law elements in Locke's work and criticizes the social contract ideas (Nussbaum 2006, pp. 48–51).

David Hume (1739–1740, 1751, 1777) describes the circumstances under which justice is possible and necessary, inspiring Rawls. Hume bases his vision on justice on convention rather than contract thinking. Mutual benefit is again the key to the emergence and continuation of justice. According to Hume, justice is only possible in cases of a limited but not extreme lack of resources, where people are simultaneously selfish and competitive, and charitable to some extent, yet capable to impose limits to their behavior. He considers this to be the human situation in reality. Egoism is not all-powerful, but kindness is unbalanced and partisan, mostly in favor of one's own family and less favorable to more remote relations. Justice is a convention whose usefulness depends on the physical and psychological circumstances, including a global equality of capabilities between people. Hume excludes animals, people with severe mental or physical disabilities, and women from justice because they do not have more or less the same capabilities as healthy men in the society in which they live. Humane treatment of these outsiders would not be based on justice but on charity and hence would be unreliable (Nussbaum 2006, pp. 51–55).

In his essay "Über den Gemeinspruch Das mag in der Theorie richtig sein, taugt aber nicht für die Praxis" (1793) and in "Metaphysik der Sitten" (1797), Kant makes a combination of moral philosophy and social contract thinking. Nussbaum is interested in the tension inherent in his work, because Kant's moral philosophical notion that people must always be treated as goal in oneself and never as a means to an end is a core element of Rawls' theory of justice. Kant's theory of the social contract is essentially the same as Locke's. The natural state is characterized by natural, egalitarian freedom. The social contract is closed when people opt for a state of distributive legal justice. The contract is needed because justified claims are uncertain in the natural state. It is not only beneficial but also morally right for all persons to join the contract. In Kant's view, the free, equal, and independent contracting parties are the same citizens whose lives are governed by the contract. He distinguishes active and passive, dependent citizens. Only active citizens are included in the contract and have political rights. Passive citizens are subordinate to the state, but still have certain prepolitical human rights, including freedom and equality. By requiring that contracting parties should be approximately equal, Kant creates two classes of citizens. Some passive citizens may become active citizens, but this does not apply to women and the disabled (Nussbaum 2006, pp. 55–57).

Nussbaum insists on developing a broader concept of justice than assumed by the social contract thinkers, but does not explain why she thinks "justice" is more applicable to questions of dealing with the disabled, poor people in developing countries, and nonhuman animals than concepts like "charity." Her capability approach is a political theory about basic rights, not an all-encompassing moral theory, and not even a complete political theory (Nussbaum 2006, p. 139). She assumes that the capabilities or basic rights are already enclosed in the notion of human dignity and humane life. Her theory converges with ethical contract thinking but does not assume mutual benefit as driver for cooperation. Instead, benefits and goals of cooperation are morally and socially inspired, and justice and participation are aims with an intrinsic value. People are connected by altruistic bonds as well as by mutual benefit. Whereas contract thinking is a procedural theory, the capability approach is aimed at results.

Nussbaum applies a political concept of the person as proposed by Aristotle: the human being is a political animal, and strives for a social form of the good, sharing complex goals with others on many levels. Her concept of dignity is Aristotelian (rationality and animal nature are a whole), not Kantian (humanity is opposed to animal nature; rationality is opposed to needs shared by humans and animals). Nussbaum requires a theory of "the good" to determine preconditions for ethical contract thinking. Capabilities are an extension of the concepts of income and poverty as measures of wellbeing. People have different individual needs. This fact necessitates a plurality of measures for wellbeing. Contrary to Amartya Sen, Nussbaum does not consider it possible to measure all capabilities in monetary terms; however, her theory requires 10 independent threshold values to determine wellbeing. A diversified form of care is a fundamental aspect of the concept of justice for all capabilities. It depends on the capability whether it is necessary to stimulate the human capability or the human functioning. Enforcing behavior should be avoided but information on beneficial behavior is welcome. Children should have more obligations than adults (e.g., in following education).

The species norm Nussbaum uses to determine who is a human being is evaluative and ethical, but contrary to her assumption, is not uncontroversial. The capability approach is a critical liberal theory, imposing limits to freedom in the interest of society.

Nussbaum compares her capability approach with other theories of international justice: two types of social contract thinking (the two-phase contract of Rawls, and the global contract of Beitz and Pogge), as well as economic utilitarian development models. Her theory aims for human development in agreement with Grotius' natural right, taking human rights as basis for international justice. Rawls' two-phase contract theory takes the state as a virtual person and contract party. The internal affairs of a state are independent of foreign relations and unchanging. International law only covers war and peace. This assumption is not in agreement with present-day reality where multinational companies and international NGOs are of importance. The current inequality between states and redistribution of wealth also does not fit Rawls' assumption.

Nussbaum does not agree with Rawls' idea of a veil of ignorance at the time of designing the contract because the parties need to know in which age they live and what the (technical) circumstances are in order to be able to determine what will be a fair agreement in those circumstances.

### 13.2.4 Martha Nussbaum's Capability Approach

The capability approach concentrates on what people are capable of. It is expected to give more robust guidelines for jurisdiction and government policies than other theories of justice. Whereas Sen applies the capability approach to comparative measurement of the quality of life, Nussbaum uses it to give a philosophical foundation to a vision on essential human rights that ought to be respected and implemented by governments of all nations, as an essential minimum of what respect for human dignity requires. This notion leads to a list of 10 essential human capabilities, which are all implicitly present in the idea of a life in accordance with human dignity. These capabilities are the source of political principles for a liberal pluralist society. The capabilities should be pursued for each individual who is treated as a goal in himself and not as a means to an end. The capability approach assumes a threshold level for each human capability, below which normal human functioning is not possible. Government policies should aim to lift citizens above this threshold level (Nussbaum 2006, pp. 71–72).

The basic intuitive notion that forms the starting point of Nussbaum's capability approach is a concept of human dignity and a dignified human life and functioning. The central notion is the capabilities someone has to undertake activities rather than resources available to him because different individuals have different needs for resources to undertake the same activities (Nussbaum 2006, pp. 74–75).

The essential human capabilities according to Nussbaum (2006, pp. 76–77) are as follows:

- *Life.* Being able to live to the end of a human life of normal length; not dying prematurely, or before one's life is so reduced as to be not worth living.

- *Bodily health.* Being able to have good health, including reproductive health; to be adequately nourished; to have adequate shelter.

- *Bodily integrity.* Being able to move freely from place to place; to be secure against violent assault, including sexual assault and domestic violence; having opportunities for sexual satisfaction and for choice in matters of reproduction.

- *Senses, imagination, and thought.* Being able to use the senses, to imagine, think, and reason—and to do these things in a "truly human" way, a way informed and cultivated by an adequate education, including, but by no means limited to, literacy and basic mathematical and scientific training. Being able to use imagination and thought in connection with experiencing and producing works and events of one's own choice, religious, literary, musical, and so forth. Being able to use one's mind in ways protected by guarantees of freedom of expression with respect to both political and artistic speech, and freedom of religious exercise. Being able to have pleasurable experiences and to avoid nonbeneficial pain.

- *Emotions.* Being able to have attachments to things and people outside ourselves; to love those who love and care for us, to grieve at their absence; in general, to love, to grieve, to experience longing, gratitude, and justified anger. Not having one's emotional development blighted by fear and anxiety. […]

- *Practical reason.* Being able to form a conception of the good and to engage in critical reflection about the planning of one's life. […]

- *Affiliation.*
    i.  Being able to live with and toward others, to recognize and show concern for other humans, to engage in various forms of social interaction; to be able to imagine the situation of another. […]

ii.  Having the social bases of self-respect and nonhumiliation; being able to be treated as a dignified being whose worth is equal to that of others. This entails provisions of nondiscrimination on the basis of race, sex, sexual orientation, ethnicity, caste, religion, national origin, and species.

- *Other species.* Being able to live with concern for and in relation to animals, plants, and the world of nature.
- *Play.* Being able to laugh, to play, and to enjoy recreational activities.
- *Control over one's environment.*
  i.  *Political.* Being able to participate effectively in political choices that govern one's life; having the right of political participation, protections of free speech, and association.
  ii.  *Material.* Being able to hold property (both land and movable goods), and having property rights on an equal basis with others; having the right to seek employment on an equal basis with others; having the freedom from unwarranted search and seizure. In work, being able to work as a human, exercising practical reason, and entering into meaningful relationships of mutual recognition with other workers.

The capability approach is a type of universal human rights approach, which respects pluralism in six forms:

1. The list is open-ended.
2. The items must be specified in an abstract and generalizable way, to allow for national differences in implementation.
3. The list is a freestanding "partial moral conception," only used for political goals and without metaphysical foundation.
4. The right political target is the human capability rather than the corresponding functioning.
5. Pluralism protecting freedoms such as freedom of opinion, assembling, and of conscience are central items on the list.
6. Problems of justification and of implementation should be separated. State sovereignty should in principle be respected (Nussbaum 2006, pp. 78–79).

### 13.2.4.1 International Capability Approach

In her international capability approach, Nussbaum assumes that people possess an ethical reason and sociability. Cicero, the Roman Stoics, and Grotius have also assumed this before her. Humans are beings with a common good, striving to live together in a way that is ordered by the measure of their moral intelligence (human dignity, sociability, and human needs). There is discussion on what should have priority: rights (capabilities) or responsibilities. Also, there is no agreement on what counts as the basis for being entitled to certain rights: rationality, intelligence, or the fact that there is life. Are the rights prepolitical or an artifact of laws and institutions? The capability approach takes the existence as a human being as basis for rights, and assumes prepolitical rights. It also pleads for a proactive government role, not only withholding itself from intrusion on the rights of citizens but also actively promoting freedom. Nussbaum is against a world state because of the risk of a dictatorship without outside countervailing force. She favors national autonomy with foreign intervention. The responsibility for maintaining a threshold level for all capabilities should be assigned to institutions that can enforce cooperation from individuals (taxes, legislation). Above this threshold, individuals may follow their own conscience or group norms. Essential human rights must be incorporated in the national constitution of each country.

On an international level, a variety of actors share in the responsibility:

1. Government organizations with responsibility for international solidarity
2. Multinationals
3. Global economic policy and organizations
4. International organizations (UN, ILO, International Court, etc.)
5. NGOs

Adapting Nussbaum's approach to sustainable (nano)technology development requires addressing a somewhat different set of actors. In addition to government organizations with responsibility for international solidarity, government organizations with responsibility for ST&I policy have to be involved. The same goes for departments of international organizations, including UNIDO, UNESCO, but also regional intergovernmental bodies such as the European Commission DG Research. In addition to multinationals and (development) NGOs, universities and research centers as well as international academic organizations have to be called upon.

The international capabilities approach distinguishes 10 principles for a just global structure:

1. A plurality of actors should be held responsible.
2. National sovereignty should be respected within boundary conditions of human capabilities.
3. Rich countries should give a substantial part of their BNP to poor countries.

4. Multinationals should stimulate human capabilities in the regions they are active in.

5. The main structures of the global economy should be fair for poor and developing countries.

6. All should strive for a limited, decentralized but powerful global open space.

7. All institutions and (most) individuals should pay attention to problems of the deprived in each country and region.

8. The global community should emphasize care for the sick, the elderly, children, and people with disabilities.

9. The family is valuable but not private.

10. Everyone must support education to emancipate the deprived and to make them self-supporting (Nussbaum 2006).

## 13.3 Applying Capability Approach to Sustainable Nanotechnology Development

As discussed above, Nussbaum recommends 10 principles for a just global structure. In this chapter, this approach is applied to sustainable nanotechnology development, but not all 10 of Nussbaum's principles are relevant to this. The international capabilities approach should be adapted to ST&I policy. This leaves us with the following set of principles:

1. *Public engagement:* A plurality of actors should be held responsible for decisions on ST&I policy in each country, including not only the traditional triple helix of natural science, industry, and government, but also representatives of other stakeholders such as members of the parliament, NGOs, and social and human scientists. Where foreign aid is given to developing countries, government and international organizations responsible for ST&I should cooperate with those responsible for development aid policies.

2. *National sovereignty* should be respected within boundary conditions of human capabilities. Thus, foreign actors should cooperate with the national government on ST&I policies, and not undermine national policies, as long as such cooperation does not undermine the human capabilities of the population in the country in question.

3. *Foreign investment:* Rich countries should invest a substantial part of their BNP in stimulating the development of a knowledge economy in poor countries.

4. *Private investment:* Multinationals should invest in the national knowledge economy in the regions they are active in.

5. *Fair structures of the global knowledge economy:* The main structures of the global knowledge economy (including intellectual property rights, mobility of knowledge workers, and trade agreements) should be fair for poor and developing countries.

6. *Access to higher education and research jobs:* The global community, national governments, and all research institutions and individual researchers should enable access to higher education and research jobs for the deprived.

7. *Target research to poverty and health-related problems:* The global community, national governments, and all research institutions and individual researchers should target a substantial part of their research to poverty and health-related problems.

8. *Environmental sustainability:* Apart from social development, environmental aspects should also be included in international cooperation in ST&I.

Principles 6 and 7 (access to higher education and research jobs and target research to poverty and health-related problems) include Nussbaum's principles 7, 8, and 10 (problems of deprived and care for vulnerable, education). Principle 8 is based on Nussbaum's capabilities "other species" and "control over one's environment." Nussbaum's principles 6 and 9 about global governance and the family are not relevant to ST&I policy.

### 13.3.1 Relationship of Criteria with Current Debate on Nanoethics

1. *Public engagement:* Public engagement in decision making on nanoscience and technology is currently a hot topic, at least in Europe. This is not only apparent in the recent public dialogues on nanotechnology policies in countries such as the United Kingdom, Belgium, the Netherlands, and France, and at the level of the European Union (EU), but also in projects stimulating discussions between natural scientists and the general public about the priorities in research (e.g., Bonazzi 2010; ObservatoryNano 2011).

2. *National sovereignty:* Primarily, each national government is of course responsible for its own national policy on ST&I. However, in international research cooperation involving research groups and companies from different countries, differences in national legislation and policies can constitute a challenge that may jeopardize the outcome of the project. Respecting the sovereignty of the national government is thus not only an ethical norm but also a pragmatic necessity, helping partners in international projects to prevent wasting

valuable resources. It also attributes responsibility to this national government for the quality of its ST&I policy. There are two aspects to the boundary condition. It can be interpreted as a warning against cooperation in ST&I with the governments of countries that do not respect basic human rights of their citizens, or as an incentive to look for cooperation with nongovernmental actors such as academics or private companies. General business ethics concepts such as Responsible Care include elaboration of possible ways for ethical behavior in such countries. The benefits for the population of a country as a whole from such nongovernmental foreign investment in ST&I in such countries could contribute to the development of an open-minded academic elite in the long term. However, such nonstructural research cooperation is unlikely to add up to substantial socioeconomic benefits for the country as a whole. For the latter, a clear innovation policy of the own government is an essential prerequisite.

3. *Foreign and private investment:* A major bottleneck in many developing countries is the lack of financial resources available for investment in ST&I. Following a global justice approach, rich countries and multinational companies share in the responsibility for investing in the capabilities of poor countries to develop their own knowledge economy. Most economic value is added in knowledge-intensive sectors of the economy. One of the foreseen implications of nanotechnology is that natural resources, including fossil fuels and raw materials, can be used more efficiently (Meridian Institute 2007). Therefore, it is even more urgent for countries mainly depending on exports of such commodities to develop their own knowledge economy.

4. *Fair structures of global knowledge economy:* The main structures of the global knowledge economy, including intellectual property rights, mobility of knowledge workers, and trade agreements, should be fair for poor and developing countries. The current global dialogue on responsible nanotechnology development organized by the American National Science Foundation (NSF) and the European Commission (Cordis 2008) and in Organisation for Economic Co-operation and Development (OECD) circles (OECD 2010a, 2010b) could be a good platform for discussing relevant measures, provided the discussions are not limited to environment, health, and safety risks and technological standards. However, most decisions on the structures of the global economy are outside the scope of such international dialogue on nanotechnology.

5. *Access to higher education and research jobs:* The global community, national governments, and all research institutions and individual researchers should give opportunities for the deprived to have access

to higher education and research jobs. Industrial uptake of nano-technology is expected to lead to a need for skilled labor force of 2 million workers worldwide by 2015 (Roco 2002). People in develop-ing countries, but also deprived people from poor families, women, and minorities need special support measures to be able to compete on this highly skilled labor market and to be able to contribute to the socioeconomic development of their country.

6. *Target research to poverty and health-related problems:* The global com-munity, national governments, and all research institutions and indi-vidual researchers should target a substantial part of their research to poverty and health-related problems. It is not clear how much money is actually being invested in nanoresearch toward those aims.

7. *Environmental sustainability:* Apart from social development, envi-ronmental sustainability should also be a condition for interna-tional cooperation in ST&I. This principle is not explicitly included in Nussbaum's principles for an international capabilities approach. Nevertheless, it is an important prerequisite for sustainable nano-technology development. Environment, health, and safety risks, and potential environmental benefits of nanotechnology are key issues in the current international debate on nanotechnology. Nussbaum's approach includes two relevant capabilities: "other species" and "control over one's environment."

## 13.3.2 Why Can These Criteria Contribute to Fairness in Nanotechnology Development?

The capability approach is a result oriented political theory on basic rights. Policies stimulating international cooperation in (nano) ST&I are not inte-grated with policies for stimulating international solidarity. This limits the chances that nanotechnology may contribute to sustainable development. Nussbaum's principles for a just global structure are intended to evaluate and direct policies of international organizations, governments, companies, and NGOs for building capacities for development in developing countries. The role of ST&I policies is not explicitly included in her approach. However, the present set of principles for sustainable (nano)technology development can be considered an adaptation of Nussbaum's principles to a specific case, just like she has done for people in developing countries, disabled persons, women, and nonhuman animals (Nussbaum 2006).

The principles for sustainable (nano)technology development can be used to analyze factors influencing the chances that poor people in developing countries may benefit from nanotechnology development. The scheme is thus more an evaluative framework for assessing policies than a normative framework determining morally sound policy aims. The motivation why people in developing countries should benefit from nanotechnology is given to some extent in Rawls' Theory of Justice and Sen's Idea of Justice.

Examining each of the above-mentioned principles for sustainable nanotechnology one by one, it becomes clear that they highlight different aspects of the international innovation system that may stimulate or hamper equal opportunities to benefit from nanotechnology.

1. *Public engagement:* The question of who should be engaged in setting priorities in nanotechnology development features on the international political agenda. Views on the matter range from the traditional triple helix of science, industry, and policy making to direct democracy involving all citizens. Nussbaum states, "a plurality of actors should be held responsible" without specifying which kinds of actors or what they should be held responsible for. This criterion can be used to analyze which actors are engaged in some form in the debate or decision making on priorities in nanotechnology in international cooperation and individual countries, what role each group plays, and what the connections between the different actors are. This allows for factual comparison rather than moral evaluation of good or bad practices.

   Sen's concept of democracy as deliberative governance implies that more rather than less relevant stakeholders and even impartial observers should be heard to enable more just decision making.

2. *National sovereignty:* In international cooperation in (nano) ST&I, respect for national sovereignty implies that foreign investors or cooperation partners refrain from undermining national policies. Again this appears to be more a pragmatic guideline to avoid wasting resources than a moral rule. As the case studies of nanotechnology in Argentina, Brazil, and Mexico below will demonstrate, without a deliberate policy of the national government, the chances that investment in nanotechnology research in or for the country will eventually benefit the national socioeconomic development can be considered low.

3. *Foreign and private investment:* The demand that governments of rich countries and multinational companies invest in building up a knowledge economy in developing countries can be considered a genuinely moral rule. More than vague declarations of good intentions, it implies transferring hard cash and other resources from serving a country or company's self-interests to supporting the development of countries that lack the resources to develop themselves. From the case studies of Argentina, Brazil, and Mexico, it appears that the European Commission and national governments of other countries are making available resources for nanoscience and nanotechnology in these countries. On the other hand, investment by

industry in R&D in Latin America is lagging behind private investments in North America, Europe, and Oceania. Thus, apart from
being a moral rule, the criterion demanding foreign investment in a
knowledge economy in less developed countries can also be used to
identify factors that need improvement.

4. *Fair structures of global knowledge economy:* The call for fair structures of the global knowledge economy is again a moral rule, which
may suffer from the fact that the term "fair structures" is not well
defined. As for international cooperation in nanotechnology, the
relevant structures of the global knowledge economy are mainly
outside the scope of those responsible for such nano-cooperation.
For example, the TRIPS agreement on intellectual property rights
in the World Trade Association and bilateral free trade agreements
between countries are greater determinants of who will benefit from
investment in nanoscience in Latin America than any foreign investment in the nanoresearch in the countries. Thus, again, this criterion
helps identify relevant dynamics rather than giving guidelines for
nanoresearch activities and policies.

5. *Access to higher education and research jobs:* A substantial part of the
benefits nanotechnology is expected to bring is in high-technology
employment and economic benefits for the companies selling products made with nanotechnology. On the down side, nanotechnology
is expected to reduce the demand for commodities and may make
unschooled labor superfluous. A precondition to participating in
the economic benefits nanotechnology is expected to bring is therefore access to higher education, especially in nanotechnology, and
at least in the near future to research jobs. In addition to allowing
students and researchers from less developed countries to study or
work in research in Western countries, investment in high-quality
(interdisciplinary) education and research infrastructure in less
developed countries is mandatory. As the case studies on nanotechnology in Argentina, Brazil, and Mexico show, the actual situation
needs improvement both for all students and researchers from those
countries and for deprived groups inside the countries. This criterion is again a moral rule.

6. *Target research to poverty and health-related problems:* Apart from the
question of who gets access to jobs and economic benefits thanks to
nanotechnology, the choice for which applications will eventually be
enabled or improved thanks to nanotechnology can also be evaluated from a perspective of fairness. Nussbaum's capability approach
prescribes a clearly moral choice for targeting the limited resources
for research to problems that benefit the weakest groups in society: the poor and sick. Assessing the priorities in nanotechnology
research in Argentina, Brazil, and Mexico, it appears that relevant

research is indeed supported, but maybe not getting a major part of the resources. This criterion can thus be considered to be a moral rule stimulating changes in funding priorities.

7. *Environmental sustainability:* In line with the philosophical concept of human beings as rational animals, a fair development of nanotechnology should prevent endangering other species as well as human beings. Risk governance of engineered nanomaterials should therefore be aimed at reducing environmental as well as health risks. The debate on how to accomplish such nanorisk governance is ongoing; however, it appears that there is currently more attention for health risks than for environmental risks. In most developing countries and emerging economies, risk assessment research and debate on regulation of engineered nanomaterials is lagging behind compared with Western countries. On the other hand, there is some discussion on potential environmental benefits of applications of nanotechnology for sustainable energy, remediation, environmental monitoring, and resource efficiency. Whether the actual investment in nanotechnology for stimulating environmental sustainability is enough and well targeted is a matter for debate. These developments may contribute to the capability "control over one's environment."

## 13.4 Applying Capability Approach to Nanotechnology Policies in Latin America

The present chapter makes use of conceptual analysis of national nanotechnology policies in several Latin American countries, including Argentina, Brazil, and Mexico. Information on these policies has been compiled mainly in the EU-funded projects Nanoforum, NanoforumEULA, and ICPC-NanoNet from the literature, Internet, interviews, and participation in events. The countries take different positions in the UN HDI (ranking between 46th and 70th out of 179 countries), but none of them is among the 50 Least Developed Countries (Table 13.1).

### 13.4.1 International Cooperation Involving Latin American Countries

International cooperation in nanotechnology research is stimulated in a number of cooperation agreements between Latin American countries (e.g., MERCOSUR, Common Market of the South), and with other continents (e.g., EU–Latin American framework agreements). The research question for this section is whether these international cooperation activities contribute to the principles for a just global structure for ST&I.

**TABLE 13.1**

Scores and Positions of Latin American Countries in the HDI

|  | Argentina | Mexico | Brazil |
| --- | --- | --- | --- |
| HDI-2006 (179 countries) | 0.860 (46th) | 0.842 (51st) | 0.807 (70th) |
| HDI-2006, Life expectancy at birth (years) | 75 (49th) | 75.8 (42nd) | 72 (80th) |
| HDI-2006, Adult literacy rates (% ages 15+ years) | 97.6% (28th) | 91.7 (59th) | 89.6 (70th) |
| HDI-2006, Combined primary, secondary, and tertiary gross enrollment ratio (%) | 88.6 (35th) | 80.2 (54th) | 87.2 (39th) |
| HDI-2006, GDP per capita (PPP US$) | 11,985 (60th) | 12,176 (59th) | 8949 (77th) |

*Source:* UNDP 2006, Website: http://hdr.undp.org/en/ (last accessed August 27, 2010).

1. *Public engagement:* Decisions on international cooperation in nanotechnology in MERCOSUR and between the EU and Latin America are taken on a political level. MERCOSUR is an economic cooperation agreement between Argentina, Brazil, Paraguay, and Uruguay, to which Chile and Venezuela are candidate members. The MERCOSUR Action Plan of Buenos Aires (2006) aims to advance scientific research and development, including nanotechnology, through establishing a web of centers of excellence (Chinacone et al. 2008). The current ST&I Programme for MERCOSUR 2008–2012 includes "Nanotechnology and New Materials" as one of five priority areas. The EU is cooperating in science and technology not only with MERCOSUR but also with the Andean Community (Bolivia, Colombia, Ecuador, and Peru) and six Central American countries (Costa Rica, El Salvador, Guatemala, Honduras, Nicaragua, and Panama), as well as with the Latin America and Caribbean region as a whole (EU–LAC) and in bilateral cooperation with each individual country. In these EU–Latin American regional cooperation agreements, nanotechnology is not explicitly prioritized (Malsch 2009).

   Social scientists from different Latin American countries have organized themselves in the ReLANS Latin American network for Nanotechnology and Society. They tend to criticize the lack of integration of nanotechnology research policy in national development policies from the perspective of people who are not involved in decision making (e.g., Foladori and Invernizzi 2007). International NGOs—including the ETC group, Meridian Institute, Friends of the Earth, and the International Union of Agricultural Workers—have published statements on nanotechnology, mainly focusing on risks, but also on factors affecting the socioeconomic development of developing countries (e.g., commodities markets, intellectual property). It appears that on the international level, a plurality of actors are engaged in the debate on nanotechnology for developing countries, but it is not clear which actors actually influence decision making on investing in nanoresearch in Latin America.

2. *Respect national sovereignty:* Since interregional and bilateral cooperation agreements are decided upon by governments, national sovereignty should in principle be respected, as long as the less developed countries are not forced to agree to unfair conditions because they have no viable alternative.

    In the case when research groups from Latin American countries participate in EU-funded nanoresearch projects, contractual obligations of the EU—including those on intellectual property—may conflict with the laws or interests of Latin American countries. A minor investment of European funding in high-quality research in a Latin American university could lead to European ownership of the results of a much bigger and longer-term prior investment of public funding in the Latin American country. Such transfer of intellectual property from South to North would contradict the principles of global justice. It is important to be aware of such potential conflicting interests before agreeing on R&D contracts.

3. *Foreign and private investment in stimulating a knowledge economy in poor countries:* The EU has opened up the Framework Programme for Research and Technological Development to participants from International Cooperation Partner Countries, including Latin American countries. This is a bottom–up, researcher-driven process for North–South investment by rich countries in a knowledge economy in poor countries, without a predetermined budget. In addition, the EU and individual countries, including Mexico, have made cooperation agreements stipulating budgets for nanotechnology research cooperation where each of the partners invests 50%.

    In general, private investment in R&D in Latin America is considerably below the global average. This is around 65% of the total investment in R&D in North America, around 55% in Europe, around 50% in Oceania, and around 40% in Latin America and the Caribbean (RICYT, Estado de la Ciencia 2008).

    According to UNESCO (2009), the importance of foreign government investment and private industry investment in different Latin American countries varied considerably in 2007. Total foreign investment was highest in Panama (almost 60%), Guatemala (about 40%), El Salvador (more than 20%), Paraguay and Bolivia (around 15%), and less than 10% in other countries. All business investments ranged between 40% and 50% in Mexico, Chile, and Brazil; around 30% in Argentina, Peru, Uruguay, and Costa Rica; and between 20%

and 30% in Trinidad and Tobago, Bolivia, Colombia, and Ecuador. In other Latin American countries, business investment was insignificant (UNESCO 2009). Nanotechnology research in Latin America suffers from the same lack of private investment, according to researchers.

4. *Fair structures of the global knowledge economy:* The structures of the global knowledge economy influence the chances that nanotechnology development will contribute to socioeconomic development of Latin America. However, these structures fall outside the scope of international cooperation agreements on nanotechnology. For example, since 1994, international and bilateral agreements on intellectual property rights are more and more in favor of multinational companies from highly developed economies (Pacon 2009). Latin American organizations have thus far applied for very few nanopatents. Under these circumstances, the results of Latin American public investment in nanoscience and technology could well end up benefiting companies from industrialized countries.

5. *Access to higher education and research jobs:* Cooperation agreements between the EU and Latin America include access for Latin American students to higher education and research jobs in Europe. However, if this is not complemented by return grants and investment in higher education and research infrastructure in Latin America, the resulting brain drain will hamper the development of a knowledge society in Latin America. This is especially bad because Latin American countries are not characterized by universal access to higher education.

The percentage of all researchers in the world who work in Latin America and the Caribbean has increased from 2.9% to 3.6% between 2002 and 2007, placing this whole region between Germany and France. In 2007, there were 460 researchers per million inhabitants in Latin America and the Caribbean (625 in Brazil and 464 in Mexico). For comparison, there were 4262 researchers per million inhabitants in Oceania, 2515 in Europe, 2013 in the Americas, 742 in Asia, and 169 in Africa. In Latin America and the Caribbean, 46% of researchers were women, which is much better than the world average of 29% (UNESCO 2009).

Taking a closer look at nanotechnology, the development of nanotechnology curricula in higher education in Latin America is still in a very early stage and investment in world-class research infrastructure for doing nanotechnology research is a major problem in R&D in most Latin American countries.

6. *Target research to poverty and health-related problems:* There are projects aiming to develop nanotechnology for poverty and health-related

problems including agrifood, water purification and desalination, sustainable energy, and nanomedicine for infectious diseases. However, the percentage invested in such "nano for the poor" appears to be modest compared with investments aimed at enhancing the competitiveness of leading economies, including the United States, Europe, and Japan.

7. *Environmental sustainability:* In international discussions on responsible nanotechnology development coordinated by the OECD, risk governance of nanomaterials is a big issue and several European countries have announced considerable investments in nanorisk research (10% or 15% of future national public funding for nanotechnology). However, in Latin American nanoresearch, it is hardly addressed at all. The European Commission is stimulating debate on responsible nanotechnology research not only inside the EU but also in international cooperation, including with Latin American countries. No figures on the budgets for applications of nanotechnology in sustainable energy and resource saving are available.

### 13.4.1.1 Summary of International Cooperation

Applying the capability approach to international cooperation in nanotechnology helps clarify which factors are important for improving the chances that investment in nanotechnology R&D will contribute to sustainable nanotechnology. Many different actors are engaged in the public debate on nanotechnology on a global level, but the decision-making process could be more transparent. To strengthen the national sovereignty of less developed countries, awareness should be raised on potential conflicts of interest before signing R&D contracts. Foreign government and private investment in nanotechnology vary considerably between Latin American countries. The structure of the global knowledge economy influences the chances of success of international cooperation in nanotechnology. However, these structures are mostly out of reach of the actors engaged in such nanocooperation. Access to higher education and research jobs is important for getting a share in the expected socioeconomic benefits of nanotechnology. However, such access is limited for Latin Americans in general and the deprived population in that continent in particular. Women appear to have more than the global average access to research jobs in Latin America; however, this may be distorted if it turns out that more male researchers migrate to Western countries. No data on migration of knowledge workers have been found. Poverty, health, and environmental sustainability are the subject of some research in nanotechnology, but it is not clear how big a percentage of the total this is.

In the following, nanotechnology policies in the three Latin American countries that are most active in nanoscience and technology are analyzed, to identify bottlenecks for sustainable nanotechnology development in those countries and what role international cooperation could play.

### 13.4.2 Argentina

The Argentinean government has developed prospective "Bases for a Strategic Medium Term Plan in ST&I" (SECyT 2005) in a stakeholder dialogue involving hundreds of experts and stakeholders. The main aim of this exercise was to develop a strategy for sustainable development. Its feasibility depends on the generated willingness to rethink the country, based on equality, responsible use of natural resources, technological development, and strengthening education on all levels. This scenario is the preferred middle road between a pendulum scenario characterized by large swings in the economy and society without real development and a scenario of compulsive opening as tried in the 1990s. Nanotechnology is included as one of the technological areas with emphasis. Nanotechnology research in Argentina is still in an early stage of development. Therefore, the main priorities in policy are to develop basic research capacities for nanotechnology in networks inside Argentina as well as in MERCOSUR and in international cooperation.

Applications of nanotechnology include

- Molecular electronics (logic and energy storage)
- Advanced and intelligent materials (e.g., screens and displays)
- Sensors and biosensors (especially for food quality, environment, medicine, and bioterrorism)
- Diagnostics and medical therapy
- Cosmetics

The experts and stakeholders proposed several measures for improving the innovation system for nanotechnology, including strengthening and articulating networks and creating and revising interface mechanisms with the productive sector (SECyT 2005).

Nanotechnology is among the thematic priority areas for scientific and technological development in the Bicentennial Strategic Plan 2006–2010, one of the plans following from the bases–scenario exercise. Nanotechnology is expected to contribute to five out of nine problem-opportunity areas:

- Competitiveness of industry and modernization of its production methods
- Competitiveness and sustainable diversification of agricultural production
- Knowledge and sustainable use of natural renewable resources and protection of the environment

- Energy infrastructure: rational use of energy
- Prevention and attention for health

Only under "competitiveness of industry and modernization of its production methods" is the contribution expected from nanotechnology explicitly specified, "Nanotechnology; Development and Application of Micro and Nanodevices" (SECyT 2005).

Responsible nanotechnology development is an explicit aim of the Argentinean government. The minister for ST&I, Dr. Lino Barañao, is addressing these issues personally. The National Committee on Ethics of Science and Technology (CECTE 2008) is developing a code of conduct for responsible nanotechnology research, inspired by the European Commission code of conduct (EC 2008), and organized an international conference on this in 2008.

According to patent analysis by CAICyT (2008), Argentinean nanotechnology appears to be biased toward nanomedicine and nanobiotechnology (9 out of 11 patents).

1. *Public engagement:* Public engagement with decision making on nanotechnology in Argentina appears to be relatively extensive compared with what is known about other Latin American countries. In June and July 2005, the government organized the above-mentioned public consultation on prospective bases for a strategic medium term plan in ST&I, to which citizens were also invited to participate. In 2005, a presidential decree installing the Argentinean Foundation for Nanotechnology (FAN) with an investment of US$10 million and investment of US defense funding bodies in nanotechnology research in Argentina gave rise to heated debate in the congress, the Argentinean Physics Association, the Committee for Ethics in Science and Technology (CECTE), and in the media.

   Whether this apparent openness actually gives different stakeholders influence on decision making on nanoresearch is contested by some nanoscientists in personal communication. There are complaints about corruption on public investments in research. In the International Property Rights Index 2009, Argentina scores 4.3 out of 10, and ranks 80th out of 115 countries in the world and 12th out of 20 Latin American countries. This index consists of criteria measuring the legal and political environment (including corruption and political stability), physical and intellectual property rights, and gender equality.*

   According to Transparency International (2009), Argentineans considered their country's public and private institutions to be more

---

* See http://www.internationalpropertyrightsindex.org/.

corrupt than the global average (scoring 4 out of 5 compared to 3.6 out of 5 on average). Political parties (4.4), public officials/civil servants (4.3), and the judiciary and parliament/legislature (both 4.2) were considered more corrupt than the business/private sector (3.7) and the media (3.3) (TI 2009).

2. *Respect national sovereignty:* The Argentinean government is playing an active role in nanotechnology policy making; however, a major bottleneck is the lack of funding, especially for research infrastructure and instrumentation. This makes nanoscientists dependent on international cooperation, which may undermine national sovereignty. A case in point is the heated debate on US military investment in nanoscience and other research in Argentina in 2005 (c.f. Foladori 2006). The EU policy allowing non-European scientists to participate in EU-funded projects under the Framework Programme for RTD could also have an unintended undermining effect of Argentinean ST&I policy. The development of an Argentinean code of conduct for responsible nanoresearch may counteract such undermining effects. The current government led by President Christina Kirchner has made investment in nanotechnology a priority, installed a separate Ministry for Science and Technology (MinCYT) led by the biologist Lino Barañao, and planned to increase the percentage of the GDP for R&D from 0.66% in 2007 to 1% in 2010 (Dalton 2008).

3. *Foreign and private investment in stimulating a knowledge economy in poor countries:* The World Bank is investing US$150 million in research infrastructure in Argentina in several strategic areas, including in nanotechnology. Furthermore, Argentina has research cooperation agreement with the EU as well as individual countries including the United States, Germany, and Brazil where nanotechnology is explicitly mentioned (Malsch 2009).

   Investment by multinational companies in research in Argentina, including in nanotechnology, is low. In 2006, Argentina invested 0.49% of the GDP in R&D, including 29.4% from companies. Especially the private investment is considerably low compared with North America (~65%), Europe (~55%), Oceania (~50%), and Latin America and the Caribbean (~40%) (RICYT, Estado de la Ciencia 2008).

   In general, foreign direct investment in Argentina has decreased considerably after the financial crisis of 2001. Confidence in the Argentinean government and banking sector among foreign investors has only been increasing gradually since then. The lack of investment is not due to a lack of valuable human and natural resources in Argentina.

4. *Fair structures of the global knowledge economy:* As in other Latin American countries, patenting research results is not a very common

practice in Argentina. The Argentinean economy is still mainly dependent on export of commodities, including agricultural products and raw materials. Almost two-thirds of exports are agricultural or food products (EVD 2009). One aim of the national nanotechnology activities is to increase the value added to exports, but it is unclear how international structures influence the success in achieving this goal.

5. *Access to higher education and research jobs:* Globally, Argentina ranks 35th on the HDI "Combined primary, secondary, and tertiary gross enrolment ratio," with 88.6%; thus, in general, the population has access to education. In nanotechnology, the current nanotechnology networks offer employment to hundreds of nanoscientists and in the Interdisciplinary Centre for Nanoscience and Nanotechnology (CINN), 60 PhD students will be trained. This is sufficient to fill the research jobs in nanotechnology in academia but not to fulfill potential demand for trained staff in industry (Nanotechnology in Argentina, Malsch 2008a). The main bottleneck appears to be a lack of funding. There is no information on access to higher education and research jobs for deprived groups in Argentina.

6. *Target research to poverty and health-related problems:* Nanotechnology development in Argentina focuses on applications in health care. Diagnostics and medical therapy, and (bio)sensors for food quality, environment, medicine, and biosecurity are among the foreseen application areas of nanotechnology. Nanotechnology is expected to contribute to sustainable agrifood production, and prevention and attention for health. Most Argentinean nanotechnology patents are in nanomedicine and nanobiotechnology. It is not so clear how much of it will benefit the poor.

7. *Environmental sustainability:* In Argentina, nanotechnology is expected to contribute to knowledge and sustainable use of natural renewable resources and protection of the environment; however, the actual investment in such applications appears to be modest. It is not clear whether the Argentinean government will be able to protect the environment and consumers against potential risks of products made with nanomaterials. Also, the budget for risk assessment of nanomaterials is unknown and it is unclear whether and how much rich countries will contribute to protecting less developed countries from potential risks of nanomaterials.

### 13.4.2.1 Conclusions for Argentina

In this section, the nanotechnology policy in Argentina has been analyzed to identify bottlenecks for sustainable nanotechnology development and what role international cooperation could play. Whereas public participation in the debate on nanotechnology since 2005 has been abundant in comparison with other countries, there are concerns that corruption in the public sector may reduce the level to which investment in nanotechnology will benefit the whole population. The Argentinean government is taking a leading role in nanotechnology development and international cooperation, which will increase the chances that national sovereignty will be respected. Foreign government and private investment in R&D in Argentina is currently lower than the average in Latin America. It is unclear how structures of the global knowledge economy influence the chances that Argentina may reap the benefits of nanotechnology investment in the country. Educating students is part of the national activities in nanotechnology; however, the numbers are relatively low owing to a lack of funding. Whereas health and environmental applications are among the priorities for nanotechnology research, it is not clear how much poor people and the environment will benefit.

### 13.4.3 Brazil

Nanotechnology is included in the Action Plan for Science, Technology and Innovation (PACTI 2007–2010) (MCT 2007), action line III: Research, Development, and Innovation in strategic areas. It is one of two future carrying areas together with biotechnology. A wide range of economic sectors relevant to the country are expected to benefit from applications of nanotechnology. The action plan includes strategy development, investment in R&D, higher education and research infrastructure for nanotechnology, and innovation support and technology transfer from academia to industry. Concrete, measurable milestones are included that enable evaluation of the policy. The total budget for nanotechnology in PACTI is R$69.99 (~€23) million in 4 years, from MCT/FNDCT (National Fund for Scientific and Technological Development) and MCT/other actions PPA.

1. *Public engagement:* The network on Nanotechnology, Society, and Environment—RENANOSOMA aims to stimulate public dialogue on the implications of nanotechnology for society and the environment. This network is the initiative of social scientists and not included in the national nanotechnology program. Brazilians involved in nanoscience and in RENANOSOMA give evidence of limited cooperation between the social scientists cooperating in this network with Brazilian nanoscientists and technologists. The public or stakeholder debate on nanotechnology and society in Brazil appears to be rather polarized (Martins et al. 2007).

2. *Respect national sovereignty:* The Brazilian government plays a clear leading role in planning and managing nanotechnology research in the country. International cooperation including North–South as well as South–South collaborations is an integral part of this policy.

The government looks after Brazil's national interests in these international agreements. In direct contacts with nanoscientists, they appear to be interested only in international cooperation with active support from the Ministry of Science and Technology (MCT). The complicated Brazilian legislation imposes barriers for international cooperation in ST&I.

3. *Foreign and private investment in stimulating a knowledge economy:* Brazil is an emerging economy. Nanotechnology is included in international cooperation agreements in science and technology with the EU, Germany, and Argentina. The EU is investing €30.5 million in scholarships and capacity building in higher education in Brazil, and Brazilian scientists can participate in projects funded by the EU Framework Programme for RTD, including in nanotechnology. It appears that international cooperation helps build a knowledge economy in Brazil.

   In 2006, Brazil invested 1.02% of GDP in R&D, the highest in Latin America. Companies were responsible for 47.9% of investment in R&D, more than the average in Latin America. This is a result of the Brazilian government policy obliging companies to invest a percentage of their profits into sectorial funds for Research and Development (RICYT, Estado de la Ciencia 2008). There are no separate statistics for investment in nanotechnology in Brazil.

4. *Fair structures of the global knowledge economy:* Patenting results of nanotechnology research is still not very common in Brazil. Brazilian organizations only hold 89 nanopatents registered in the period between 2000 and 2007. This is very low compared with Western countries. In the current structures of the global knowledge economy, this lack of patenting is a disadvantage.

5. *Access to higher education and research jobs:* In the HDI-2006, Brazil's combined primary, secondary, and tertiary gross enrolment ratio is 87.2%, ranking 39th in the world. In nanotechnology, the Brazilian government aimed to train 100 nanoscientists in the period between 2007 and 2010, under the PACTI action plan for ST&I. In the 10 nanotechnology research networks funded under the same scheme, 1000 nanoscientists are employed. It is not clear if deprived groups have access to nanoeducation or research jobs, but the federal government actively promotes networking in nanotechnology research, including in less developed regions of the country (Malsch 2009).

   In general, one of Brazil's weaknesses is that access to the higher education system is low for deprived groups. There is currently a shortage of skilled technical manpower. The main challenge is therefore generating manpower by, for example, repatriating Brazilian scientists from abroad and offering basic education in order to overcome inequality (Bound 2008, p. 44).

6. *Target research to poverty and health-related problems:* Food production is among the application areas of nanotechnology in PACTI (2007–2010) (MCT 2007). The National Institute for Science and Technology is funded in nanobiopharmacy and other research targets medical applications, including infectious diseases. It is unclear how much of these innovations will benefit poor people in Brazil. RENANOSOMA is very skeptical that nanotechnology development in Brazil will benefit the poor in any way (Martins et al. 2007).

7. *Environmental sustainability:* Sustainable energy and environmental monitoring are among the application areas developed by PETROBRAS, INPA, etc. Nanosensor technologies are being developed for environmental monitoring.

### 13.4.3.1 Conclusions for Brazil

In this section, nanotechnology policy in Brazil has been analyzed to identify bottlenecks for sustainable nanotechnology development and what role international cooperation could play. The government, especially the MCT, is playing a leading role in nanotechnology policy and research in the country. One of their priorities is to build up a research capacity for nanotechnology in less developed regions, to stimulate employment and socioeconomic development. It remains to be seen how successful this strategy will be. Social scientists are also actively discussing nanotechnology, taking mainly a critical position. There appears to be a gap between proponents and opponents and little communication between them. The government is successful in enforcing respect for its national sovereignty; however, the complicated Brazilian legal system imposes barriers to successful international cooperation. Brazilian organizations are still not very active in patenting nanotechnology inventions, which is a disadvantage in the current structures of the global knowledge economy. Education and employment in nanotechnology is stimulated but the capacity is limited. In general, deprived groups have limited access to higher education. Whether poverty, health, and the environment are priorities of nanotechnology funding is contested by RENANOSOMA.

### 13.4.4 Mexico

Mexico is a Latin American middle-income country with 110 million inhabitants and a per capita income of US$10,000. It has been a member of the North American Free Trade Agreement (NAFTA) since 1994 and of the OECD. It has Free Trade Agreements with the EU, Japan, and several other countries. Nanotechnology is mentioned as a strategic technology in one of 10 lines for improving competitiveness (2008–2012) by the Secretariat for Economy. The general aim of the policy is to contribute to more and better employment, enterprises, and entrepreneurs. The application areas for nanotechnology are mining, (sustainable) energy, housing, and added value to natural resources (metals, minerals, and agrifood) (Malsch 2008a).

1. *Public engagement:* The federal government has not published its national strategy for nanotechnology development, even though it was announced in 2007. Activities in nanoscience and nanotechnology in the country seem to be more the result of a bottom–up process. Natural scientists are beginning to cooperate in nanotechnology networks and they appear to be in favor of a more centralized strategy for nanotechnology development. Social scientists cooperating in ReLANS (see Section 13.8.1) lobby for a national nanotechnology policy. It is not clear to what extent natural and social scientists are talking to each other.

2. *Respect national sovereignty:* Since the Mexican federal government has not published a strategy for nanotechnology development thus far, there are no mechanisms to control the influences international cooperation in nanoscience and nanotechnology might have on national policy.

3. *Foreign and private investment in stimulating a knowledge economy:* Mexico is collaborating in nanotechnology research with the EU as well as individual countries in Europe, North and South America, and Asia. Mexican researchers can participate in the EU Framework Programme for RTD, and Mexico and the EU have agreed to invest both about 5 million euro in common projects in nanotechnology for construction. The main bottleneck hampering socioeconomic benefits from foreign public investment is the lack of a clear government policy fostering innovation and the Mexican culture where networking and cooperation is still underdeveloped.

   In 2006, Mexico invested 0.46% of GDP in R&D, ranking fourth in Latin America behind Brazil, Chile, and Argentina. Companies were responsible for 41.5% of this (RICYT, Estado de la Ciencia 2008). Few public research organizations participate in academia–industry cooperation in nanotechnology.

4. *Fair structures of the global knowledge economy:* In the period between 2000 and 2007, Mexican organizations and individual patent holders registered only 28 nanotechnology patents (RICYT, Estado de la Ciencia 2008). This is very low compared with Western countries. In the current structures of the global knowledge economy, this lack of patenting is a disadvantage.

5. *Access to higher education and research jobs:* The Mexican higher education system is still mainly discipline oriented, and interdisciplinary education including in nanoscience is only just emerging. According to HDI-2006, the combined primary, secondary, and tertiary gross enrolment

ratio is 80.2%, ranking 54th worldwide. There is great variety in quality of higher education in Mexico with great differences between public and private universities. There are no data on access to higher education and research jobs in nanotechnology for deprived groups in Mexico.

6. *Target research to poverty and health-related problems and environmental sustainability:* The housing sector is interested in applications of nano-technology. In the diagnostic report on nanotechnology in Mexico and other advisory reports, applications including water purification, cheap housing, etc., are mentioned; however, no data are available on how much effort is really deployed to achieve those aims (Nanoforumeula 2007).

### 13.4.4.1 Conclusions for Mexico

In this section, nanotechnology policy in Mexico has been analyzed to identify bottlenecks for sustainable nanotechnology development and what role international cooperation could play. There is a lively debate on nanotechnology policy in Mexico, in which federal, regional, and local governments, and natural and social scientists participate. However, this debate has not yet been translated in an official government strategy. The government does not enforce respect for its national sovereignty in international cooperation in nanotechnology, which limits the chances that foreign investments benefit the socioeconomic development of the country. Patenting nanoinventions by research organizations in Mexico is not done on a large scale. This is problematic because the structures of the global knowledge economy benefit organizations possessing IPR. Nanotechnology education does not appear to be a national priority. There is reference to poverty, health, and environmental sustainability in the discussion about nanotechnology; however, there is no separate funding budget set aside for achieving these priorities. To conclude, the lack of a national nanotechnology policy in Mexico is the main bottleneck hampering sustainable nanotechnology development in the country.

## 13.5 Conclusions

To conclude, the theory of justice and its practical application in the form of the capabilities approach makes it possible to develop a framework for assessing which factors influence the chances that national policies and international cooperation in nanotechnology will contribute to sustainable nanotechnology development. It is not only suitable for making the dynamics of the activities of actors inside nanotechnology research and policy making visible, but also to identify relevant external bottlenecks that should be addressed to improve the chances of success of such nanotechnology policies. Comparing Argentina, Brazil, and Mexico, the main bottlenecks in Argentina appear to be a lack of financial resources and a lack of trust in especially public institutions. The strengths of Argentina include good human and natural resources, and well-established national and international networks. The main bottlenecks in Brazil appear to be a lack of access to higher education among deprived parts of the population and the complicatedness of the national legislation. The strengths of Brazil include the strong federal government policy on nanotechnology development, strong networking inside the country and internationally, and very rich natural resources. The main weaknesses in Mexico include the lack of a formal federal government policy and the lack of networking among research groups inside the country, as well as academic–industrial cooperation. The strengths of Mexico include the availability of high-quality research infrastructure and world-class researchers and a wealth of natural resources. All three countries are weak in patenting nanotechnology inventions and hence are disadvantaged in the current structure of the international knowledge society.

## References

Anand P, Santos C, and Smith R. The measurement of capabilities, in Basu K and Kanbur R (eds.), *Festschrift for Professor Amartya Sen*, Oxford University Press, Oxford, 2008.

Arrow, Kenneth J. Social Choice and Individual Values, Wiley, New York, 1951.

Bonazzi, M. Communicating Nanotechnology; Why, to whom, saying what and how? European Commission, Brussels, 2010, http://cordis.europa.eu/nanotechnology/src/publication_events.htm.

Bound K. Brazil, the natural knowledge economy, in *DEMOS Atlas of Ideas*, 2008, http://www.demos.co.uk/publications/brazil.

CAICyT, Estudio de Inteligencia Estratégica en Nanotecnología, (Strategic Intellicence Study on Nanotechnology) CAICyT, Buenos Aires, 2008.

CECTE, 2008, Web site: http://www.cecte.gov.ar/conferencias-seminarios-ytalleres/#conferencia-internacional-para-la-investigacion-responsable-en-nanociencia-ynanotecnologia.

Chiancone A, Chimuris R, and Garrido Luzardo L. Nanotechnology in Uruguay, in Foladori G and Invernizzi K (eds.), *Nanotechnology in Latin America*, Rosa Luxemburg Stiftung Manuskripte 81, Karl Dietz Verlag, Berlin, 2008.

Condorcet, Essai sur l'application de l' analyse à la probabilité des decisions rendues à la pluralité des voix (essay on the application of analysis to the probability of majority decisions) Paris: de l' imprimerie royale, 1785.

Cordis, 2008, Web site: http://cordis.europa.eu/nanotechnology/src/intldialogue.htm (last accessed 09-04-2010).

Dalton R. Argentina: The come back, *Nature* 456, 441–442, 2008, http://www.nature.com/news/2008/081126/full/456441a.html.

EC, "Recommendation on a code of conduct for responsible nanosciences and nano-technologies research," Commission Recommendation of 07/02/2008, Brussels.

EVD, Website of Dutch Export Voorlichtingsdienst, 2009, http://www.evd.nl/home/landen/landenpagina/land.asp?land=arg.

Foladori, Guillermo, Nanoscience and Nanotechnology in Latin America, Nanowerk, 2006, http://www.nanowerk.com/spotlight/spotid=767.php.

Foladori, Guillermo & Invernizzi, Noela, "Agriculture and food workers challenge nanotechnologies," Rel-UITA website, 2007, http://www.rel-uita.org/nanotecnologia/trabajadores_cuestionan_nano-full-eng.htm.

Grotius, H. De Jure Belli ac Pacis (The law of war and peace) Paris, Nicolaum Buon, 1625.

Hobbes, T. Leviathan or The Matter, Forme and Power of a Commonwealth Ecclesiaticall and Civil, Clarendon Press, Oxford, 1651.

Hume D. *A Treatise of Human Nature*. London, John Noon, 1739.

Hume D. *An Enquiry Concerning the Principles of Morals*, originally published 1751. Republished: Oxford University Press, Oxford, 2006.

Kant, I. "Über den Gemeinspruch: Das mag in der Theorie richtig sein, taugt aber nicht für die Praxis," in *Berlinische Monatsschrift* (September 1793), pp. 201–84. [Ak. 8:275–313] "On the Common Saying: 'That may be correct in theory, but it is of no use in practice'."

Kant, I. *Die Metaphysik der Sitten in zwei Teilen* (Königsberg: Friedrich Nicolovius, 1797); 2nd edition: 1798. [Ak. 6:205–355, 373–493] "The Metaphysics of Morals."

Malsch I. Social and economic contexts; making choices in the development of bio-medical nanotechnology, in Malsch NH (ed.), *Biomedical Nanotechnology*, CRC Press, Boca Raton, FL, 2005.

Malsch I. *Comparing Needs in Nanotechnology Research Cooperation between Mexico, Argentina and Brazil*, Nanoforumeula, November 2008a, www.nanoforumeula.eu.

Malsch I. Nanotechnology solutions looking for developing problems, in *The Broker*, 2008b, www.thebrokeronline.eu.

Malsch I. *First Annual Report on Nanoscience and Nanotechnology in Latin America*, ICPC-NanoNet, June 29, 2009, www.icpc-nanonet.org.

Martins, Paulo Roberto, Premebida, Adriano, Dominguez Dulley, Richard, Braga, Ruy, "Revolução invisível; desenvolvimento recente da nanotecnologia no Brasil," Xamã, São Paulo, 2007.

MCT, Science Technology and Innovation for National Development Action Plan 2007–2010, summary document, Ministry for Science and Technology, Brasilia, 2007, http://www.access4.eu/_media/Action_Plan_ST_Brazil.pdf.

Meridian Institute, International Dialogue on Responsible Research and Development of Nanotechnology, 2004.

Meridian Institute, International Workshop on Nanotechnology, Commodities and Development, Rio de Janeiro, Brazil, May 29–31, 2007.

Mnyusiwalla A, Daar AS, and Singer PA. Mind the gap; Science and ethics in nano-technology, in *Nanotechnology 14*, R9–R13, Institute of Physics Publishing, London, 2003.

NanoforumEULA, Sector Diagnosis of Nanotechnology in Mexico, Enschede, 2007, www.nanoforumeula.eu.

Nussbaum MC and Sen A (eds.). *The Quality of Life*, Clarendon Press, Oxford, 1993.

Nussbaum MC. Frontiers of Justice: Disability, Nationality, Species Membership; The Tanner Lectures on Human Values, Harvard University Press, Cambridge, MA, 2006.

ObservatoryNano, "Relevant ongoing and finished projects in Europe," ObservatoryNano website, Societal issues, 2011, http://www.observatorynano. eu/project/catalogue/4LP/ (last accessed 08-02-2011).

OECD, 2010a, Web site: Working Party on Nanotechnology, http://www.oecd.org/ sti/nano (last accessed 09-04-2010).

OECD, 2010b, Web site: Working Party Engineered NanoMaterials, http://www.oecd. org/department/0,3355,en_2649_37015404_1_1_1_1_1,00.html (last accessed 09-04-2010).

Pacon, Ana Maria, The role of intellectual property rights. Paper presented at EULAKS Summer School. The role of social sciences in the construction of knowledge-based societies: Latin American and European perspectives. 17–30 August 2009, Mexico D.F.

Rawls J. *Een Theorie van Rechtvaardigheid*, Lemniscaat, Rotterdam, 2009 (original title: *A Theory of Justice* (Revised Edition 1999), Harvard University Press).

RICYT, El Estado de la Ciencia 2008. Principales indicadores de ciencia y tecnología iberoamericanos/interamericanos, (The State of Science 2008. Principal indicators of iberoamerican and interamerican science and technology) Red de Indicadores de Ciencia y Technología Iberoamericana y Interamericana, Buenos Aires, 2008.

Roco M. Nanotechnology—A frontier for engineering education, *International Journal of Engineering Education* 18(5), 2000 pp. 488–497.

Salamanca-Buentello F, Persad DL, Court EB, Martin DK, Daar AS et al., Nanotechnology and the developing world, *PloS Medicine* 2(4), e97, 2005.

SECYT, "Bases para un plan estrategico de mediano plazo en ciencia, tecnologia y innovacion, 2005–2015," SECYT, Buenos Aires, Argentina, 2005.

Sen A. *Commodities and Capabilities*, Oxford University Press, Oxford, 1985.

Sen A. *Development as Freedom*, Knopf, New York, 1999.

Sen A. *The Idea of Justice*, Allen Lane, Penguin Books, London, 2009.

TI, Global Corruption Barometer 2009, Transparency International, 2009, http://www.transparency.org/whatwedo/pub/global_corruption_report_2009.

UN General Assembly, United Nations Millennium Declaration, Resolution adopted by the General Assembly (A/55/L.2), United Nations, New York, 18 September 2000.

UNDP, 2006, Web site: http://hdr.undp.org/en/ (last accessed 08-27-2010).

UNESCO, Fact Sheet No. 2, *A Global Perspective on Research and Development*, UNESCO Institute for Statistics, Paris, October 2009, http://www.uis.unesco. org/ev.php?ID=7793_201&ID2=DO_TOPIC.

# Conclusion

## Claude Emond and Ineke Malsch

As discussed in this book, nanotechnology is a complex and multidisciplinary science. Chemists, biologists, toxicologists, medical doctors, engineers, and social scientists need to take part in this development because if one of these disciplines is missing, it can result in an incomplete understanding of this complex field. However, this does not mean that we always need to work together as a group, because usually our research question is a small portion of a larger picture, and this is particularly true for nanotechnology. However, it is essential that representatives from each field review the questions with attention and from that point interact with other scientists in a multidisciplinary fashion.

In this book, collaborators from many disciplines have come together to discuss their knowledge of their fields, especially the sections that relate to nanotechnology. The nanoparticle characterization chapters discussed the importance of well characterizing the nanoparticles. As discussed in this book, the smaller the nanoparticles, the larger the reactivity surfaces might be. In addition, an important part of characterization is standardization. As presented in Section I, there are too many different types of characterization tests that have been developed. The problem with having too many characterization tests is that when attempting to compare similar experiments, we cannot be sure that the nanoparticles are similar if the tests are not the same.

In Section II on biomedical nanotechnology, the author of one chapter discussed the pseudoinactivity of gold metal, which becomes active and begins to exhibit some toxicity behavior at the nanosize level. The second chapter discussed the application of nanoparticles in medicine, including engineering tissues and bone reconstructive composites.

Section III also presented two chapters on nanotechnology and agrofood and water. Agrofood represents an important market for nanotechnology because many important applications can result from this technology, including pesticides, food additives, or intelligence packaging. At the same time, both chapters informed the reader of the importance of public investment and collaboration and of transparency or environmental and health issues, which will facilitate the public investment in nanotechnology. In the second chapter, the authors emphasized the similitude between nanotechnology and genetically modified organisms. In addition, the authors discussed the importance of not letting the market or industry decide what will be on the market.

Section IV, titled *Bionanotechnology and the Environment*, highlighted the new potential resources' link to nanotechnology and how this new technology can improve the quality and remediation capacities. More research on nanotechnology is needed, but there is definitely potential in this science.

Section V presented observations related to the potential toxicity or the risk from nanoparticles. The first chapter, on nanotoxicology, reviewed some technical protocols that are used in *in vitro* approaches starting from the cell lines or primary cultures. This chapter also emphasized the importance of investigating these toxicity mechanisms. The *in vitro* approach is useful for comparing different families of nanoparticles because it is a fast and low-cost method to study preliminary classifications. However, an understanding of the global aspect of the exposure is required in order to complement the *in vivo* approaches. The second chapter, on toxicokinetics, reviewed the different phases of absorption, disposition, metabolism, and excretion. The chapter provided an overview of what is happening biologically to these small particles when they cross the membrane. This was followed by an eco-toxicological chapter, which described in detail the environmental fate of nanotechnology. This last chapter discussed the different types of nanoparticles and their interaction with ecotoxicological models, as well as the factors affecting the toxicities.

Section VI focused on the life cycle assessment relating to nanoparticles. Here, all of the aspects of the interaction were discussed, from the production to the disposal of nanoparticles.

Finally, Section VII outlined the ethical and social implications of nanotechnology. This section contained the most important information because today, society is more critical about technology and as a society, we need to question ourselves about the importance of new technology. This section complemented Section III because it discussed what we want and what we do not want in a new technology.

Nanotechnology is probably the most important technology because we believe that it is important to improve our quality of life while simultaneously addressing concerns from the population and the nongovernmental organization who want to make informed decisions. This book is for professionals, not necessarily specialists, who want to understand more about the advantages and disadvantages of the technology and gain more of an understanding of other nanotechnology issues. I hope that this book will be very useful to you.

# Index

Page numbers followed by f and t indicate figures and tables, respectively.

Printed and bound by CPI Group (UK) Ltd, Croydon, CR0 4YY

22/10/2024

01777857-0001